The Ultimate Volumetrics Diet

ALSO BY BARBARA ROLLS, Ph.D.

The Volumetrics Weight-Control Plan
The Volumetrics Eating Plan

The **Ultimate Volumetrics Diet**

Smart, Simple, Science-Based Strategies for Losing Weight and Keeping It Off

Barbara Rolls, Ph.D.

with Mindy Hermann, R.D.

Photographs by Ben Fink

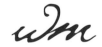

WILLIAM MORROW
An Imprint of HarperCollins*Publishers*

This book is written as a source of information only. The information contained in this book should by no means be considered a substitute for the advice of a qualified medical professional, who should always be consulted before beginning any new diet, exercise, or other health program.

All efforts have been made to ensure the accuracy of the information contained in this book as of the date published. The authors and the publisher expressly disclaim responsibility for any adverse effects arising from the use or application of the information contained herein.

HarperCollins books may be purchased for educational, business, or sales promotional use. For information please write: Special Markets Department, HarperCollins Publishers, 10 East 53rd Street, New York, NY 10022.

FIRST EDITION

Designed by Ashley Halsey

Library of Congress Cataloging-in-Publication Data has been applied for.

ISBN 978-0-06-206064-8

12 13 14 15 16   WBC/RRD   10 9 8 7 6 5 4 3 2 1

To Arabella, Cecilia, Charles, Henry, and William—
Hoping you eat your vegetables

Contents

Ultimate Volumetrics Recipes

Desserts—Fruit Desserts

Desserts—Fruit Salads

Appendix

Acknowledgments

Special thanks go to Mindy Hermann, R.D., who has been my partner in writing *The Ultimate Volumetrics Diet*. Her experience as both a dietitian and a writer has been invaluable in helping create this practical, evidence-based weight-management plan. She developed and tested many of the delicious Volumetrics recipes, and she worked with the photographic team to ensure that the beauty of healthy eating makes your mouth water. Along the way, my lab manager, Jennifer Meengs, R.D., contributed her dietetic expertise and Penn State–friendly recipes, while she made sure the charts and numbers added up.

My literary agent, Alice Martell of The Martell Agency, knows that without her continual support, enthusiasm, and nudging this book would not have been written. My thanks also go to my editor Cassie Jones for knowing how to make our Volumetrics foods and messages appealing.

Many thanks to photographer Ben Fink for his talent, vision, and expert eye behind the camera, and to digital technician Jeff Kavanaugh for his technology know-how. Food stylist Libbie Summers brought invaluable expertise, a can-do attitude, and creativity in staging the magnificent photos in this book. Her kitchen assistant, Andrew Erbschloe, was a pleasure to work with. Robert, Lori, and Sarah Horowitz, who lent their home for the photo shoot, were wonderful and gracious hosts. Many thanks to Eric Zaidins and Jon Hermann for their assistance with logistics.

Family and friends who contributed favorite recipes have helped make Volumetrics meals even more delicious: Alexandria Blatt, Juliet Bostock, Kim Cavanagh, Anne Corr,

Kitti Halverson, Pao Ying Hsiao, Jennifer Meengs, Melissa Rolls, Mary Serdula, Diane Sweetland, and Jacqueline Vernarelli.

I appreciate the contributions of my colleagues who generously gave of their time and expertise: Steven Blair, P.E.D.; Adam Drewnowski, Ph.D.; Anne M. Fletcher, M.S., R.D.; Emily Fonnesbeck, R.D.; Delia Hammock, M.S., R.D.; Terry Hartman, Ph.D.; Marion Hetherington, D.Phil.; James O. Hill, Ph.D.; Chor San Khoo, Ph.D.; Michael Lowe, Ph.D.; Traci Malone, M.H.S., R.D.; Juliet Mancino, M.S., R.D.; Megan Mc-Crory, Ph.D.; Christine Pelkman, Ph.D.; Xavier Pi-Sunyer M.D.; Paul Rozin, Ph.D.; Christopher N. Sciamanna, M.D.; Bonnie Taub-Dix, M.A., R.D.; Brian Wansink, Ph.D.; Hope Warshaw, M.M.Sc., R.D.; and Jill Weisenberger, M.S., R.D.

I would like to extend sincere thanks to Kristie Bundro, Anne Kapinus, Ric Keller, Jill O'Nan, Darryl Slimak, and Sabrina Staedt for sharing their personal Volumetrics stories.

Thank you to copy readers Alexandria Blatt, Juliet Bostock, Kitty Broihier, Kim Cavanagh, Kitti Halverson, Susan Light, Susanne Marder, Jennifer Meengs, Susan Raab, Liane Roe, Julie Sherman, Maureen Spill, Nancy Tringali, and Rachel Williams for their invaluable feedback and suggestions.

Penn State University continues to provide the facilities and stimulating environment for our studies, while funding from the National Institute of Diabetes and Digestive and Kidney Diseases keeps it going. I thank them and my dedicated staff and students who continue to believe that we can fight the obesity epidemic with knowledge.

Thanks to my family and friends who have sampled lots more of my cooking than usual and who by now know that when I am writing a book, I will be spending much more time with my computer than with them. I appreciate your understanding and support!

Introduction

Welcome to the Ultimate Volumetrics Diet, a scientifically backed approach to managing your weight while eating satisfying and nutritious foods. If you are a newcomer to Volumetrics, I look forward to teaching you how to put together delicious, filling, calorie-conscious meals. To those of you who are familiar with my previous books, *The Ultimate Volumetrics Diet* brings you new discoveries and new recipes, combined with the same solid science.

A Brief History of Volumetrics

My previous books, *The Volumetrics Weight-Control Plan* and *The Volumetrics Eating Plan*, adhere to the most fundamental principle of weight management, calorie control and the calorie balance equation. In order to lose weight, you have to eat fewer calories than your body uses as fuel. And to maintain weight, you have to continue to match calorie intake to calories burned. Volumetrics offers a positive approach to managing calories. You will learn how to make smart food choices that fill your day with plenty of enjoyable, healthful foods and leave you feeling full and satisfied. This involves choosing foods that pack fewer calories into each bite—that is, they are lower in calorie density.

When we published *The Volumetrics Weight-Control Plan* in 2000, everyone was talking about fad diets and overly restrictive food plans that cut out particular foods or entire food groups. Because Volumetrics is about filling up on fewer calories without eliminating foods, you can imagine how different it was! In fact, I was told that I shouldn't write a book that was about calories because people were not interested in calorie control.

As it turned out, people did want to know how to manage their calories while still eating satisfying amounts of food. *The Volumetrics Weight-Control Plan* was named the top diet in the country by *Self* magazine. Since its release in 2005, *The Volumetrics Eating Plan* has been rated as the best diet by *The Daily Beast* and a leading national consumer publication, and was cited among the best on CNN.com, fncimag.com (Fox News), and usnews.com (the website for *US News & World Report*, where it also was a featured cover story). Both books made the list of *New York Times* best sellers.

How Volumetrics Fits into Weight Loss Today

The science that was new in the year 2000 has stood the test of time. In fact, the fundamentals of choosing foods with lower calorie density are so solid that they have been incorporated into weight-loss studies, centers, and programs around the world, and have been embraced by health agencies and policy makers tackling the biggest health challenge we have ever faced—the obesity epidemic.

Have you noticed that revolutionary new diets are making the headlines less often these days? A lot has happened in the seven years between my second book and this one. My colleagues and I now agree that managing weight is about eating a variety of nutritious foods that help control calories. Forget about just cutting the fat or carbohydrates, or cutting out whole food groups. The key to success is finding positive strategies that will lead to sustainable, healthy eating and activity patterns that fit your lifestyle. The box on the following page summarizes the fundamentals not only of Volumetrics but of any sound weight management plan.

The Science Behind Volumetrics

As a professor of nutritional sciences who studies eating behavior and how it affects body weight, I have a lot of information to share about the latest research on weight management. The science behind Volumetrics comes from labs around the world, as well as from my own at The Pennsylvania State University. The lab, described by *US News & World Report* as my "quirky culinary empire," is a custom-built kitchen for developing and preparing the tasty foods that we use in our studies. My staff and students know food and

The Ultimate Volumetrics Diet

- Focuses on thinking positively about what you *can* eat.
- Is based on sound nutritional advice widely accepted by health professionals.
- Emphasizes that the only proven way to lose weight is to eat fewer calories than your body uses as fuel for your activities.
- Stresses that when you are managing calories, it is more important than ever to eat a good balance of food and nutrients.
- Teaches you to make food choices that will help control hunger and enhance satiety.
- Shows you how to fit your favorite foods into your diet.
- Reinforces eating and activity patterns that you can sustain for a lifetime of achieving your own healthy weight.

love to cook, and most are dietitians. Each week they cook for and feed dozens of volunteers who agree to eat their meals at the lab so that we can study their eating behavior when we change portion size, calories, or nutrients. We work hard to serve foods that they will like—and I have included some favorites in this book.

Keep in mind that we are looking for ways to help people feel full, so we ask participants to rate their hunger and fullness before and after eating. They also tell us how much they enjoyed their meal—after all, taste and pleasure are the top reasons that people eat the foods they do. In order to track your own satisfaction, you'll be doing much the same, keeping a Volumetrics diary for your own personal weight management plan.

Calorie Density and the Foods You Choose

In the Ultimate Volumetrics Diet, the basics are simple—you will learn to choose foods that give you satisfying portions without overloading you with calories. This involves lowering the calorie density (CD) of foods. Foods vary in the number of calories they pack into each bite. Reduce the calories per bite—that is, the CD—and you can eat the same amount of food (bites) while saving calories. Research shows that lowering the CD of foods will help you feel full while eating fewer calories. (If you followed my previous

Volumetrics plans, you may be wondering if calorie density is the same as "energy density," the term I used previously. They are the same; readers tell me that calorie density is an easier term to understand.)

So what will your meals look like? Your plate will be full of nutrient-rich foods, with plenty of vegetables, fruits, soups, and salads, and more modest portions of important foods such as lower-fat dairy products and meat. And I will show you how to do this without sacrificing taste! There will even be room for your favorite indulgences—in moderation.

What's Included in *The Ultimate Volumetrics Diet*

This book is written for you, whether you are trying to lose weight or are happy where you are. The Volumetrics lessons you'll learn will help you establish the habits that are associated with eating well for optimal health.

The Ultimate Volumetrics Diet is about your personal preferences. You can read the book from cover to cover, go straight to the weekly plans, jump ahead to the recipes, or read those sections that interest you most. *The Ultimate Volumetrics Diet* offers a lot of options to choose from:

TWELVE-WEEK DIET PROGRAM. Lasting weight loss involves developing eating habits that are nutritionally sound, satisfying, and sustainable. I have divided the basics of how to do this into a twelve-week structured plan that you can personalize to fit with your lifestyle. Each week presents the best available scientific evidence on a unique aspect of the food you eat. You will learn which types of foods give you the most satisfying portions for the calories, different ways to fill your plate, how to sneak in vegetables and fruits, and strategies to manage your food environment both at home and when eating out. Every week also includes these features:

- Key Points: The most important take-away information for the week
- Let's Get Physical: Guidance on incorporating walking and physical activity into your day
- Head and Habits: Attitudes and behaviors to support your weight management efforts

Typical or Volumetrics Dinner: Which Is More Filling?

Here's the type of satisfying meal you'll be eating. Take a look at these "before" and "after" dinners. Each contains 500 calories, which for many people is an appropriate number of calories for dinner. The typical meal below includes foods that pack lots of calories into each bite, such as fried chicken, steak fries, and a regular soda. You don't get much food for your 500 calories. The large Volumetrics meal gives you the same number of calories in much larger portions because the foods—*Baby Arugula Salad* (page 210), *Chicken and Seasonal Tomatoes in a Packet* (page 271), melon balls, and unsweetened iced tea—have fewer calories per bite. Which would you find to be more filling?

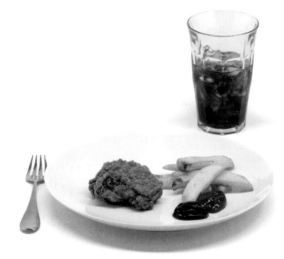

Typical Dinner

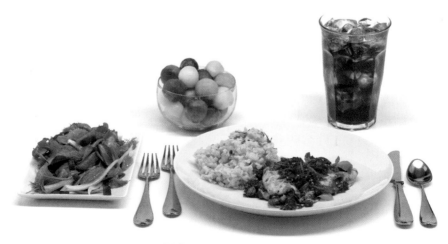

Volumetrics Dinner

- **To Do This Week:** Suggested weekly goals to use as a starting point for checking your progress, adjusting your goals, and customizing your action plan for the next week.

THE MENU PLAN. The Ultimate Volumetrics Diet eating plan is easy to adapt to your preferences. I worked with registered dietitian Mindy Hermann to create four weeks of sample meals and menus. Some meals are based on one or more of the 105 recipes created for this book by Mindy and me, along with registered dietitians Jennifer Meengs and Alexandria Blatt, and our friends and family members. Other meals are quick-fix combinations that require little or no cooking. While we organized the meals into sample menus, we have made these "modular" so you can mix and match to suit your taste and lifestyle.

ULTIMATE VOLUMETRICS RECIPES. Volumetrics recipes show you how appealing healthy eating can be. The recipes are organized into thirty-five categories based on type of dish—salads, soups, sandwiches, stews, and others—or type of occasion, including parties and celebrations. I know that you are busy and that it is easiest to grab prepared food while on the run, but much of that quick food is so calorie dense that it is easy to eat too many calories. That's why I encourage you to get back into the kitchen—it's one of the best (and most affordable) weight-management strategies! The recipes in this book show you how to cook the Volumetrics way, with tasty ingredients and delicious flavors. I chose a combination of classics and newer favorites with an international flair and then adapted them for Volumetrics by lowering the CD to give you more food for the calories. Before-and-after photos show that Volumetrics dishes can be highly filling and satisfying. I also include plenty of tips on how to modify your favorite recipes in ways that use CD-lowering ingredients without sacrificing flavor.

MODULAR FOOD LISTS. This section of the book organizes hundreds of foods into easy-to-use categories that you can mix and match to create your own Volumetrics meals and personalize Volumetrics into a plan that is right for you.

Are you ready to get started? Week 0 guides you through setting your eating, activity, and weight-loss goals. This is your time to get ready for the weeks to come. I look forward to helping you achieve lasting weight loss and good health.

The **Ultimate Volumetrics Diet**

Week 0
Getting Started

My dietitian helped me determine how many daily calories to eat; Volumetrics showed me how to feel full at that calorie level.—Ric, Florida

It's time to get started on your personal Ultimate Volumetrics Diet for managing your weight! You will notice immediately that the Ultimate Volumetrics Diet is different from others you may have tried in that it doesn't tell you to eat less food. You'll be eating satisfying amounts that allow you to feel full and manage hunger *while you're losing weight.* Throughout the twelve weeks of this program, we will be working together to make lasting changes in your eating habits and lifestyle. The Ultimate Volumetrics Diet is an approach to food that shows you how to be in charge of your meals and snacks and your lifestyle so that the pounds don't come back.

How many times have you tried the latest trendy diet, only to find that it didn't work for you? The foods may have been too different from the ones you usually eat, or the diet was complicated and hard to follow. Maybe it had so little food that you couldn't stick with it because you were hungry all the time. That is why weight-loss programs have to be individualized to your likes and dislikes and to what is feasible and sustainable for you.

I will be working with you to create an eating plan that is just for you. It will be based on who you are today—how much you weigh, your weight-loss goals for the next few months and long term, the foods you like to eat, and the activities that fit your lifestyle. That is why I am asking you to spend a bit of time gathering important baseline information before we begin. Just as you wouldn't ask for driving directions without knowing your starting point and destination, you shouldn't start on your Volumetrics journey without noting where you are today, where you want to go, and how you will get there. Before you start, discuss any health concerns, special diet requirements, changes in medication, and other considerations with your doctor and get the okay to begin a weight-loss program.

Your Weight

How much weight would you like to lose? Maybe you're hoping to shed enough pounds to fit into a favorite pair of jeans or get back to a former weight. Is your goal realistic? It is if your goal weight is sensible, achievable, and appropriate for improving your health. Let's start by taking a look at where you are today.

The first step is to get on the scale. Love it or hate it, the scale can be your friend when you're trying to lose weight. It doesn't lie. The scale tells you how you're doing right now. Watching the numbers go down over time also is a great motivator. In a study at the University of Minnesota, adults who weighed themselves most often lost the most weight over a two-year period. Daily weighing also helped a group of successful "losers" make quick adjustments in their diet and exercise as soon as the number on the scale went up even a little, so that they could nip weight gain in the bud and get right back on track. This is why I encourage you to weigh yourself every day.

Remember to weigh yourself on the same scale at the same time of day, preferably in the morning when your weight is at its lowest. Go to the bathroom first, and wear the same amount of clothing—or no clothing at all—to get the most consistent and encouraging number.

Although frequent weighing is an effective tool for managing weight, some people find that getting on the scale is too stressful. If you prefer to weigh less frequently, or not at all, consider other ways to monitor your progress, such as belt notches or how your clothing fits.

Your Weight and Your Health

Knowing just your weight doesn't give a detailed enough picture of how your weight relates to your health. For that, you need two additional numbers: body mass index (BMI) and waist circumference.

BMI is a number that indicates whether your weight is appropriate for your height. You can calculate your BMI using a calculator and a formula (see Calculating Your BMI below), with the online National Heart Lung and Blood Institute calculator at www.nhlbisupport.com/bmi/ or the BMI charts on the Centers for Disease Control and Prevention (CDC) website at www.cdc.gov/healthyweight/assessing/index.html, or with a smartphone app. You will need your current weight and height without clothing or shoes to determine your BMI.

Calculating Your BMI

1. Multiply your height in inches by itself. For example, if your height is 5 feet 5 inches (65 inches), multiply 65 times 65, equaling 4,225.
2. Divide your weight in pounds by that number. If you weigh 160 pounds, divide 160 by 4,225, equaling 0.038.
3. Multiply that number by 703. So your BMI is 0.038 times 703, equaling 26.7.

Your BMI tells you whether your current weight is at a healthy level and if you should make weight loss a priority. Write your BMI on the Personal Daily Record Form (page 7) and periodically check it as you lose weight.

- **BMI under 18.5:** You're underweight, so there's no need to lose. Use this book to help you choose healthy meals for yourself and your family.
- **BMI 18.5 to 24.9:** You are at a healthy weight. Keep up the good work by following the eating and exercise suggestions in this book.
- **BMI 25 to 29.9:** You are overweight (unless you are a muscular person who is lean but weighs a lot) and can use this twelve-week program to work toward losing enough to drop your BMI into the healthy weight range.
- **BMI 30+:** Your weight puts you in the obese range and increases your disease risk. Let's work together over the next twelve weeks to bring your weight down to a lower level while improving your health and providing you with a diet framework to keep going beyond the twelve weeks.

Next, measure your waist. If you have extra weight around your middle—that is, you are apple-shaped—your chances of developing heart disease, stroke, diabetes, and high blood pressure are greater, even if your BMI indicates that your weight is healthy. Take this measurement on your own or ask a friend to help. Wrap a tape measure around your belly across the top of your hipbones and below your belly button, exhale—no cheating by sucking in your gut—and hold the tape snug but not too tight. A measurement of over 35 inches if you're a woman or 40 inches if you're a man means you need to slim down. As with BMI, check your waist measurement every month or so to see how you're doing.

The Foods You Eat

We need a starting point for building on and modifying the foods that you enjoy. This means first keeping a record of everything that you eat—types of foods, portion sizes, and approximate calories—for the next few days before you start the Ultimate Volumetrics Diet. (See the Personal Daily Record Form on page 7 for the type of information you might include, or make copies of this form to fill out.) You won't have to count calories long-term but I am asking you to track them for now to get an idea of your calorie intake. Once you understand where calories are in foods and in your diet, you will be better able to choose a nutritious balance of foods that are filling and satisfying without excess calories. You can find calorie information on food labels or use online tools such as ChooseMyPlate.gov, websites, or phone apps.

Ideally, I would like you to have a week's worth of records before you start this program. But if you are excited about getting started as soon as possible, write down what you eat over the next three days. Include every bite—nobody is going to judge you or grade your diet. You may find that merely writing everything down makes you think twice about some of your food choices. Keep your pre-Volumetrics food records in a convenient place so that you can refer back to them for planning meals with the healthy foods that you and your family already eat.

Personal Daily Record Form

Date_____ Weight_____ BMI_____
Goal weight_____ Daily calorie goal_____ Step goal_____
My personal goal for today_____

Time/Meal	What and how much I ate	Calories	Hunger and fullness	Notes

Today I ate based on hunger and fullness ☐ Yes ☐ Mostly ☐ Need to improve

Time	Activity	Duration	Notes

Total step count:

Strategies used to achieve my goals _____
_____
_____

I encourage you to continue writing down what you eat for at least the next twelve weeks. Whether you use a Volumetrics record sheet, plain sheet of paper, computer, or smartphone app, keeping track of what you eat on a daily basis can help you lose more weight. You don't need anything fancy. Any system that works for you boosts your chances of success. Get into the habit of recording your meal or snack immediately after you eat so that you don't forget it. Even seemingly insignificant nibbles can tip you off regarding eating behaviors you may want to change.

Once you settle into your new way of eating, you may not need a detailed record each day. Some people keep a few days' worth of records only during challenging times such as holidays, when it can be difficult to maintain a healthy lifestyle. I try to jot down short notes every day just to remind myself to pay attention. Ric, whom you met at the beginning of this chapter, still maintains a daily diary. "Keeping a simple journal helps me stay on track. I jot down what I ate at each meal and snack and note whether I exercised. It doesn't require much thinking and I keep myself accountable by writing everything down."

Now that you're geared up to keep track of your eating, let's gather the rest of your baseline information.

Satiety: The Missing Ingredient in Weight Management

Over the next twelve weeks, you will learn a lot about satiety. It's the feeling of fullness that comes with having eaten enough and not being hungry anymore. Satiety is so important to dieters that food companies are dedicating research teams to the search for ingredients that enhance fullness. But achieving satiety is more complicated than just turning to specific foods.

Satiety works as a tool for managing your weight if you pay attention and respond appropriately to your body's feelings of hunger and fullness. You may be surprised to discover that some foods don't fill you up much at all, even though they have a lot of calories—think chips, pretzels, cookies—while others with fewer calories such as soups and salads are very filling. Track your hunger and fullness levels before and after each meal and snack, noting which foods help you control hunger and feel satisfied with fewer calories.

Get In Touch with Feelings of Hunger and Satiety

Have you lost touch with what your body is trying to tell you about when to eat and how much to eat? If so, I am going to show you how to start listening again. Begin by slowing down at each meal and paying attention. Before each meal it is appropriate to feel hungry. Most people describe hunger as stomach growls and stomach aches. You should not get so hungry that you feel dizzy and light-headed, or that you lose control of your eating. While you are eating, hunger should decline and you should feel pleasantly but not overly full. If you don't recognize or experience this cycle of hunger and fullness, try the following:

- For two days this week, ask yourself before each meal, "Am I hungry?"
- Use the scale below to rate your hunger on a scale of 1 to 10, 1 being painfully ravenous and 10 being so full you couldn't eat another bite.

Am I Hungry?

Ravenous   1 2 3 4 5 6 7 8 9 10   Completely full

- As you eat, periodically pause and ask yourself again, "Am I still hungry?"
- If your rating has reached 5, it may be time to stop eating. Ratings in the middle of the scale indicate that you are no longer hungry nor are you overly full—you should be comfortable.
- If you are starting to feel full and satisfied, stop eating and wait for several minutes to give yourself time to recognize your body's satiety signals.
- If you still feel hungry, continue eating while monitoring your feelings of hunger and fullness.
- If you are really out of touch with hunger and satiety, try a routine. Eat breakfast, lunch, and dinner on a regular schedule for several days and don't snack. You should feel hungry before meals and satiated after meals. Use the rating scale before each meal and pay attention to how you feel. Remember these feelings and use them to guide your future eating.

Thus far, we've been looking at one half of your weight balance equation—the foods you eat. Now let's consider the other half, physical activity.

The Calories You Burn

You may be wondering if activity makes a difference when you're trying to lose weight. Some experts are skeptical about the role of exercise, saying that it can increase hunger, doesn't burn enough calories for you to lose weight, and may lead you to reward yourself with foods that have more calories than you've burned off. Major magazines have gone as far as suggesting that exercise is a bad idea for weight management. I disagree. Physical activity is a must for everyone because its benefits go far beyond weight loss.

Exercise can improve both your physical and emotional health by lifting your mood, helping you feel more energetic, and reducing anxiety. Dr. Steven Blair of the University of South Carolina points out:

> Daily physical activity allows you to take advantage of all of these benefits rather than trying to use exercise for weight loss alone. The government's recommendation of 150 minutes per week, or a little over twenty minutes each day, is a realistic goal. It may even help you lose and maintain weight, as long as you are eating sensibly. Even half that amount of activity will improve your health and energy levels.

Dr. Blair also notes that activity goals apply to children and teens, too, and can help them avoid problems with their weight.

How much activity do you get in an average day? Do you think you come close to the government recommendation of about twenty minutes per day? You'll find out when you record physical activity in your daily journal. If you fall short, there's no need to wait until you start the Ultimate Volumetrics Diet to increase your activity. My favorite form of exercise is one that you can consider doing now: walking.

Here's why I recommend walking as your main activity. It is part of your routine every day. You walk in your house, to your car, at work, and when you're shopping. Walking doesn't require a lot of money, a gym membership, or fancy equipment. You can do it indoors or outside, in good weather or bad, and on your own or with other people. And walking at a brisk pace counts as the type of physical activity that the government recommends. To keep track of your progress, you need a simple step counter (pedometer) for counting your daily steps and writing them in your daily record. The Personal Daily Record Form includes a section on activity, or you can create your own form.

You don't have to limit yourself to just walking. Explore other activities that match your interests and abilities, including swimming, water aerobics, and stationary cycling. You can use the Shape Up America! Physical Activity Selector at www.shapeup.org /interactive/phys1.php for information on different types of exercises. Strength-building exercises at least twice a week in addition to walking and other activities can help tone muscles and improve your physical well-being. The American Heart Association offers guidance at www.heart.org/HEARTORG/Conditions/More/CardiacRehab/Strength -and-Balance-Exercises_UCM_307384_Article.jsp.

Setting Your Goals

Once you know where you are currently—weight, diet, hunger and fullness, and activity level—you're ready to think about your destination, that is, your goals. The Ultimate Volumetrics Diet is based on goals in three areas—weight loss, daily calories, and daily steps—and I include space on your Personal Daily Record Form for each so that you'll be reminded of them every day.

You may be really motivated and have ambitious goals in mind. The problem is that if you don't meet these goals, you may become discouraged and give up. That is why your goals need a reality check to make sure they're right for you. The following guide-lines can help:

- Make goals *specific*, such as "I will walk for 30 minutes on at least three days of the week."
- Set *measurable* goals that you can keep track of—for example, adding 150 steps a day.
- Find the balance between a weight loss that is *attainable* and your dream weight. Divide big goals into smaller steps. For example, rather than trying to lose your extra pounds all at once, set goals in attainable ten-pound increments.
- Choose *realistic* goals and personalize them to fit into your lifestyle. A goal to

walk for one hour every day is not realistic if you are just getting started or your days are too busy.

- Make your goals *forgiving* rather than all or nothing. Leave yourself wiggle room for occasionally missing the mark—for example, eating a piece of cake at a friend's party or running out of time for activity. Just get back on track the next day.

- Set *timely* goals that make sense for you now. Also give yourself enough time to accomplish them.

Let's start with your overarching goal: the amount of weight you want to lose. If you are overweight or obese, experts recommend losing 5 to 10 percent of your current weight as a realistic and attainable first step that also can help your health by lowering blood sugar and blood pressure and improving blood cholesterol levels. To calculate your first weight goal, multiply your current weight by 0.1 for a 10 percent loss or 0.05 for a 5 percent loss and then subtract that number from your current weight. For example, if you weigh 200 pounds, 10 percent would be 20 pounds and 5 percent would be 10 pounds, and your first weight goal would be 180 pounds for a 10 percent loss or 190 pounds for a 5 percent loss.

Now you are ready to determine the number of calories you should eat each day so that you have a calorie goal to help guide your food choices. You can estimate your needs using the chart, Your Calorie Needs (Calories per Day), that was developed from the Institute of Medicine guidelines. It recommends daily calorie levels based on age, gender, and level of physical activity, which I've described in terms of daily steps (you'll learn more about steps shortly). You also can visit the website www.choosemyplate.gov, click on "Get a personalized Plan," and enter your age, sex, and current physical activity.

The suggested calories are a reasonable approximation of your daily needs to maintain your weight. To lose weight at a rate of one to two pounds per week, subtract 500 to 1,000 calories from this number. So if the chart says a person of your age, sex, and activity level should eat 2,000 calories to maintain weight, your new goal for losing is eating 1,500 calories. I don't recommend that you drop below 1,200 calories per day, because it becomes too difficult to meet all of your nutrition needs. These calorie goals are not precise—calorie needs are different from person to person and weight loss is very indi-

Your Calorie Needs (Calories per Day)

AGE	ACTIVITY LEVEL		
	Sedentary (< 3,600 daily steps)	Moderate (3,600 – 10,000 daily steps)	Active (>10,000 daily steps)
19–30 years, female	1,800–2,000	2,000–2,200	2,400
19–30 years, male	2,400–2,600	2,600–2,800	3,000
31–50 years, female	1,800	2,000	2,200
31–50 years, male	2,200–2,400	2,400–2,600	2,800–3,000
51 + years, female	1,600	1,800	2,000–2,200
51 + years, male	2,000–2,200	2,200–2,400	2,400–2,800

vidual. You may need to adjust calories up or down a bit to maintain a steady loss or to find a level that helps you manage hunger and is sustainable.

You will learn how much you can eat to meet your calorie goal by following the four-week sample menus (pages 156–163), using Meal and Snack Strategies by Calorie Level (page 154) to adapt the meals and snacks to your calorie goal. Over the next twelve weeks, I will introduce you to foods and tools that will help you learn what and how much to eat so that you can move away from counting calories.

You'll be measuring your activity in terms of number of daily steps, with an ultimate activity goal of at least 10,000 steps a day, or a total of four to five miles. You'll work toward this goal by adding 1,000 daily steps each week. Rather than increasing by 1,000 steps all at once, I suggest that you add 150 steps each day until you reach your 1,000 extra steps. The 1,000 steps take less time than you think, about seven to ten minutes, and they add up to about half a mile. It's as simple as walking around when you have a bit of free time or while you're texting or talking on the phone. Or you can bump up your steps doing other types of physical activity.

Overcoming Challenges

There are as many excuses for not trying to change your habits as there are minutes in the day—maybe even more. And I guarantee that you will encounter challenges along the way. But you can overcome them if you're ready to make the necessary adjustments to your lifestyle. Before you begin the Ultimate Volumetrics Diet, ask yourself these few simple questions to determine whether now is the time for you to start.

1. Am I ready to change my eating and activity habits?
2. Can I make changes that will fit into my routine and lifestyle?
3. Can I stick with the program long enough to learn new habits?
4. Can I make a commitment to keep food and activity records?
5. Will I make time in my busy schedule for physical activity?
6. Am I willing to take action to avoid or overcome the triggers that affect my food and activity decisions?
7. Can I develop personal strategies for solving problems that may affect my eating?
8. Do I have friends and family members who can be my support and help me stay motivated?

If you answered "yes" to all or most of these questions, you're mentally prepared to embark on our journey together. If most of your answers are "no," consider how you might adjust your mindset in a way that changes your answers, one at a time, to "yes."

Your Next Steps

Week 1 is just around the corner! Keep your daily records handy as I will be asking you to refer back to them as you learn how to modify your lifestyle in a Volumetrics way. For your diet, I suggest choosing from among the four weeks of sample menus on pages 156–163 for at least the first several weeks. Each full day provides a set number of calories, and Meal and Snack Strategies by Calorie Level (page 154) offers instructions on how to adjust them to your daily calorie goal. The purpose is not to count calories but instead to learn what your meals should look like at that calorie level. Menus include a combination of different types of meals made from the recipes in the book, simple combinations of foods, convenience items, and restaurant fare. You can follow them exactly as written, or mix and match choices from other menus. Meals are at set calorie levels—400 calories for breakfast and 500 each for lunch and dinner—that you can use as is or modify as needed as a guide to how much food to eat.

Once you get started, here is the way that I would like you to keep track of your daily progress over the next few weeks.

- Write down the foods you eat at each meal and snack. You may want to circle the Volumetrics dishes that you like best.
- Rate your hunger and fullness at the beginning and end of each meal. You will be pleased to see how satisfied you feel even though you are eating fewer calories.
- Record your daily steps and other types of physical activity that you choose to include in your day.
- Step on the scale daily if you can, but not more than once a day and not less than once a week. Remember not to be discouraged if your weight goes up and down from day to day; that's normal. If your weight hits a plateau, check the amount you're eating and your activity level to make sure you're not getting more calories or moving less than you had planned. You may need to lower your daily calorie level and increase your steps.
- Keep track on the Personal Daily Record Form (page 7) of the strategies you've used to reach your weekly goals. They can be as simple as packing your lunch instead of buying it at work or calling a friend to take an afternoon walk.
- Include notes on your mood, emotions, or other factors that may have affected your eating.

In each of the next twelve weeks, you'll learn about Volumetrics principles and how to put them into action through the food you eat, new behaviors and habits, and steps toward being more active. I recommend that you follow along week by week, but feel free to read ahead if you like.

Week 1
Calorie Density Basics

Volumetrics is my personal eating plan. I've never been a "small portion" girl and am no good at pushing myself away from the table before I'm totally satisfied. So the only way I can control calories is by choosing foods that incorporate lots of water and fiber.—Delia Hammock, M.S., R.D.

Chances are that you have been down this road before, looking for a simple way to lose weight and keep the pounds off for good. What derailed you in the past? Did you feel too hungry? Deprived because you had to give up favorite foods? Unsatisfied from skimpy meals? Then you will love Volumetrics, a positive, scientifically proven approach to weight management that focuses on what you *can* eat.

When you are managing your weight, eating a satisfying amount of food for the right number of calories is a priority. Who wants to be overly hungry and unsatisfied when you can feel full and lose weight? People who learn to eat in a Volumetrics way are thrilled that they can eat ample portions while cutting calories. Kristie, who participated in a research study that included a Volumetrics eating plan, says, "When trying to lose weight in the past, I would eat smaller portions and feel hungrier. Volumetrics opened my eyes to the fact that I didn't have to eat less and be hungry; I just had to make some smart substitutions."

Why Losing Weight Is Not Just About Calories

One of the first things I asked you to do to get started was to determine how many calories to eat each day. While having an understanding of your calorie requirements and appropriate food choices is important, you also need to learn how to choose foods that satisfy your hunger and meet your nutritional needs. The photo in Similar Calories and Macronutrients, Different Foods shows two meals with similar calories and percentages of calories from the macronutrients protein, fat, and carbohydrate. As you can see, the types and amounts of food are completely different—relatively small portions of snack foods on the left, compared with foods chosen according to Volumetrics principles on the right. The Volumetrics meal is satisfying—with more than three times the amount of food. Can you guess the "magic" ingredient that accounts for the difference in meal size? You'll learn the answer shortly.

Similar Calories and Macronutrients, Different Foods

This photo shows that even if you focus on calories and the balance of fat, carbohydrate, and protein, you can end up with a very different selection of foods in your diet. Each of these meals provides about 500 calories, 30 percent of calories from fat, 60 percent of calories from carbohydrate, and 10 percent from protein. The meal on the left, which looks like a snack, includes 1½ tablespoons of peanuts, 2 ounces of pretzels, and a little more than a cup of lemon-lime soda. Portions are skimpy and the meal is lacking nutritionally. In the Volumetrics meal, you get a large bowl of soup, a side salad with oil and vinegar dressing, pita chips, a large bowl of melon balls, and a glass of water. This meal provides large portions and better diet quality.

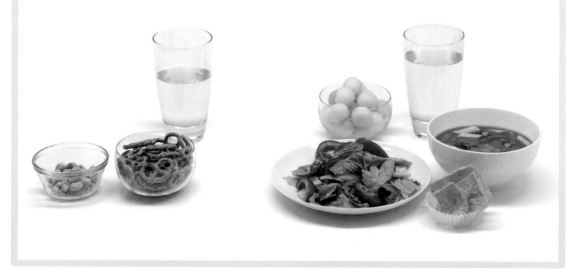

This week and next are devoted to a fundamental property of food called *calorie density* (CD), which reflects the calories in a given portion of food. A food that has a high CD has lots of calories in a small amount of food. The opposite is true for low-CD foods. They have fewer calories relative to their weight, so you can eat a bigger portion for the same calories.

What Affects the Calorie Density of Food?

Everything you eat or drink is a combination of the macronutrients fat, carbohydrate, and protein, as well as water and sometimes alcohol. Together these determine the calorie content of foods and the CD (see Where the Calories Are).

- Fat has a CD of 9 calories per gram and packs the most calories into a bite, more than twice as many as protein or carbohydrate.
- Alcohol has a CD of 7 calories per gram, almost as high as fat.
- The CD of both carbohydrate and protein is 4 calories per gram.
- Fiber, a type of carbohydrate, has a lower CD than other carbohydrates, only 2 calories per gram, because it is not fully digested and absorbed by the body.
- Water is like a "magic" ingredient in food because it adds weight and volume without any calories. The CD of water is zero. So the "wetter" the food, the lower its CD and the more food you get for your calories.

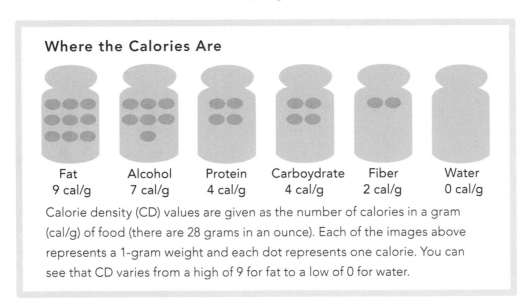

Where the Calories Are

Fat	Alcohol	Protein	Carboydrate	Fiber	Water
9 cal/g	7 cal/g	4 cal/g	4 cal/g	2 cal/g	0 cal/g

Calorie density (CD) values are given as the number of calories in a gram (cal/g) of food (there are 28 grams in an ounce). Each of the images above represents a 1-gram weight and each dot represents one calorie. You can see that CD varies from a high of 9 for fat to a low of 0 for water.

When asked to guess which of these components has the biggest effect on the CD of foods, most people don't think of water. Foods with a high water content help fill you up since water bulks up food, giving you bigger portions without more calories. The soup, salad, and melon in the photo Similar Calories and Macronutrients, Different Foods (page 17) all are water-rich foods, while the pretzels and peanuts have almost no water.

In contrast to water, fat is calorie dense. The higher the fat content of foods, the smaller the portion you get for your calories. But I don't want you to eliminate all fat. Volumetrics focuses on healthy fats and how to use just enough to give you delicious flavor along with fat's nutritional benefits.

You can vary the proportions of water, fat, carbohydrate, and protein to lower the CD of many foods. For example, if you substitute a lower-CD nutrient such as carbohydrate for one higher in CD such as fat, you lower the CD of the food. That is why a serving of reduced-fat cheese has fewer calories and a lower CD than regular cheese; some of its fat has been replaced by carbohydrate, protein, and water. We will talk more about fat and the other nutrients in foods in later weeks.

I want you to learn to choose more foods that are low in CD so that this becomes your preferred eating pattern. You will find that as you eat more of the lower-CD foods and less of those higher in CD, your daily calorie intake will go down and you will feel full and satisfied. I will show you how to recognize foods that provide the most satisfying portions for the fewest calories. Let's start by looking at the nutrition label on food packages.

Two Important Numbers That Matter Most for Calorie Density

Turn to the back of any package of food in your cupboard or refrigerator and you will see a panel labeled "Nutrition Facts." This panel contains useful and important information on the food's calories and nutrients and how they compare to daily recommendations. This week, let's focus on two numbers near the top of the panel, calories and serving size.

In order to manage your weight, you need a basic understanding of how many calories are in different foods. When you look at calories on the Nutrition Facts panel, keep in mind that the number refers to the calories in the suggested serving size. This may well be much smaller than your idea of a serving and also much smaller than the amount in the package. The standard serving of frozen yogurt as listed on the Sample Frozen Yogurt Nutrition Facts Panel is a puny half cup, while the carton contains four half-cup servings. If you eat the entire carton—four servings—you will have consumed 640 calories rather than the 160 in a single serving!

Sample Frozen Yogurt Nutrition Facts Panel

The Nutrition Facts panel on food packages includes calories and serving size information that will help you choose lower-CD, satisfying foods that fit into your daily calorie goal.

Serving Size: The suggested serving size of the food, and, in parentheses, the weight in grams

Calories: The calories in the suggested serving of food

Nutrition Facts

Serving Size 1/2 cup (98g)
Serving Per Container 4

Amount Per Serving

Calories 160   Calories from Fat 25

Servings Per Container: The number of servings in the package

$$\frac{\text{Calories per serving}}{\text{Grams per serving}} = \text{calorie density (CD)}$$

Now let's see how to use the panel to determine a food's CD. It is calculated using the two numbers near the top of the label, calories per serving and serving size in grams. Grab any packaged food that's handy and check the Nutrition Facts panel, or follow along with my frozen yogurt example. Find the weight of the serving size in grams and the calories in that serving. Now divide the calories by the weight. In my example, 160 calories divided by 98 grams equals 1.6, meaning that the calorie density of this frozen yogurt is 1.6 calories per gram.

CD will vary between 0 calories per gram for pure water to 9 calories per gram for pure fat. Next week, you will be introduced to charts that categorize foods based on their CD. These categories will serve as a guide to help you learn which foods have so few calories per gram that you can eat almost unlimited portions, as well as those that have a higher CD and need more moderation. For now, keep this quick rule of thumb in mind:

- If a food has more grams than calories in a serving, it is relatively low in CD and can be eaten in satisfying portions.
- When a serving contains more calories than grams, use portion control.

CD is particularly useful for comparing two brands or varieties of a similar food to decide which gives the biggest portion for the calories. Suppose you are in the mood for a snack and you want to treat yourself with a 100-calorie preportioned snack food. To get the most for the calories, pick the one with the greatest weight for those 100 calories—it has the lowest CD.

Now that you understand the basics of CD, I want to share with you some of the research in our lab that got us excited about CD as a tool for cutting calories and helping people lose weight and keep it off.

Why Low Calorie Density Equals Lower Calorie Intake

Early studies in my lab, as well as in colleagues' labs, revealed a fascinating finding. At a meal, or even over a day or so, people decide how much of a food to eat more by its portion size than by its calorie content. This is surprising since our bodies have a system for adjusting how much to eat based on the number of calories we need. Indeed much of the research on eating behavior is geared toward understanding the body's systems for regulating calorie intake and body weight. But when you are deciding how much to eat at a meal, you will be guided more by how much you think you should eat than by your biology.

To see this in action, let's visit my lab and imagine that you are a participant in one of our studies. Participants come to the lab to eat lunch once a week for three weeks in a row. Each week they are offered a large dish full of a baked pasta casserole with tomato sauce. It might look like the same casserole each week, but behind the scenes we tweaked the casseroles to change the CD. One week's casserole is high CD and the others have CD lowered by 12 or 24 percent. We do this by substituting chopped or puréed vegetables (remember, veggies are mostly water) for some of the pasta. Our study participants rarely notice the change. They eat the same amount of the casserole each week, with fewer calories when CD is lower—and don't feel hungrier or compensate by eating more later. This shows that people decide how much food to serve themselves based more on what they judge as an appropriate amount than by its calorie content.

Volumetrics Helps with Weight Loss

Here is another benefit of eating the Volumetrics way: several trials show that it can help you lose weight. In one such study, obese women completed a one-year weight-loss program. All of them met regularly with a dietitian to learn how to trim fat from their diet. Half of the women also were taught how to lower the CD of their diet by eating more water-rich foods, including vegetables and fruits. Unlike participants in many weight-loss programs, the women were not given a specific daily calorie goal.

We found that over the year on the diets, the advice to eat less fat was associated with decreased CD and weight loss. But the women who were advised also to eat *more* vegetables, fruits, and water-rich foods did even better by:

- reducing CD more and losing about 33 percent more weight after six months
- feeling less hungry
- weighing less at the end of the year.

THE BOTTOM LINE. This study is exciting because it shows that teaching people how to make food choices that lower the CD of their diet helps them lose weight—without counting calories. The group that was told to eat more vegetables, fruits, and other water-rich foods was encouraged to think positively about what they could eat rather than what they had to give up. That is what I want you to do.

How Calorie Density Can Help You Manage Your Weight

As you go through this twelve-week plan and explore the recipes in the book, choosing satisfying portions of low-CD foods most of the time while still enjoying small portions of foods higher in CD will become second nature. Traci Malone, M.H.S., R.D., shared with me the reactions she gets when teaching weight-loss classes that use the principles of Volumetrics: "People always comment that the meals have so much food that they don't think they can eat it all. The amount of food in their meals is very satisfying and filling."

Now it's your turn to put your knowledge of CD to use. I know you're anxious to get a running start on your new way of eating, so this week's meals are planned out for you to show you how to make food choices that fit your calorie goals. Turn to Your Personal Ultimate Volumetrics Diet Plan (page 153) to select your meals for the coming week. You'll get to taste the Volumetrics way of eating firsthand.

Key Points

- Calorie density (CD, or calories per gram) is the amount of calories (energy) in a specific amount of food.
- A high-CD food gives you lots of calories in a small amount of food, while a low-CD food has fewer calories for the same amount of food.
- For the same number of calories, you can eat a larger portion of a low-CD food than of a food higher in CD.
- Water is the "magic" ingredient that lowers CD.
- Over a day, people generally eat a similar amount of food by weight. Choosing foods with a lower CD will allow you to eat your usual amount of food while reducing your calorie intake.

Let's Get Physical

Using your baseline number of steps as a starting point, you will be adding an extra 150 steps, less than a tenth of a mile, each day until you reach an additional 1,000 steps or about half a mile by the end of this first week. Remember to keep track in your daily record. Your ultimate goal is 10,000 daily steps, but you don't need to get there all at once! Here are some tips to get you started.

- Walk around while you're talking on the phone.
- Play with your kids in the yard or challenge them to a game of tag.
- While your kids are playing sports, take a walk with a few of the other parents or on your own.
- Walk to a friend's house when you want to chat, instead of calling, emailing, or texting.
- Swap screen time in front of the television or computer for walking time.

- Make a daily appointment with yourself to walk, whether around the house or around the block.

Head and Habits

This week's focus is identifying the Volumetrics habits you already have. Take out the food record that I suggested you keep before starting Week 1.

- Circle the meals that have plenty of vegetables and fruits. Vegetables and fruits that have a very low CD should be included in every meal.
- Look for meals that contain a salad or noncreamy soup. These water-rich foods help fill you up without too many calories.
- Check for meals and snacks where you've included lower-fat alternatives to foods high in fat. Fat increases the CD of foods, so making a switch can cut calories and CD.
- Pat yourself on the back if some meals include no snack food, candy, or dessert, or you've limited yourself to just a small portion. Calories add up quickly with these high-CD foods, so limiting portions is necessary.

To Do This Week

- ☐ Get the okay from your doctor to start Volumetrics after discussing any health concerns, special diet requirements, changes in medication, and other considerations.
- ☐ Choose your meals for the coming week from the menu plan (page 156). Then make a shopping list and shop for those meals.
- ☐ Weigh yourself at least once during the week.
- ☐ Keep track in your daily record of everything you eat and drink, your hunger and fullness ratings, and any notes on emotions or other factors that affected your eating.
- ☐ Write down strategies that have helped you work toward your goals.
- ☐ Wear your step counter and keep track of your steps each day, adding 150 steps a day until you have added a total of 1,000 daily steps by the end of the week.

Week 2

More on Calorie Density

My clients say what they like best is feeling full and eating more food while cutting calories.—Juliet Mancino, M.S., R.D., C.D.E.

Last week, you learned how the nutrients in foods affect CD. This week you will begin learning how to use CD to decide what to eat. Dr. Brian Wansink at Cornell University says that we make several hundred food-related decisions each day. Understanding how the CD of foods influences how much you eat will help you make these decisions wisely. In this second week, you will learn which foods have such a low CD that they are virtually "free"—you can eat about as much as you want—and which others are so important nutritionally they should be eaten every day, even though they are higher in CD. I will also help you decide how and when to include high-CD foods and indulgences in your diet.

Choosing Your Foods Based on Calorie Density Categories

I have divided foods into four categories, based on their CD. These categories group foods together in a way that serves as a guide for meal planning and portion control. The chart of Calorie Density Categories on page 26 provides a summary.

CATEGORY 1 (VERY LOW CD). Category 1 foods are your go-to foods for feeling full on fewer calories. The vegetables and fruits in this category offer two major benefits: a lot of food for the calories and plenty of nutrients. If you're like most people, your diet falls short of the recommendations in the Dietary Guidelines for Americans, so try to fit these Category 1 foods into meals and snacks wherever you can.

- Think large—make big very-low-CD salads, put plenty of vegetables on your plate, and look for ways to add extra vegetables and fruits to favorite recipes.
- Enjoy lots of naked vegetables and fruits. When you clothe them in fatty or sugary toppings, dressings, or sauces, they are no longer "free" foods.
- Pay attention to the amount it takes to fill you up, and stop when you reach that limit. Although I describe this category as "free," that doesn't mean it is okay to eat ten apples at one sitting! That's too many calories.

Calorie Density Categories
Use these four CD categories to guide your food choices and meal planning.

CATEGORY	CD DESCRIPTION	CD RANGE	HOW TO EAT	EXAMPLES
1	Very-Low CD	Less than 0.6	"Free" foods to eat any time	Almost all fruits and nonstarchy vegetables, and broth-based soups
2	Low CD	0.6–1.5	Eat reasonable portions	Whole grains, lean proteins, legumes, and low-fat dairy
3	Medium CD	1.6–3.9	Manage your portions	Breads, desserts, fat-free baked snacks, cheeses, and higher-fat meats
4	High CD	4.0–9.0	Carefully manage portions and frequency of eating	Fried snacks, candy, cookies, nuts, and fats

CATEGORY 2 (LOW CD). Round out your meal or snack with selections from Category 2. Many of these foods are the core of healthy eating, nutritious staples to eat every day for a varied and balanced diet. I encourage you to select foods from the low end of this CD range; as CD goes up, you will need to start moderating portion size to control calories.

- Select from whole grains, lower-fat protein foods, starchy vegetables, legumes (beans and peas), and low-fat mixed dishes.

- Make choices that give you more nutrients—brown rice instead of white rice and cereals rich in fiber and whole grains rather than sugar and fat.

CATEGORY 3 (MEDIUM CD). Pick carefully from Category 3. While the foods in this category are commonly included in meals, they can have a lot of fat, sugar, and calories for the portion size. Eating them often and in large portions can push your daily calories too high.

- Consider alternatives that are lower CD.
- Keep portions modest and pair them with larger portions of Category 1 and 2 foods.

CATEGORY 4 (HIGH CD). Limit your choices and portions from Category 4, but you don't need to cut them out altogether. Research shows that restricting high-CD foods or just anticipating having to give them up can make you want them more. That is why we will work together to fit in your favorite treats—chocolate, sweets, snack foods—so you don't feel deprived.

- Create your own personal strategy for managing indulgent high-CD foods, whether it's buying just small amounts, setting aside a daily portion, or removing all indulgences from your house. We will be looking more closely at your eating environment in Week 11.
- Include small portions of Category 4 foods such as nuts and olive oil that contain healthy fats and provide important nutrients.

Now let's dig a little deeper into how to use CD to choose specific foods that ensure you are eating nutritious and satisfying meals and snacks while controlling calories.

An Introduction to Calorie Density Charts

The charts on the next few pages, along with the comprehensive Modular Food Lists (pages 357–371) in the back of the book, include the CD for hundreds of different foods. But don't think that I am going to ask you to keep track of the CD of every food you eat. The purpose of the charts is to help you pick a variety of lower-CD foods whenever possible to bring down the CD of your overall diet. Be sure to check label information as serving size, calories, and, therefore, CD can vary by brand.

Calorie Density Charts

Category 1: Very-Low-CD Foods
(less than 0.6 calories per gram)

FOOD	CD
SOUPS	
Chicken broth, regular	0.17
Vegetarian vegetable soup	0.29
Tomato soup, prepared with water	0.30
Chicken noodle soup	0.31
Lentil soup	0.57
VEGETABLES	
Celery	0.12
Cucumber	0.12
Tomato, raw	0.16
Spinach, raw	0.17
Zucchini, steamed	0.17
Salad greens	0.18
Asparagus, cooked	0.22
Broccoli, raw	0.29
Mushrooms, raw	0.29
Greens beans, cooked	0.31
Bell pepper, red, raw	0.33
Carrots, raw	0.33
Winter squash	0.38
FRUITS	
Watermelon	0.29
Strawberries	0.33
Cantaloupe	0.34
Peach	0.40
Orange	0.46
Raspberries	0.52
Apple	0.53
Blueberries	0.57
Pear	0.58
DAIRY	
Yogurt, light (nonfat, low-calorie sweetener)	0.44
Yogurt, Greek-style, nonfat, plain	0.53
Yogurt, nonfat, plain	0.56
CONDIMENTS	
Salsa	0.33
Italian dressing, fat-free	0.50

Category 2: Low-CD Foods
(0.6 to 1.5 calories per gram)

FOOD	CD
SOUPS	
Clam chowder, prepared with milk	0.62
Split pea	0.71
VEGETABLES, LEGUMES (BEANS AND PEAS)	
Tofu, firm	0.72
Sweet potato, baked or mashed	0.76
Green peas, cooked	0.81
Beans, kidney	0.85
Corn, boiled, drained	0.90
Potato, baked, with skin	0.91
FRUITS	
Grapes	0.69
Banana	1.1
DAIRY	
Yogurt, low-fat plain	0.68
Cottage cheese, 1% fat	0.70
Yogurt, low-fat fruit	1.1
CEREALS, GRAINS	
Bran flakes, with fat-free milk	1.1
Shredded wheat, with fat-free milk	1.2
Rice, brown, long-grain, cooked	1.2
Spaghetti, whole-wheat, cooked	1.2
MEAT, POULTRY, FISH	
Shrimp, steamed	1.2
Tuna, light, canned in water	1.2
Tilapia, cooked	1.3
Turkey breast, roasted, no skin	1.4
Ham, extra lean	1.5
MIXED DISHES	
Spaghetti with meatballs	1.1
Chili con carne with beans	1.2
Macaroni and cheese, prepared from frozen	1.2
CONDIMENTS	
Pasta sauce, tomato-based	0.72
Mustard, Ketchup	1.0
Black olives	1.1
Ranch dressing, fat-free	1.2

Category 3: Medium-CD Foods
(1.6 to 3.9 calories per gram)

FOOD	CD
VEGETABLES, LEGUMES (BEANS AND PEAS)	
Hummus	1.8
Potatoes, french-fried	2.9
FRUITS	
Avocado, California	1.6
Raisins	3.1
DAIRY	
Cream cheese, light	2.0
Cheese, feta	2.5
Mozzarella cheese, part-skim	2.8
Cheese, Swiss, reduced-fat	3.0
BREADS	
Tortilla, corn	2.2
Pita, whole-wheat	2.5
Bread, white	2.7
Bread, whole-grain	2.8
MEAT, POULTRY, FISH, EGGS	
Chicken breast, roasted, no skin	1.6
Egg, hard-cooked	1.6
Sirloin steak, lean, broiled	1.8
Salmon, farmed, baked	2.1
Pork chop, center loin, broiled	2.2
Ground beef, lean, broiled	2.2
MIXED DISHES	
Cheese pizza, thin crust	3.0
Cheeseburger, fast food	3.0
Biscuit with egg and sausage	3.2
DESSERTS, SNACK FOODS	
Frozen yogurt, soft serve	1.6
Apple pie	2.6
Ice cream, premium	2.8
Hard pretzels	3.5
CONDIMENTS	
Ranch dressing, reduced-fat	2.0
Italian dressing, full-fat	2.8
Mayonnaise, light	3.3
Cream cheese, full-fat	3.3

Category 4: High-CD Foods
(4.0 to 9.0 calories per gram)

FOOD	CD
DAIRY	
Cheese, Parmesan	4.5
Butter	7.0
BREADS, CRACKERS	
Cinnamon Danish pastry	4.0
Graham crackers	4.0
Croissant	4.2
Wheat crackers	4.3
MEAT	
Pork spareribs, braised	4.0
Bacon, cooked	5.2
DESSERTS, SNACK FOODS, CANDY	
Carrot cake, cream cheese frosting	4.0
Popcorn, caramel	4.0
Brownie	4.1
Donut, cake	4.1
Trail mix	4.3
Creme-filled chocolate sandwich cookies	4.4
Potato chips, baked	4.5
Tortilla chips, regular	4.7
Granola bar, hard	4.8
Milk chocolate	5.0
Potato chips, regular	5.2
Chocolate chip cookies, homemade	5.2
Cheese puffs, fried	5.3
Dark chocolate	5.7
NUTS	
Peanut butter, reduced-fat	5.0
Almonds, dry-roasted	5.9
Peanuts, roasted	6.1
Peanut butter, regular	6.3
Pecans, dry-roasted	6.8
CONDIMENTS	
Jam	4.0
Ranch dressing, full-fat	4.8
Mayonnaise, regular, full-fat	6.7
Margarine, stick	7.0
Oil, olive	8.8

You can use the charts to choose foods and ingredients that have a lower CD than those you might otherwise select—for example, extra lean ham (CD 1.5) instead of a lean burger patty (CD 2.2) or grapes (CD 0.69) in place of raisins (CD 3.1). Practice choosing lower-CD alternatives to foods that you typically ate before starting Volumetrics by pulling out your three days of food records from Week 0 and looking through the CD charts for foods to swap into your meal in place of higher-calorie, high-CD items. Some swaps will lower CD by only a small amount but will make positive changes in nutrition. The chart Making High-CD/Low-CD Swaps provides other ideas to lower CD and save calories.

Making High-CD/Low-CD Swaps

These examples show how swapping foods can lower CD and save calories while providing satisfying amounts of food.

INSTEAD OF THESE FOODS			TRY SUBSTITUTING THESE			CALORIE SAVINGS
Higher-CD	CD	Calories	Lower-CD	CD	Calories	
Croissant (1 medium)	4.2	230	*Blueberry Lemon Breakfast Loaf (1 slice)*	1.9	170	60
Granola (1 cup) with fat-free milk (½ cup)	2.4	570	Wheat bran flakes cereal (1 cup) with fat-free milk (½ cup)	1.1	170	400
Low-fat fruit yogurt (6 oz)	1.0	185	Light yogurt (6 oz)	0.44	80	105
Ranch dressing (2 tbsp)	4.8	145	Fat-free ranch dressing (2 tbsp)	1.2	35	110
Premium ice cream (½ cup)	2.8	290	Frozen yogurt (½ cup)	1.3	110	180

THE BOTTOM LINE. It's okay if some CD changes are not very big; large and small decreases in CD add up over the course of the day to have a positive effect on calories and the amount of food you can eat. In one of our studies, people who decreased the CD of their daily diet by just 0.5 calories per gram ate two-thirds of a pound more food, cut out 500 calories per day, and lost weight!

What About Beverages?

Did you notice that beverages are missing from the lists? That's because beverages don't affect hunger and fullness the same way food does. You could drink a lot of beverage calories without making a difference to how hungry you are. For example, if you have a large regular soft drink, are you full or do you still have room for food? Studies show that you will likely eat just as much food when you have the soda as when you don't. The beverage calories add on to the calories from food. Another reason I list beverages separately is that their high water content gives them a relatively low CD that should not be compared with foods (see the Beverage chart on page 370). Because we drink large amounts of beverages, their calories add up quickly. A 16-ounce cola, for example, has a CD of only 0.42 but over 200 calories! So think before you drink. You will be learning more about how to make wise beverage choices in Week 9.

Calorie Density and Nutrition

The CD charts can help you make food choices based on CD and nutrition in ways consistent with widely agreed-upon recommendations for a healthy diet. The 2010 Dietary Guidelines for Americans (www.dietaryguidelines.gov), a government policy that affects individuals, agencies, restaurants, food manufacturers, and retailers alike, call for a diet based on nutrient-rich foods—vegetables, fruits, whole grains, fat-free or low-fat milk products, and lean and meatless proteins. These are the foods at the core of Categories 1 and 2. The Guidelines also encourage cutting back on some higher-fat foods, while including small amounts of nuts, seeds, and other nutrient-rich foods that are higher in calories. You will find these foods in Categories 3 and 4.

What's Next?

In the coming weeks, you will learn how to use the CD of foods to help you eat satisfying portions while you lose weight. I will show you specific strategies, based on research from my lab, that allow you to cut calories and still enjoy a full plate of food, add a first course to your meal to get more food but fewer calories, and change the proportion of food on your plate for a more satisfying meal.

As a first step, I encourage you to get into what I call a "CD state of mind." Delia Hammock, R.D., the former nutrition director of the Good Housekeeping Research Institute, describes the way that she approaches every meal:

> My goal is to get the most food and nutrition out of every calorie. Personally, I don't want to feel hungry or deprived. So whether I am planning my own meals or creating a meal plan for readers, I always consider ways to make food satisfying. Thinking about food in a Volumetrics way has become a habit.

Key Points

- Foods can be divided into four categories based on their CD for purposes of meal planning and portion control. Those in Category 1 are virtually "free" but as CD goes up in Categories 2, 3, and 4, the need to manage portion size increases.

- As you look at a day's meals that you ate during Week 1 using the sample menus as a guide, notice how Category 1 foods take up a lot of space on the plate, with Category 2 choices to round them out, small portions of Category 3 foods, and Category 4 foods used sparingly.

- Within each category, foods with a lower CD are usually preferable to those with a higher CD for managing calories. Make changes to what you usually put on your plate by swapping high-CD foods for those that are lower on the CD charts.

- Don't get bogged down with the numbers. Instead, look through the CD charts to see how CD varies in different types of foods. Think about how you can use the charts to lower the CD of your meals.

- Leave room for your favorite high-CD foods—I have my own personal list of foods that are too delicious to give up (hint: this includes chocolate), so I include them on occasion, and in small portions purely for enjoyment. Giving them up isn't necessary.

Let's Get Physical

Have you been able to add steps to your day? For this week, I suggest that you continue adding about 150 steps a day until you have increased your total daily steps for this week by 1,000, bringing you closer to the 10,000-step goal of this program. These suggestions can help you step up your steps around town.

- Don't take the closest parking space.
- Use stairs whenever possible in parking lots, stores, and malls.
- Treat the dog to a nice, long walk.
- Walk instead of driving to run an errand.

Head and Habits

It's important to reward yourself for your accomplishments with small, nonfood gifts and activities that mean something to you. You could buy yourself a small item—a book, new walking shoes, a clothing accessory—or treat yourself to a favorite activity such as a massage, walk with a friend, or relaxing bubble bath.

To Do This Week

- ☐ Choose your meals for the coming week, mixing and matching from among those that have the same number of calories. Then make a shopping list and shop for your menu.
- ☐ Weigh yourself at least once during the week.
- ☐ Keep track in your daily record of everything you eat and drink, hunger and fullness ratings, and any notes on emotions or other factors that affected your eating.
- ☐ Write down strategies that have helped you work toward your goals.
- ☐ Wear your step counter and keep track of your steps each day, adding 150 steps a day until you have added a total of 1,000 daily steps by the end of the week.
- ☐ Create a list with at least five small, nonfood rewards that will help keep up your motivation and reinforce your successes.

Week 3
Portion Size:
When Bigger Is Better

We all like big portions and most people are eating too much. The Volumetrics approach gives a positive message—foods to eat more of rather than foods to avoid.—Bonnie Taub-Dix, M.A., R.D.

We live in a super-sized world. It is not unusual these days to be served pasta on a plate that is too big to hold with one hand or soda in a bucket-sized cup. Portions are huge because we like them that way and restaurants, fast-food outlets, and movie theaters know it. We appreciate what looks like good value—lots of food for our money. The reality is that oversized portions are poor value if they lead us to eat more than we need. If you are like most people, you eat what you are served. In my lab, we have found over and over that the bigger the portion, the more people eat.

- Men ate a whopping 350 more calories when we served a 12-inch submarine sandwich compared with when we served one that was half as big.
- Serving a larger portion of macaroni and cheese at lunch increased intake by 30 percent—and most people in the study didn't even notice the difference in portions.

I know that when you eat a big meal, you have good intentions to cut back on the next one. It makes sense that you expect to be less hungry and to adjust your calories for the day. The problem is that in our super-sized environment the next meal and the one after that are likely to provide too much food as well, and this sets us up to keep on overeating. Big portions are so compelling that they overwhelm the biological regulatory systems that should signal us to eat less after several days of overeating. This happened in our lab—when we increased portions by 50 percent for eleven days, both men and women ate over 400 extra calories each day and a total of more than 4,600 extra calories over the eleven days! Remember, it takes approximately 3,500 calories to gain a pound.

THE BOTTOM LINE. Large portions affect everyone—lean and obese, young and old, members of the clean plate club, and those of us who leave food behind. And large portions are sneaky. In our studies, most people don't notice the difference when we increase the size of the portions offered.

Are Big Portions Really to Blame?

There have been huge increases in the size of the portions of many calorie-dense foods at home, outside the home, and in cookbooks since the 1970s. Oversized portions have borne much of the blame for the recent rise in obesity rates. Indeed, two of the top six messages for consumers in the U.S. Department of Agriculture (USDA) 2010 Dietary Guidelines for Americans (www.dietaryguidelines.gov) focus on managing portions.

- Enjoy your food, but eat less.
- Avoid oversized portions.

While I agree that managing portion size is important, I don't want you to do it simply by eating less. Cutting down to skimpy portions of all foods may work in the short term, but over time you're likely to go back to eating the amount of food you have grown accustomed to. That is why this week focuses on how to make strategic and sensible portion size decisions that can help you feel satisfied and stay within your calorie goal.

Portion Size Does Not Have to Be the Villain

Not all big portions will derail your diet. Big portions of calorie-dense foods are the problem. If your diet consists mostly of foods from Categories 3 and 4, you'll have to eat smaller portions to cut calories, and that's hard to do. The amount of food you can eat to lose weight, or even to avoid gaining weight, will be too small to satisfy your hunger. Your plate will be half empty (see How to Have a Full Plate When Cutting Calories). Instead, if you lower the overall CD of your diet, by eating mainly very-low- and low-CD Category 1 and 2 foods, you'll have a full plate with satisfying portions.

How to Have a Full Plate When Cutting Calories

You don't have to have a half-empty plate to manage portions. But calories add up quickly when you fill your plate with calorie-dense foods. The plate on the left—rib-eye steak, a baked potato with butter and sour cream, and broccoli—has 800 calories, about half your calories for the entire day. Portions are not very large because most of the foods are high in CD. If you want to decrease the meal to a more reasonable 400 calories, you could eat half-size portions of the same foods (the middle plate) but the meal wouldn't be satisfying—it doesn't have enough food. In contrast, the Volumetrics plate on the right is full and yet gives you only 400 calories. The portion of steak is more moderate, while the portions are bigger for lower-CD foods that are more filling such as the vegetables and the baked potato topped with light sour cream.

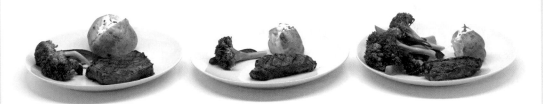

| 800 Calories, Higher CD | 400 Calories, Higher CD | 400 Calories, Lower CD |

Eating More to Eat Less

Our studies have shown that portion size has a powerful and consistent effect on intake—the bigger the portion, the more people eat. Why not harness this effect to help you eat *more* of the low-CD foods that will control calories? We have been testing whether this approach works. Here's what our results suggest you should do.

- *For your first course:* Start your meal with plenty of vegetables or fruits from Category 1 foods. A big bowl of soup, a salad, or a piece of fruit at the start of the meal can give you more food for fewer calories by filling you up so that you eat less later in the meal.
- *For your main course:* Fill your plate by substituting Category 1 vegetables for some of the higher-CD ingredients or foods. I will give you the specifics on how to do this in Weeks 4 and 5.

The Volume in Volumetrics

You probably noticed that we talk about CD in terms of the weight of foods rather than their volume. Why is that? The weight of solids is easier to measure precisely than the volume, so most of our studies are based on weight. But the volume of food and how big it looks can influence hunger, fullness, and how much you eat.

You can trick your mind into thinking you have eaten more food when the portion is aerated to increase volume or piled up to fill the plate or bowl. Studies in my lab show that if you perceive that you are getting a big portion, you are likely to feel fuller.

- We served three variations of a strawberry smoothie with the same ingredients and number of calories but different amounts of air to make their sizes appear different. People who drank the biggest smoothie—that is, the one with the most air—felt fuller and ate less at the lunch that followed.
- When study volunteers could eat as much as they wanted of two different cheese puff snacks with the same CD—one compact and the other puffed up with extra air—they ate fewer calories of the puffier version.

Try high-volume foods—air-popped popcorn, mousse-style yogurt, rice cakes, puffed and flaky cereals, lower-fat frozen desserts, smoothies. See if "big" portions will help fill you up, but be sure to keep your calorie goals in mind.

Now that you recognize how portion size can work for you—more low-CD food, fewer calories—you need the tools for figuring out how much food to eat to meet your daily calorie goals.

Your Portion-Control Toolkit: The Nutrition Facts Panel

In an ideal world, you would be able to lower the CD of your diet by choosing most of your foods from Categories 1 and 2 and you wouldn't have to worry about managing portion size. But realistically, our environment continually tempts us with oversized portions of tasty, calorie-dense foods. Often these are the only foods available. So you need a plan.

By now, you know how to read a Nutrition Facts panel to determine the calories per serving and the CD (see page 20). The panel also can help you manage portion size. You should get in the habit of checking the panel for servings in a package and calories in a serving. You can eat the suggested serving, or you may decide to eat a bigger or smaller portion, depending on what the food is and how it fits into your meal plan and Volumetrics goals.

The Nutrition Facts panel helps you compare similar products—for example, two snack foods with different serving sizes. You can calculate and use CD to choose the lower-CD snack that will give you a bigger portion for the calories. There's no need to calculate CD if you choose sweet or salty snacks in 100-calorie packages. The Nutrition Facts panel tells you the weight of food you get for those 100 calories. Usually it is not much—most of these snacks fall into Categories 3 and 4, where CD is high and portions for the calories are small.

Your Portion-Control Toolkit: Serving Size Guide

The Dietary Guidelines offer another tool for helping you eat a healthier diet—eating plans that group foods together and suggest how much to eat based on daily calories. For each food group, the Dietary Guidelines list the size of a serving and recommended number of servings per day for different daily calorie levels. A summary chart of Suggested Food Group Servings (page 372) in the Appendix shows serving sizes and recommended numbers of servings per day from each food group for diets of 1,400 calories, 1,600 calories, 1,800 calories, and 2,000 calories. You may find this chart useful for making sure that you're choosing the right balance of foods. For example, if you're eating 1,600 calories, the Dietary Guidelines recommend three to four daily servings of vegetables. When you follow Volumetrics, you already will be eating in a way that is consistent with these Dietary Guidelines.

Your Portion-Control Toolkit: Convenient Portion Tools

If you were a scientist interested in people's eating patterns and habits, you would find that getting people to tell you how much they have been eating is challenging. It's hard to estimate portion sizes, but tools such as measuring cups and spoons, pictures of foods in different portions, or a kitchen scale can help. Let's consider the available tools so you can decide which will help you.

Weighing and measuring: Weighing and measuring using simple tools like a kitchen scale and measuring cups and spoons can help you get to the point where you know almost on autopilot how much food to eat without a lot of hassle or number crunching. I suggest that you continue to use the kitchen scale not only to give guidance on how much to eat, but also as a handy tool for measuring ingredients when you are cooking. Most scales allow you to switch between ounces and grams so you can become comfortable with both measures. The recipes in this book list ingredients in both household measures and gram weights. Over time, you will become familiar with the look of common volumes—for example, a cup of cereal or half-cup of rice—but the scale will be useful when cooking from Volumetrics recipes.

Comparison to everyday objects: You may find it useful to relate common measurements to everyday household items.

- Deck of cards = about 3 ounces (meat portion in a meal)
- Lipstick tube = 1 ounce (cheese)
- Baseball = 1 cup (cereal)

For more examples, visit the Weight-control Information Network at www.win .niddk.nih.gov/publications/PDFs/justenough.pdf. You can also devise your own list of familiar objects, but be sure that their size accurately represents the measurement or you might end up eating portions that are too big.

Hands: A few years ago, Italian scientist Michele Sculati visited my lab and shared a secret with me about a different way to visualize appropriate portions. He and his father developed a system based entirely on the hand. For example, your fist (unless you have huge hands) is about the size of a cup. The palm of your hand can be used to remind you of the amount of meat that should be in your meal. This type of hand-based approach is so simple, it has been shown to improve fifth graders' portion size knowledge. Come up with your own equivalents based on the size of your hand and fingers. Using your hand is certainly convenient!

Plates and bowls: As portions have grown, so have plates, bowls, and even cup holders in cars. Use measuring cups to determine how much your plates, bowls, cups, and glasses hold. This way, you can eyeball portions based on how they look when you dish them out.

Electronic and mobile applications: If you want to include an electronic or mobile application in your portion-control toolkit, you can choose from numerous websites, blogs, and software options for computers, smartphones, tablets, and other mobile devices. Products are available to help you keep track of your daily calories, compare your portions to photos of different foods, scan bar codes on food packages, and, most important, track your progress. The number of offerings is so large and growing so quickly that it is impossible for me to make specific recommendations. I suggest that you try out different options to find the one that works best for you and fits into your lifestyle.

How to Manage Portion Distortion

Out-of-control portions are driving up calorie intake. However, if you choose very-low-CD Category 1 foods, you won't need to worry about the size of your portions. These are the type of foods I want you to eat more of. But as the CD of food increases, portion control becomes critical for weight management. Here are additional strategies to help you manage portions.

- Use portion-controlled frozen entrées or preportioned meals and snacks as a tool for learning about the amount of food you can eat for different amounts of calories. Not only do they give you a guide to portion size, but they can be kept on hand for a quick lunch or dinner when you're on the go or eating at work. You may need to add extra vegetables, fruit, and low-fat dairy products as necessary to meet your calorie and food group goals for the meal.
- If you usually prepare more food than you need, learn to cook less, plan to use extras for lunch or other meals, or portion leftovers into single-serving freezer/microwave containers for your own customized preportioned meals. Wrap up extra right away to avoid temptation.

- If someone serves you a portion that is just too big, decide how much you should eat and leave the rest or request a doggy bag.
- Assess your hunger and fullness while you are eating (see Get In Touch with Feelings of Hunger and Satiety on page 9). Rather than automatically cleaning your plate or reaching for seconds, relax for several minutes to see if you are still hungry.
- Eat slowly, experiencing the flavors and textures of your food, rather than racing through your meal. Your meal will be more enjoyable and satisfying, and you will find it easier to stop before you've eaten too much.

It's your turn . . .

Are you comfortable with your knowledge of how much to eat? Test whether you are portion savvy with these online quizzes:

- Size Up Your Servings and Calories
  www.fda.gov/Food/LabelingNutrition/ConsumerInformation/ucm114022.htm
- Portion Distortion! Do You Know How Food Portions Have Changed
  in 20 Years?
  hin.nhlbi.nih.gov/portion/ (This quiz also tells you how much physical activity you will need to burn off the extra calories from oversized portions.)

Key Points

- If you choose mostly Category 1 and Category 2 foods, you can be less concerned about restricting your portions. These are low in CD, so you get satisfying amounts for the calories. At the same time, manage portions of foods from Categories 3 and 4 because they're more calorie dense.
- Your portion-control toolkit—the Nutrition Facts panel, serving size guides, tools for weighing and measuring, dishes, and applications for electronic devices—can help you learn to control portions. By trying these tools, you can determine which give you the best guidance for putting together meals so you have your own personal system to remind you to eat appropriate portions.

Let's Get Physical

Over the past several weeks you've worked toward a weekly goal of adding 1,000 more steps to your day. Remember to reward yourself for a job well done! Add variety to your day by increasing your steps at work or during your daily routine: park farther away or get off the bus one stop earlier and enter the office building, mall, or school at the farthest entrance. Stop by a colleague's desk or walk to a neighbor's house rather than calling, emailing, or texting. Walk the long way. Go outside rather than to the vending machine or kitchen to combat midafternoon slump. Take the stairs whenever you can. Get up from your computer and take a five-minute walk several times a day. Invite the people you work with to take a walk with you. Look for opportunities to add to your daily step count wherever you can.

Head and Habits

Before you started this program, how often did you go into the kitchen and grab something to eat even though you weren't hungry? Eating based on emotions instead of hunger is pretty common. That is why your daily record sheet includes space to write down your feelings. You can learn a lot about emotions and feelings that trigger eating by looking through your daily records from the past two weeks. Do you eat when you are bored or tired? Does nervousness or tension send you into the kitchen? Which foods, if any, do you turn to after an argument or disagreement with a loved one? What happens to your eating habits when you're under stress?

Now think about ways you could deal with your emotions without turning to food. Choose distractions that you find enjoyable, such as chatting with a friend if you're lonely, exercising if you're restless, or doing something to occupy your hands if you're bored.

To Do This Week

- ☐ Choose your meals from the menu plan for the coming week. Make a shopping list and shop for those meals.
- ☐ Use at least one portion management tool for a full day's meals and snacks.

- ☐ Weigh yourself at least once during the week.
- ☐ Keep track in your daily record of everything you eat and drink, your hunger and fullness ratings, and any notes on emotions or other factors that affected your eating.
- ☐ Write down strategies that have helped you work toward your goals.
- ☐ Wear your step counter and keep track of your steps each day, finding new ways to add 150 steps a day until you have added a total of 1,000 daily steps by the end of the week.
- ☐ Identify on your daily records three occasions when emotions affected your eating. Use your Personal Daily Record Form to list strategies that can substitute for food, and try at least one this week.

Week 4
Putting Together Satisfying Meals

The effects of eating soup made a big impression on me when I participated in a calorie density study. Starting my meal with soup makes me feel full, and that helps me eat less of foods that are higher in calories. Sometimes I even take a short break between soup and my main course until I get hungry again.—Anne, Pennsylvania

We have become a nation of grazers. Among the hottest new products are foods and beverages that can be eaten on the run without time away from our overly busy lives. While we all find ourselves in situations where we are grateful for these convenience foods, their high CD makes it hard to manage calories. More important, if these become your staple foods, you miss out on the satisfying meals with family and friends that are among the most pleasurable of human activities.

What is a meal? You and I could have very different definitions. What and when we eat is influenced by where we live, who we eat with, our lifestyle, culture, family tradition, and dozens of other factors. Some of us, for example, live in a region where grits are served for breakfast, while others of us start the day with a bagel topped with cream cheese and lox. We eat differently with family and friends than we do when packing a lunch to bring to work. Holiday meals look different from everyday meals. Mastering the principles of Volumetrics means that you can enjoy satisfying meals anywhere and at any occasion while managing your weight.

Let's look at a day of "three square" meals, starting with breakfast and including first courses, entrées, and desserts at lunch and dinner. In a few weeks, we will move on to the beverages you include in your meals and the snacks you eat in between.

The Breakfast Bonus

I am surprised when people tell me that they skip breakfast as a way to cut calories and lose weight. The math may seem to make sense—not eating in the morning could free up calories for the rest of the day. But the numbers don't add up the way you might think. Going without breakfast appears to undermine weight loss success; breakfast skippers often make up the calories later in the day with foods that are less nutritious.

Whether you're a man, woman, teen, or child, eating breakfast is linked to a healthier body weight. The connection between breakfast and body weight is so strong that the 2010 Dietary Guidelines for Americans recommend eating a nutrient-rich breakfast as part of a healthy eating plan for weight loss and weight maintenance. Breakfast is particularly important if you're trying to keep pounds off. Over three-quarters of the participants in the National Weight Control Registry—several thousand men and women who have kept off thirty pounds or more for at least a year—say that they eat breakfast every day. Their breakfast is not complicated or time consuming—most eat cereal, milk, and fruit.

Do you still need convincing? Here are even more good reasons to eat breakfast.

- Adults who eat cereal for breakfast say they feel good physically and emotionally.
- Children who have breakfast are more alert in school, perform better, and have fewer discipline problems.
- Breakfast is the easiest meal to put together in a healthy way because typical breakfast foods such as whole-grain cereals and breads, fruits, and low-fat and fat-free dairy products are rich in vitamins, minerals, and fiber without being overly high in calories.

You can pick from a number of different types of breakfast food to help you manage your weight. Ready-to-eat or hot whole-grain or high-fiber breakfast cereals and whole-grain breads can help fill you up, and people who eat them tend to have healthier body weights than those who include fewer whole grains. (You'll learn more about fiber and whole grains in Week 6.) If you like eggs, you may find that having them for breakfast is more satiating than the same number of calories from a high-carbohydrate food such as a bagel. Several studies suggest that eating eggs for breakfast can help you cut calories at lunch and over the rest of the day. To have a nutritious meal that helps keep your hunger at bay through the morning, try one or more of these options.

- For a quick meal, go with ready-to-eat breakfast cereal topped with fruit and fat-free or low-fat milk, or whole-grain toast, fruit, and yogurt. You can have a generous bowl of a flaked or puffed cereal, while compact cereals such as granola require a skimpier amount for the same calories. For guidance on how much cereal to pour for the calories, look at the serving size and calorie information on the Nutrition Facts panel.
- A delicious yogurt parfait (pages 186–190) takes just minutes to make, but if you want to save time in the morning, prepare it the night before so you just grab it from the refrigerator.
- If you find that eggs enhance your satiety best, choose one of the breakfast egg recipes on pages 180–185 or create your own meal that fits into your breakfast calorie limit. Use whole eggs, whites, a combination, or egg substitute, whichever you like best, but note the difference in CD and calories (see Eggs on the Menu [page 47] for a comparison).
- Choose wisely when eating out or on the go; stick with basics such as whole-wheat toast, oatmeal, poached or boiled eggs, and ready-to-eat cereal. You might find that bars made with granola, cereal, dried fruit, or nuts are convenient for travel, but be aware that these Category 3 and 4 foods all have a relatively high CD.

THE BOTTOM LINE. The breakfast that is best for you is one that fits your schedule, is nutritious, includes foods that you like to eat, fills you up, and works into your calorie goals.

Eggs on the Menu

Whole eggs are nutrient rich, with high-quality protein, vitamin D, and choline. Although egg yolks are high in cholesterol, eating one whole egg a day isn't likely to increase heart disease risk. You can use whites or egg substitute in place of whole eggs for less cholesterol and a lower CD. Here is a simple chart to help you decide which option to choose when looking for the equivalent of one large egg:

TYPE OF EGG	CALORIES	CD	BEST USES
Large egg	80	1.5	The standard for eating, cooking, and baking
Whites of 2 large eggs	34	0.51	Work well in muffins and quick breads, and in combination with whole eggs for scrambling and omelets
¼ cup egg substitute	30	0.50	For baking

Lunch and Dinner: Eating More to Eat Less

I separated breakfast from lunch and dinner because it differs from them in the types of foods usually eaten and it tends to be lower in calories. Lunch and dinner are grouped together, with similar foods and the same Volumetrics meal strategies applying to both.

Consider the traditional lunch or dinner. The meal may start with an appetizer, followed by an entrée and perhaps some accompanying side dishes. It usually ends with something sweet such as fruit, dessert, or chocolate. Lunch is eaten around midday, following breakfast by several hours, and dinner is enjoyed in the evening. This timing and structure of meals has evolved over centuries with a primary goal in mind: to encourage us to eat for the calories we need to fuel our bodies. At lunch and dinner, the succession of courses and plates filled with a variety of meats, vegetables, and grains with different tastes, colors, textures, and aromas encourages us to keep eating. As we tire of one sensory experience, there will be others that keep the food appealing. With meals that have evolved to encourage us to eat, how can we structure them to help us eat fewer calories?

APPETIZERS. Let's start at the beginning of the meal with appetizers. The words "appetizer" and "appetite" sound similar for a reason. Appetizers are meant to rev up your appetite for the meal, but in my lab we have found that starting a meal with a big, low-CD first course from Category 1 or 2 can do the opposite. You'll notice that Volumetrics appetizers are different from familiar high-fat, high-CD restaurant menu starters like fried mozzarella sticks and breaded fried onions. The delicious appetizers in this book—Crudités with Cilantro-Lime Ranch Dip (page 317) and Volumetrics Spinach-Artichoke Dip with carrot sticks and pita wedges (page 324), to name just two—give you a reasonable number of calories in a satisfying portion, while greasy fried appetizers contain hundreds of calories in a small serving. You will quickly see how much bigger portions are when you choose a low-CD Volumetrics appetizer.

Lots of studies from my lab show that a low-calorie, low-CD appetizer helps you manage the calories in your meal. It takes the edge off hunger and fills you up so that you can better control the calories from your main course. The types of appetizers recommended in this book—salads, broth-based soups, and lower-CD dips with a variety of veggies—will help you eat fewer calories.

- Start with a big, low-CD green salad. In my lab, women who began their lunch with a 3-cup 100-calorie salad appetizer cut more than 100 total calories from their meal—they ate less of the main course after filling up on salad.
- Dip vegetables rather than chips into salsa or another low-CD dip.
- Enjoy a large bowl of soup. Whether it's chunky, smooth, or somewhere in between, starting your meal with soup will help you eat fewer total calories—up to 20 percent less, according to studies in my lab. For a satisfying portion for the calories, choose soups with a broth or tomato base rather than cream—the comparison soup photo on page 197 shows the big difference in portion size between a higher-CD and The Volumetrics Soup.

THE BOTTOM LINE. Of all the Volumetrics strategies that I recommend, *filling up first* is the one that both colleagues who run weight-loss clinics and dieters tell me is the easiest and most effective dietary change. Have a filling first course whenever you can, but no matter which Category 1 or 2 appetizer you pick—soup, salad, vegetables, or fruit—

keep your portion to 100 to 150 calories or this strategy could backfire, increasing rather than decreasing total calories at the meal. Bigger is better—think a large bowlful—so long as you keep calories and CD low.

SPOTLIGHT ON SOUP. In Asia, soup is a food people turn to if they want to lose weight. I first heard about this from my colleague Dr. Chor San Khoo, former vice president of global nutrition and health at the Campbell Soup Company. In her home country, Malaysia, people know to add water to foods and eat soups to help them feel fuller. When liquids are combined with solid foods in a soup or casserole, your body treats the whole thing as a solid, triggering the many biological systems that tell your brain to feel satisfied: your eyes see a filling portion, your senses of taste and smell are stimulated, and your stomach feels full. In my lab, a generous bowl of soup at the start of a meal worked better than the same calories from a puny portion of cheese and crackers to help people eat less at lunch.

Researchers began looking at the connection between soup and weight loss in the 1980s. They were encouraged by the results of an early study: people who ate soup at least four times a day cut calories and lost more weight than those who had soup less often. But you don't have to eat four cups a day to see results! Volunteers in my lab who had a low-CD soup twice a day rather than a high-CD snack with the same number of calories lost 50 percent more weight.

Soup studies suggest that the effects of eating a water-rich food are different from drinking water. My colleagues and I found that drinking a glass of water along with food didn't fill people up as much as eating water that was cooked into food to make soup. Be sure to try the recipe for The Volumetrics Soup on page 196. In one of our studies, eating this soup as a first course reduced total lunch calories by 20 percent.

You'll find several other simple first-course soup recipes on pages 198–200. I encourage you to try them all. Freeze leftovers in single-serve portions so that you can have a soup appetizer whenever you want. You also can improvise, using the Build a Soup chart (page 50) to get started. Once you've finished your bowl of soup, it's time to move on to the look of your main course plate.

Build a Soup

Add your own signature soups to the delicious soups in this book. Start with a base of vegetable, chicken, or beef broth and choose from the ingredients listed in each CD category, or select others that you like.

CD CATEGORY	CUISINE		
	Italian	Mexican	Chinese
1 (unlimited)	Canned tomatoes Fresh tomatoes Red and green bell peppers	Fresh tomatoes Bell and chile peppers Onions	Cabbage Carrots Green onions (scallions) Mushrooms
2 (add satisfying amounts)	Cannellini beans Kidney beans Whole-wheat pasta	Black beans Kidney beans Corn	Tofu Shrimp Noodles
3 (use portion control)	Chicken breast Part-skim mozzarella cheese	Chicken breast Lean beef Reduced-fat Jack cheese	Lean ham Lean pork
Seasonings	Garlic Basil Oregano	Cilantro Cumin Lime juice Oregano	Garlic Ginger Hot pepper Sesame Soy sauce

Making Over Your Plate

Think about a typical lunch or dinner plate filled with food. Chances are that it has an ample portion of meat, chicken, or fish, a decent grain portion, and maybe just a garnish of vegetables. While many people have been eating this way for years—heavy on protein and starch and light on vegetables—health organizations and government agencies suggest that Americans fill up half the plate with vegetables and fruits as a way to help control calories.

The graphic on page 52 depicts the U.S. government's latest food guidance symbol. Their recommendations are consistent with a lower-CD, Volumetrics way of eating! Here's how recent findings from my lab and others can help you remake your plate.

- Substitute low-CD vegetables for other foods. I am encouraging you to eat more vegetables, while decreasing your meat and grain portions. When volunteers in my lab were served extra vegetables without any change in the amount of meat and grain on their plate, their meal calories didn't change. Their calorie intake went down only when we substituted veggies for other foods on the plate, and we got an even bigger drop in calories when we decreased the CD of the vegetables by eliminating butter or sauce.

- Be generous with veggies. Our study meals included up to 2½ cups of vegetables, an amount that takes up about half the plate. Choose favorites and prepare them in low-CD ways by steaming, sautéing, roasting, or microwaving without adding large amounts of butter, oil, and other calorie-rich toppings. For the biggest calorie-lowering effect, your veggies have to be low-CD.

- Try different strategies for filling half your plate with vegetables and fruits. Research shows that adding a second or third vegetable works better than increasing the portion size of a single vegetable. You also can prepare a main dish that contains lots of vegetables, such as a stir-fry or casserole. The photos of How to Fill Your Plate with Veggies (page 53) show two different ways to fill half your plate with vegetables.

- Shrink down your portions of meat and grain. Each should take up about one-quarter of your plate. You will get more advice on how to do this in Week 6, when you learn about protein and fiber.

- Pay attention to your hunger and fullness sensations with the higher-veggie meal. If you're like our study volunteers, you'll feel just as satisfied after eating the vegetable-rich meal.

USDA MyPlate Icon Guides Healthier Food Choices

In 2011, the U.S. Department of Agriculture developed a new icon to help individuals put together healthy meals that include foods from the fruit, vegetable, grain, protein, and dairy food groups. Visit www.ChooseMyPlate.gov for tips and ideas.

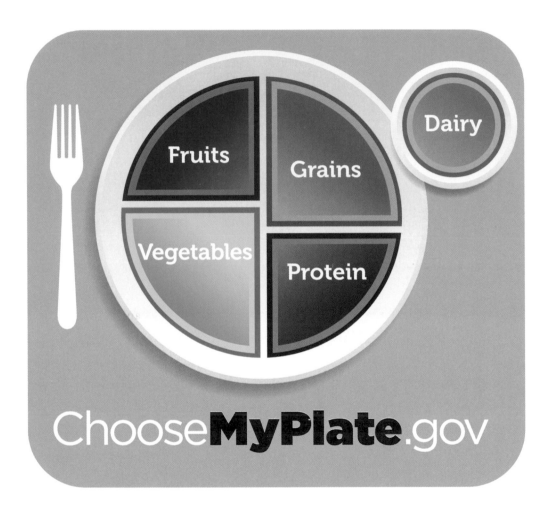

How to Fill Half Your Plate with Veggies

These two plates show you two different ways to fill half your plate with vegetables. On the left, 3 ounces of chicken breast and ½ cup of brown rice each take up one-quarter of the plate, and two separate vegetable dishes fill in the rest. The dish on the right is the same ingredients combined into a stir-fry.

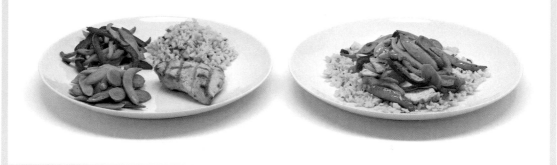

THE BOTTOM LINE. Remaking your plate with more vegetables and fruits is visually pleasing and satiating. Kitti Halverson, a dietitian in my lab, explains it best:

> Putting a lot of vegetables and fruits on the plate makes me happy. They add color and variety, and meals look more satisfying because portions are bigger for the same calories. If the plate is pretty and looks filling, think about how pleasurable the meal will be!

Next week, I will show you how to apply these "plate principles" to quick meals you can take to work or eat on the go, such as salads and sandwiches.

Bringing Your Meal to a Close

One of the questions that I'm asked most often is why we have "room" for dessert even after eating a filling meal. As with the appetizer and main courses, dessert has its distinct place in the meal. It offers a new sensory experience to enjoy when we tire of our main course, and revives our appetite. It can also serve as a signal that the meal has ended.

Do you ever find yourself opening and closing the refrigerator and cupboards looking for other foods to eat after your main course? I hope that as you enjoy satisfying Category 1 and 2 foods at your meals, you'll have less desire to keep looking for more to eat. But it may be that you need a specific signal that it is time to stop eating. For some people, nibbling on a piece of cheese or brushing their teeth helps. Others of us can stop only after having something sweet to bring the meal to a close. That's where dessert comes in. For most meals, the sweet taste of a favorite low-CD fruit is just right for a perfect dessert—think the first local strawberries in the spring or a lusciously ripe melon. But sometimes you want something that feels more indulgent—and that's okay once in a while. Cake, ice cream, pies, puddings, and even chocolate (see Managing Your Love of Chocolate) all have their place in your diet, particularly at the end of the meal.

Managing Your Love of Chocolate

If you're a chocolate lover, you might be encouraged by news that chocolate can be a health food. Many plant foods are rich in phytonutrients (also called phytochemicals), compounds that have health benefits. The phytonutrient compounds in the cacao bean, from which chocolate is made, are thought to improve heart health and increase insulin sensitivity. These compounds are most concentrated in unsweetened and dark chocolate. Studies are in progress to determine how much chocolate is needed for benefits, but keep in mind that calories add up quickly with this high-CD food.

Eat chocolate strategically by having a small amount at the end of a meal rather than having a larger portion as a snack. A piece for dessert allows you to satisfy your urge, savor the flavor, and get the most enjoyment while controlling portion size and calories.

Remember to practice moderation with high-CD treats. For a larger and more satisfying portion, try the Volumetrics desserts in this book, knowing that they were developed using strategies for lowering CD:

- Puréed fruit and extra vegetables add bulk and moisture while replacing some of the fat in the Chocolate Chip–Zucchini Squares (page 339), Alex's Three-Layer Carrot Cake (page 343), and Banana Cake (page 341).
- A generous portion of fruit helps reduce CD in the Ginger Apple Crumble (page 345) and Peach Bread Pudding (page 347).
- Sheets of phyllo dough replace higher-fat strudel dough in the Pear Cranberry Strudel (page 349).
- The flavor of naturally low-CD fruits is enhanced with a drizzle of fruit juice or liqueur in three different fruit salads (pages 350–354).

We've gone from breakfast through lunch and dinner, and from appetizers to desserts, learning to put together each meal and course in ways that fill your plate and help you keep your weight management efforts on track. This week you can continue using the sample menus, or create meals of your choosing, with a 100- to 150-calorie soup, salad, or other low-CD appetizer, a plate filled half with vegetables and fruits and one-quarter each with protein and grain, and a fruit-based dessert. Pay attention to how satisfied you feel after each course, and enjoy!

Key Points

- Start the day with a low-CD breakfast. It doesn't take a lot of time, and people who eat breakfast generally have a healthier body weight.
- To get an extra course while cutting calories, add a low-CD, Category 1 or 2 soup, salad, fruit, or vegetable appetizer. Soup is a particularly effective starter for filling you up and helping you eat fewer calories at your meal.
- To remake your plate, fill half with low-CD vegetables and fruits, either on their own or combined into a mixed dish. As you increase your vegetable portion, reduce the amount of protein foods and grains to avoid increasing calories.
- Dessert is the perfect place to fit more fruit into your day.

Let's Get Physical

You've spent the past three weeks stepping up your walking. You can continue walking as your primary exercise or mix it up with other activities. Take a quick look at your activity personality to get a sense of what you might enjoy.

I PREFER TO BE ACTIVE . . .	CONSIDER . . .
Alone or With others	Home exercise machine, swimming, pool walking, exercise DVD Exercise class, water aerobics, mall walking, play with kids or grandkids
Inside or Outside	Mall walking, gym workout, treadmill/elliptical, spinning Nature walks, gardening, bicycling
In a relaxed way or With intense exercise	Neighborhood stroll, weeding, cleaning Jogging, singles tennis, boot camp

Head and Habits

Are you reading the book week by week, or did you skip ahead? In writing this book, I decided to give you a twelve-week program to help you ease into diet and activity changes rather than overwhelming you with all the information at once. Small changes may be more achievable and easier to maintain than large ones.

Dr. James O. Hill, of the University of Colorado School of Medicine, suggests that the combination of human biology and our food and activity environment makes it difficult for people to accomplish big changes. You might be tempted to change everything at once, but that might be too dramatic for you to keep up. Dr. Hill and his colleagues have found that small changes—cutting out a reasonable number of calories, or adding 1,000 steps to an average day—help people stop or limit weight gain and empower them to continue making improvements.

Look back at how much you've accomplished over the past few weeks with gradual changes!

To Continue Doing Each Week

☐ Plan your meals using the sample menus as written or as a guide for creating your own meals. Make a shopping list and shop for those meals.

☐ Weigh yourself at least once during the week.

☐ Maintain your daily record with the information you've found to be most helpful.

☐ Write down strategies that have helped you work toward your goals.

☐ Wear your step counter and keep track of your steps each day as you move toward your goal of 10,000 daily steps. Find new ways to add 150 steps a day until you have added a total of 1,000 daily steps by the end of the week.

To Do This Week

☐ Rate your hunger at the beginning of the meal, after eating the appetizer, and at the end of the meal, and use that awareness to stop eating when you are no longer hungry.

☐ Start at least one meal a day with a low-CD appetizer.

☐ Gradually configure your plate to be half vegetables and fruits by the end of this week.

☐ Try at least one new physical activity.

Week 5

Building Your Meal Around Vegetables and Fruits

The biggest change I've made is including vegetables in every meal. I usually have mushrooms and spinach with my eggs in the morning. The soups for lunch have far more vegetables (and a wider variety) than they used to. My dinner plate is now half vegetables and has a smaller portion of meat. Making vegetables and fruit the foundation of my diet controls hunger better, and that helps keep me on track.—Sabrina, Pennsylvania

Vegetables and fruits are superstars when it comes to nutrition, but their reputation for weight loss at times has been less than stellar. Some diets make fruits taboo because of their sugar content. People tell me that vegetables remind them of rabbit food. I plan to show you that both vegetables and fruits are essential for successful and healthy weight management. Last week I described how the sweetness of fruit makes it a pleasurable way to end your meal. As for veggies, what I recommend is vastly different from living on nothing but piles of lettuce. I take a lot of my cues from culinary circles, where serving vegetables creatively is one of the hottest trends.

Much of the research in my lab now focuses on vegetables and their role in weight management. When we conducted our first calorie density studies in the 1980s, we never imagined that vegetables, and also fruits, would get us so excited. As you know, one of our earliest observations was that people tend to eat similar amounts of food over a day or two. So when we strategically incorporate vegetables to lower CD, participants in our studies eat about the same amount of food but get fewer calories, are just as full, and don't make up the calories by eating more later in the day!

We are also studying the various ways we can increase the intake of vegetables and fruits in the diets of people who like them, and sneak them into the meals of people who don't. Our strategies even nudge preschoolers, who are among the pickiest eaters of all age groups, to eat more vegetables and fruits!

Last week, I introduced you to some of our new findings on using vegetables and fruits to reduce your calories—adding a vegetable or fruit first course, filling half your plate with vegetables and fruits, and swapping vegetables for other foods in your meal. This week, we will look more closely at your first course, with a spotlight on salads, and then we'll explore more ways to make sure vegetables and fruits are on the plate, including the controversial stealth approach, which involves hiding veggies and fruits in foods. First, let's look at why vegetables and fruits are so important.

Vegetables and Fruits Boost Weight Loss

People who eat the most vegetables and fruits tend to have the healthiest body weight and gain less weight through their adult years. Eating lots of low-CD vegetables and fruits instead of other foods can help you shed pounds and keep them off.

- In a year-long clinical weight-loss trial in my lab, one group of women was encouraged to include as many servings of vegetables and fruits as they wanted as part of a low-fat diet, while the other group was told only to eat less fat. Can you guess which group lost the most weight, ate the most food, lowered the CD of their diet, and said they were less hungry? The one eating low-CD vegetables and fruits in unlimited amounts.

- We also compared the weight-loss effects of several different diets, including the veggie- and fruit-rich DASH (Dietary Approaches to Stop Hypertension) diet that is widely recommended for helping lower blood pressure. The men and women who lowered the CD of their diets the most over the first six months lost the most weight while eating more food, especially more vegetables and fruits!

We learned from these studies that giving positive messages to lower CD by eating more vegetables and fruits is a powerful tool for promoting weight loss. And eating them offers other benefits.

Vegetables and Fruits are Win-Win

Few foods offer the multitude of benefits that you get by eating more vegetables and fruits. Study after study shows that people whose diets include a lot of vegetables and fruits are less likely to develop heart disease, diabetes, high blood pressure, certain cancers, and obesity. And health professionals love veggie- and fruit-rich eating plans, including the Mediterranean diet, the DASH diet, and the Dietary Guidelines for Americans, for their numerous health benefits. As an approach to eating that is packed with vegetables and fruits, Volumetrics will help you get more of the nutritious foods you need, with fewer calories and greater satisfaction.

Knowing how important vegetables are for weight loss and for general health, my lab staff and I have determined which strategies help people boost their intake. When we combined strategies—serving ample portions of veggies as side dishes and sneaking them into main dishes—we got preschoolers to double their mealtime vegetables! These strategies can work for you, too.

Add a Course, Get More Food, Cut Calories

Adding a Category 1 vegetable or fruit first course is so important that I'm reminding you of it again this week. When you begin your meal with a generous soup, salad, or vegetable or fruit first course with 100 to 150 calories, you take the edge off hunger, feel fuller, and enjoy a lower-CD alternative to typical high-CD appetizers.

Last week, we took a look at soup. This week let's talk about salads. My idea of a salad is the type of delicious, lower-CD starter featured in this book, not the dressing-drenched, high-calorie creations that are so prevalent in supermarkets and restaurants. In my lab, we prepare low-CD salads and our study participants can't tell the difference between those and salads that have a higher CD. You can do the same.

- Fill your plate with leafy greens—lettuce; baby greens; combos with red leaf, green leaf, arugula, romaine, and radicchio; shredded cabbage—along with other colorful vegetables.

- Toss in raw and grilled vegetables that you might not ordinarily put in your salad, for color and flavor.
- Add a layer of flavor and color that contrasts with the veggies. Mandarin oranges offset the sharpness of arugula in the Baby Arugula Salad (page 210), while strawberries and pears contribute sweetness in the Mixed Greens with Strawberries, Pears, and Walnuts (page 209).
- Top with a dressing of your choice—regular, light, or fat-free—and toss well to distribute the dressing and flavor throughout. If you're using regular dressing, manage the portion and calories with just enough dressing for flavor. Anne, a participant in one of our clinical trials, adds a small amount of ranch dressing to light or fat-free vinaigrette to get creaminess with fewer calories. You also can make your own using the dressings from the salad recipes in this book (pages 206–220) as a guide, with three parts flavorful vinegar or fruit juice, one part high-quality oil—olive or canola are good choices—and seasonings. Dress the salad immediately before serving to keep it crisp.

Bulking Up Your Main Course

Salads can also be used as a veggie-rich main course. To make salad a meal, you may find that adding lean protein such as grilled chicken breast, lean beef, low-fat cottage cheese, tofu, chickpeas, or black beans to your generous plate of lettuce and vegetables helps boost satiety; you'll learn more about protein next week. Take a look at the Rainbow Chef's Salad (page 216), Chili-Rubbed Steak on a Deconstructed Guacamole Salad (page 219), and Salade Niçoise (page 220) to get you started, or be creative using the guide Build a Main Course Salad (page 62).

Eating a salad is just one of many ways to add vegetables to the main part of your meal. For example, you can fill your sandwich with as big a vegetable portion as will fit, while also substituting lower-CD ingredients for those that are higher.

- Start with whole-wheat or whole-grain bread, flatbread, or tortilla.
- Spread with plain or flavored mustard, hummus, barbecue sauce, or other high-flavor condiments in place of mayonnaise.

Build a Main Course Salad

Follow the CD category, ingredient, and seasoning guidelines to get you started on your own signature salads. Feel free to explore ingredients and flavors from other cuisines.

CD CATEGORY	ITALIAN	MEXICAN	CHINESE
1 (unlimited)	Lettuce Tomatoes Peppers Broccoli	Lettuce Tomatoes Peppers Jicama Red onion	Lettuce Cabbage Bean sprouts Water chestnuts Carrots
2 (add satisfying portions)	Whole-wheat pasta Chickpeas Cannellini beans	Corn Pinto beans Kidney beans	Rice Tofu Shrimp
3 (use portion control)	Part-skim mozzarella cheese Olives	Reduced-fat Jack cheese Ground beef Guacamole	Chicken breast Pork
4 (carefully manage)	Regular salad dressing Olive oil Parmesan cheese	Tortilla chips	Sesame oil Fried noodles
Seasonings	Basil Lemon juice Balsamic vinegar	Cilantro Lime juice Chile peppers	Rice vinegar Soy sauce

- Add a layer of vegetables. Lettuce, tomato, and red onion are standard, but be as creative as you like with options such as water-packed artichoke hearts, roasted red peppers, bell pepper slices of any color, grated carrot, cucumber slices, or a few slices of avocado.

- Top with a lower-CD filling such as lean roast beef, turkey breast, hummus, reduced-fat cheese, lower-fat tuna or chicken salad, or other favorites.
- Sprinkle with fresh herbs or additional high-flavor condiments such as hot pepper sauce.
- Add another layer of veggies.
- Top with a second slice of bread, leave open-faced, or roll into a wrap.

You also can personalize the sandwich recipes in this book. The Zesty Roast Beef and Veggie Pocket (page 230) and Hummus and Veggies Sandwich (page 229) in particular lend themselves to creative additions of vegetables. Piling on the veggies gives you a much bigger portion for your calories, as you can see in these before-and-after lunch photos.

More Variety and More Food with a 500-Calorie Volumetrics Lunch

The lunch on the left—a roast beef and cheese sandwich, coleslaw, and sweetened iced tea—is pretty standard. But look at how small and unsatisfying the portions are when they're not bulked up with vegetables and fruits. If instead you have the Zesty Roast Beef and Veggie Pocket (page 230) paired with veggie-rich Red Lentil Soup (page 200), two clementines, and iced tea sweetened with sugar substitute, you get more than double the amount of food for the calories and cut CD in half!

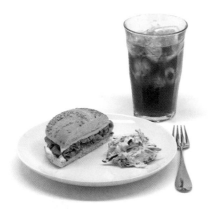

Typical Lunch

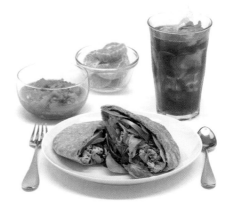

Volumetrics Lunch

You also can bump up your intake of vegetables by incorporating them into your entrée, piling them onto your pizza, and including them in side dishes. A consistent finding from a number of our studies shows that simply offering more vegetables and fruits encourages people to eat them, and the bigger the portion, the more they eat. Even kids ate more applesauce when we doubled their portion, and those who like broccoli and carrots ate more when we increased the amount served.

These tips and the others throughout this chapter, along with all the tasty Volumetrics recipes, can help you enjoy the fresh and delicious flavors of vegetables and fruits when they're in plain sight. We found that one of the most common myths about feeding kids isn't true—you *can* get them to eat more vegetables if you put appealing veggies on the plate. But sometimes sneaking them in can be an effective way to add even more. And research in my lab shows that you can sneak in a lot of vegetables without kids or adults knowing they're there.

The Stealth Approach

It's important to expose even the most reluctant eater to yummy vegetables and fruits, and to keep serving them. But what do you do if you, your kids, or loved ones refuse to eat vegetables and fruits? You can try sneaking them in. This is a *positive* strategy for getting more vegetables into a meal in a way that also makes foods flavorful and moist while lowering CD. Tucking puréed vegetables into places where they won't be noticed is a winning strategy. And I am not talking about the dainty amounts of puréed vegetables that might be recommended in other books. We add big amounts and get big results.

- Hiding four to five times the usual amount of veggies in all of the main entrées served to preschoolers over a day doubled their daily vegetable intake. You might wonder if this stealth approach had any negative effects, but let me assure you that our hidden veggies didn't cut into intake of the side dishes of green beans and broccoli that we served. Don't worry about this approach being deceptive; rather, think of it as recipe improvement. Parents change food ingredients all the time when preparing meals. Just make sure your kids know what whole vegetables are and be persistent in offering them!

- For adults, even those who reported low liking for vegetables, sneaking four and a half times the usual amount of vegetables into recipes for carrot bread, macaroni and cheese, and chicken-rice casserole increased daily vegetable intake by 80 percent. Adding veggies didn't affect liking for the foods or the amount eaten, and because the veggies reduced the CD, daily calorie intake went down by 360 calories.

When you hide chopped or puréed vegetables—fruits work, too—you'll need to experiment to find the amount that is large enough to make a difference without compromising flavor and texture. See How to Hide Your Veggies and Fruits for ideas, and to give you a head start, several recipes in this book contain hidden vegetables:

Pumpkin Cranberry Bread (page 193)
Squash Risotto (page 309)
Cauliflower Rice (page 311)
Jennifer's Buffalo Party Dip (page 314)
Volumetrics Macaroni and Cheese (page 321)

Speaking of flavor, you're likely to eat more vegetables and fruits when they're enjoyable. Variety, flavor, and convenience all are essential.

Getting the Most Enjoyment Out of Vegetables and Fruits

VARIETY. No food groups are more varied in color, flavor, texture, and nutrients than vegetables and fruits.

- Try to include vegetables of several colors, including red-orange and dark green, over the course of the day.
- Buy fresh or frozen combinations of several vegetables or fruits—for example, fresh assorted stir-fry vegetables or frozen mixed berries.
- Add a fruit or vegetable that you've never tried or one that has just come into season to your shopping cart each time you shop.

How to Hide Your Veggies and Fruits

Start with about ¼ cup of extra vegetables or fruit for each serving in the recipe. For example, if a pasta dish or meat loaf serves four, add about a cup of vegetables while reducing higher-CD ingredients. Here are some more tips.

- Hide vegetables where they blend in easily and are not noticeable, such as in mixed dishes, pastas, stews, and soups.
- Match the color of vegetable to the color of the main ingredients, especially in dishes that are light in color, such as puréed cauliflower in potato soup or puréed summer squash in macaroni and cheese.
- Sneak purées and chopped vegetables into tomato-based dishes, where they can be hidden by the strong flavor and bold color of the sauce. Cook frozen or fresh white vegetables (cauliflower, parsnip, onion), orange vegetables (carrot, pumpkin, winter squash), or even green vegetables (broccoli, spinach), and then purée or chop.
- Spice it up. Mexican-style and other spicy dishes are particularly good for hiding purées because they have such strong flavors.
- Tuck puréed squash or puréed black beans into brownie or chocolate cake batter.
- Substitute vegetable or fruit purées for half or even two-thirds of the added fat in quick breads and muffins.
- Put chopped vegetables or purées into casseroles that have ingredients of several different textures and colors.
- Add as much as you can get away with while retaining the flavor, appearance, and appeal of the original dish.

- Start a vegetable garden. You can enjoy the varied colors and flavors of homegrown tomatoes, lettuce, beans, berries, and other vegetables and fruits right outside your door. Gardening also increases your physical activity.

FLAVOR. Most people love fruits because of their sweet taste but are not as fond of vegetables. Having a choice of good-tasting vegetable dishes can make the difference between loving and not caring for them. If you're a reluctant vegetable eater, you may be particularly sensitive to their naturally bitter compounds, such as those in cabbage, Brussels sprouts, or kale. To make them tastier, pair with interesting flavors and textures, as suggested in the Vegetable Flavor Boosters chart (page 68).

Try these additional flavor tips:

- Roast them to enhance their natural sweetness.
- Sprinkle on a pinch of sugar to help counteract the bitterness.
- Avoid overcooking, and partially cover the pot rather than putting the lid on completely, to allow strong aromas to escape.
- Add a little salad dressing, grated cheese, a light drizzle of flavorful oil, butter flavoring, or light butter. If adding a small amount of fat will help you eat them, enjoy!

Keep experimenting with your recipes and dishes. Adjust the amount of seasoning, the combination of vegetables, and the cooking time until you're happy with the results. Then you'll have a great-tasting lower-CD dish!

CONVENIENCE. People often tell me that they would eat more vegetables and fruits if they didn't take long to prepare. If you don't have the time or inclination to peel and cut vegetables and fruits, you have dozens of other options from food manufacturers and your local supermarket.

- Look for peeled and precut fresh carrots, broccoli, butternut squash, onions, and other popular vegetables. They're great timesavers!
- Buy vegetables and fruits from the salad bar or packaged in bags or plastic containers. They may cost more, but they can help you put a meal on the table in minutes.
- Shop the frozen aisle. Vegetables and fruits are picked at the height of freshness and quickly frozen, preserving their flavor and nutrition. Some packages of vegetables can go straight from the freezer to the microwave to the table. What could be more convenient?
- Take advantage of canned. Canned vegetables such as corn, beans, and

Vegetable Flavor Boosters

These seasonings work well to enhance the flavor of vegetable dishes.

SEASONING	BEST ON
Basil	Eggplant, tomatoes, zucchini
Chervil	Asparagus, carrots, tomatoes
Chives	Potatoes, carrots
Cilantro	Bell peppers, carrots, lettuce
Cinnamon	Carrots, winter squash
Coriander seeds	Bell peppers, lentils
Cumin	Cabbage, eggplant, tomatoes
Curry powder	Potatoes, green beans, carrots
Dill	Beets, cucumbers, salads
Marjoram	Mushrooms, spinach, summer squash
Mint	Carrots, cucumbers, legumes
Oregano	Bell peppers, eggplant, tomatoes
Rosemary	Bell peppers, legumes, cabbage
Savory	Legumes, mushrooms
Tarragon	Fennel, mushrooms, tomatoes
Thyme	Carrots, legumes, mushrooms
Vinegar (balsamic, rice, champagne, flavored)	Salads, tomatoes, most vegetables

tomatoes are convenient for adding to soups, stews, and casseroles. To control sodium, drain and rinse before using or choose from the growing number of salt-free and lower-salt products.

As you use the various strategies in this chapter to eat more vegetables and fruits, remember to follow all the principles of Volumetrics. Even though most vegetables and fruits are Category 1 "free" foods, you need to use them strategically to reduce CD and fill up while lowering calories.

Key Points

- Eating lots of vegetables and fruits can help you shed pounds and keep them off. Plus, you can eat more food to better manage your hunger.
- Vegetables and fruits are the foundation of Volumetrics eating—they support good health, balance higher-CD foods, and boost meal satisfaction.
- Starting your meal with low-CD veggies and fruits is an effective way to manage calories while enhancing fullness.
- Be aggressive when incorporating vegetables into meals. The more you include—in plain sight as well as hidden—the more that will be eaten.
- Get the most enjoyment out of vegetables and fruits by shopping and preparing them with an eye toward variety, flavor, freshness, and convenience.

Let's Get Physical

One of the benefits of setting an activity goal in terms of steps is that you can spread your steps out over the course of the day. There's no need to worry about finding a thirty-minute block of time to take a 4,000-step walk. You can accumulate steps in five- or ten-minute increments that fit easily into your schedule. And weather never gets in the way since you can walk indoors or outside.

Do you keep a daily schedule on your computer, phone, tablet, or desk calendar? Make an activity appointment with yourself!

Head and Habits

What happens to your eating habits when you're stressed? Some people head straight for the refrigerator or snack shelf. Others find themselves eating more rapidly, without tasting their food. While these are signs that stress is disconnecting you from your satiety signals, you can take action to manage stress in a way that doesn't involve food or affect your eating.

- Minimize your time in the kitchen when stress strikes.
- Take your mind off stress, and food, by taking a walk, calling a friend, or doing an activity or hobby that you enjoy.
- Try to relax in the evening so that you can get a good night's sleep, as sleep deprivation is associated with a higher body weight.
- Work with others or on your own to come up with solutions for the problems that are causing your stress.

To Do This Week

- ☐ Include at least three different vegetables in meals, and experiment with sneaking them into at least one dish.
- ☐ Make sure that you get at least thirty minutes of activity each day, either in one block of time or divided into shorter segments.
- ☐ Write down two or three nonfood strategies for handling stress.

Week 6
Make Meals More Satisfying with Protein and Fiber

I lost a lot of weight, and what helps me keep my weight on track the most is eating protein and fiber with every meal.—Kristie, Pennsylvania

If you've tried to lose weight in the past, you may have considered diets that make attractive promises—eat more protein or fiber and you can shed pounds quickly, keep them off for good, and never feel hungry. Do they really work? If weight loss were that simple, all of us would be thin and I wouldn't be writing this book!

Protein and fiber are important for losing weight. To be satisfying and balanced, your diet needs both, and including them may help you feel fuller. This week, I will update you on the science behind protein and fiber—why they're important and what we know about their role in weight management and satiety.

Protein: Vital for Health

Our bodies contain lots of protein—it is in our muscles, blood, organs, hair, and skin. Without protein, you couldn't walk or move, digest and absorb food, or fight off infections. Eating protein is particularly important when you're losing weight; studies show that adequate protein in conjunction with increased physical activity can help retain your muscle mass. The recommended amount of protein you should include in your diet ranges from 10 to 35 percent of your total calories. This gives you plenty of scope to eat the protein-containing foods that you like in satisfying portions. But if some protein is good, might more protein be even better for losing weight?

The Connection Between Protein and Weight Loss

High-protein diets come in and out of fashion. For some of us, the prospect of eating unlimited quantities of protein-rich, high-fat foods, such as cheese and steak, while shedding pounds is irresistible. In a typical high-protein diet, you might get 30 percent or more of your calories from protein—about twice what most people eat—along with moderate to strictly limited amounts of carbohydrate. Favorite high-carbohydrate foods such as bread, potatoes, and anything with sugar are eliminated or restricted. Cutting down on such foods may seem like the right thing to do, since we enjoy them so much and feel guilty about eating them.

What has surprised me and other weight-loss researchers is that these strict high-protein diets work and may even provide health benefits—at least for a short while. Studies comparing different diets show that people following a high-protein, low-carbohydrate diet lose more weight over the first several months than people on a low-fat diet. But high-protein diets have a downside. Many high-protein foods are high in CD, so portions have to be small to control calories. Dieters on such diets don't learn sustainable eating habits that will keep the weight off, and high-protein diets have not been found to lead to long-term weight loss.

You don't need to eat high levels of protein to lose weight, but you need to make sure you get enough lower-CD protein foods to meet your body's requirements and help you hold on to muscle.

- Two daily protein servings of 2 to 3 ounces of meat, poultry, or fish, or their equivalent in beans, eggs, or nuts
- Three servings a day of milk or milk products such as yogurt and reduced-fat cheese, or foods and beverages fortified with the key nutrients in milk

The Effects of Protein on Satiety

The grocery store is filled with products—bars, powders, and drinks—that advertise their high protein content. What is the appeal of high protein? Some people hope to build more muscle, but many may turn to protein for the promise of greater fullness or satiety. Let's consider the evidence.

While some studies support the suggestion that increasing protein intake can enhance how full you feel and decrease how much you eat, this effect could relate at least in part to psychology. We think of meals as more substantial if they contain meat or other high-protein options. Ric, who has been eating according to the principles of Volumetrics for several years, explains that "meat, chicken, fish are very satiating for me. Maybe chicken breast is not as low-CD as a cucumber, but it fills me up more than straight vegetables do. Something about protein works for me."

A recent study in my lab supports the idea that the satiety response to protein may be based on our expectations. Alexandria Blatt, a dietitian and doctoral student, developed recipes that allowed her to vary the amount of protein in both a chicken casserole and a shrimp stir-fry from moderately low to moderately high. She kept the CD the same and she finely chopped the ingredients so that participants couldn't readily detect whether protein was lower or higher. These covert variations in protein content didn't affect the amount that participants ate or their ratings of satiety.

Beyond beliefs that protein is crucial for a satisfying meal, it has not been established that extra protein will boost satiety enough to give you a lasting reduction in intake. Much of the research is centered on foods that have been supplemented with hefty amounts of casein, whey, soy, or albumin protein powders. Results have been inconsistent and effects on weight loss have been disappointing. Since this is a rapidly emerging field and one that the food industry thinks holds great promise, it is possible that specific types and amounts of protein that consistently enhance satiety will be discovered.

THE BOTTOM LINE. Eating meat and other types of protein won't automatically enhance satiety and help you eat less. But if you associate satisfaction with having meat or other protein sources, include those that are relatively low in CD. Don't count on protein-enhanced products to boost satiety enough to help you resist all the high-CD foods that beckon to you to overeat.

Spreading Protein Throughout Your Day

You might be tempted to stockpile your day's protein, eating just small amounts at breakfast and lunch so that you can eat a hefty portion at dinner. Your body can better utilize protein if it is spread over the day, so try to include protein at each meal and snack.

- Incorporate low-fat or fat-free milk or milk products into breakfast, along with an egg if you find it boosts your satiety.
- Vary your proteins at lunch—for example, have beans on your salad or in your soup, or water-packed tuna or chicken in your sandwich. Take a look at the sandwich recipes on pages 221–230 for ideas on how to use vegetables and fruits to lower the CD of protein-rich sandwich fillings.
- Mix it up at dinner. You have plenty of lean meat cuts to choose from (see Protein Picks), along with poultry and fish. Vegetable protein foods, such as legumes, soy beans, tofu, and other soy products, supply both protein and fiber, have a low CD, and are quite filling.
- Choose proteins wisely to get the most satisfying portion for the calories (see the Leaner Meat, Larger Portion photo on page 76).
- At snack time, enjoy protein-rich, low-CD options such as nonfat yogurt, lower-fat cheese with fruit slices, or a bean dip with vegetables.
- Round out each meal with low-CD whole grains, vegetables, and fruits.

Protein Picks

Over the course of a week, have a variety of protein foods including lean meat and poultry, and seafood, along with beans and peas, soy products, eggs, and nuts and seeds. This chart also includes dairy products, as they are a major source of protein in the American diet.

BEEF AND PORK: To lower CD and cut down on detrimental fats, select the leanest round and loin cuts, go with "choice" or "select" grade for less fat and a lower price, and trim off visible fat. Choose ground beef that is at least 90% lean.

POULTRY: Select skinless, boneless chicken and turkey for convenience, less fat, and lower CD. If you purchase and cook poultry with the skin on, remove the skin before serving.

FISH AND SEAFOOD: Enjoy all types and try to include at least twice weekly in place of meat or poultry. Most fish and seafood have a low CD; those that have a higher CD, such as salmon, are rich in healthy fats. Avoid choices that are breaded or stuffed—they are prepared with cheese, bread crumbs, extra fat, and other higher CD ingredients.

LEGUMES: Explore the versatile world of beans and peas. The convenience of canned beans makes them an easy addition to salads, soups, and stews, and each quarter-cup is comparable to an ounce of meat, poultry, or seafood. Plus, they have almost no fat, giving you flexibility to add healthy fats to your favorite recipes.

SOY PRODUCTS: Use soy beans (edamame and mukimame), tofu, tempeh, and other soy products in place of or in addition to other protein foods. As with legumes, you get much more than protein, including fiber and beneficial plant compounds.

EGGS: A whole egg is the equivalent to one ounce of protein, and guidelines give the okay to enjoy up to an egg a day on average. Two whites provide the same amount of protein as a large egg, while having half the CD.

NUTS AND SEEDS: All types of nuts and seeds, including peanuts, almonds, and pumpkin seeds, count as protein. They have a high CD because of their fat content; manage portions and use them mainly to add flavor and texture to recipes.

DAIRY PRODUCTS: Milk, yogurt, and cheese are important protein sources that also supply calcium and vitamin D. Switch from higher-fat to lower-fat dairy products for about the same amount of protein, a lower CD, and less unhealthy fat.

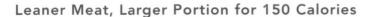

Leaner Meat, Larger Portion for 150 Calories

You don't get much for 150 calories when you pick higher-CD, fatty meats such as sausage (CD 3.5) and 80% lean ground beef (CD 2.7). Switch to the lower-CD London broil (CD 1.9), chicken breast fillet (CD 1.6), or snapper (CD 1.3) to make your calories go further. The snapper portion is almost three times the size of the sausage!

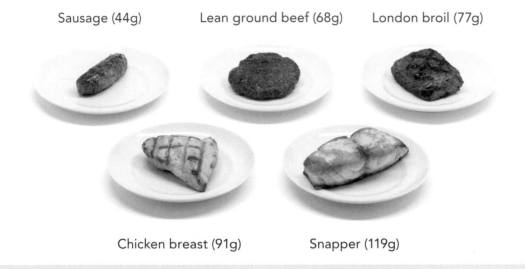

Sausage (44g) Lean ground beef (68g) London broil (77g)

Chicken breast (91g) Snapper (119g)

Your Daily Dairy

Dairy products are a major source of protein, and they supply other important nutrients including calcium and potassium. Some also are fortified with vitamin D. Calcium and vitamin D help improve bone health, and including dairy products in your diet also lowers your risk of heart disease, type 2 diabetes, and high blood pressure. Most of us need three daily servings of fat-free milk or low-fat milk and milk products, or their equivalent in fortified nondairy foods and beverages, to get enough calcium and vitamin D.

A number of studies have suggested that calcium and calcium-rich dairy products might be linked to a healthier body weight—especially for people who are not getting enough—by boosting metabolism, speeding up weight loss, and decreasing belly fat. The results of follow-up studies have been mixed. Expert panels have concluded that dairy products have not been shown to boost weight loss, although they may improve weight loss in dieters who are not eating enough calcium.

THE BOTTOM LINE. There are a lot of good reasons to include protein-rich foods on your plate—flavor, satisfaction, variety, nutrition—and they may help boost satiety. With so many choices and benefits, making foods with protein a part of every meal is an easy decision. Like protein, fiber has been part of the weight-loss promise and it, too, plays an important role in satiety and weight management.

Fiber: A Multitasking Nutrient

The growing number of high-fiber cereals, breads, pasta, and other food products on supermarket shelves is testament to fiber's importance to health. Many of these products also imply that they can help you shed pounds. This claim is backed by some studies showing that increased fiber intake can boost satiety and help people eat less. For example, people eating the most fiber in their cereal at breakfast had the greatest reduction in calories at breakfast and the lunch that followed. Could this enhanced satiety be simply because fiber lowers the CD of foods? Fiber, a type of carbohydrate, is not absorbed completely, so it has a lower CD than other carbohydrates. But in the context of your diet, the effect of fiber on CD is modest compared to that of increasing water or decreasing fat. We just don't eat fiber in quantities that are large enough to make much difference to CD. There are other reasons that fiber may enhance fullness.

- Foods with fiber tend to require more chewing, stimulating your senses in a way that can help boost satiety.
- Fiber slows down the emptying of food from the stomach and slows down absorption from the small intestine, helping you feel full longer.
- Fiber "bulks up" in the digestive system by absorbing water, and this can help reduce hunger.

Fiber for Managing Your Weight

Fiber has the potential to help you manage your weight. People who eat the most fiber tend to weigh less, and they gain less weight as they get older. What I like about fiber is the company it keeps. Foods rich in fiber (see Finding the Fiber on page 78) are the same low-CD foods that are the foundation of Volumetrics: vegetables, fruits, legumes, and whole grains. These plant-based whole foods can provide adequate fiber, so there's little need for you to seek out fiber supplements or foods with added fiber to get enough.

Finding the Fiber

The 2010 Dietary Guidelines for Americans recommend a daily fiber intake of 25 grams for women and 38 grams for men. These foods with at least 1 gram of fiber per serving can help you reach your goal.

Legumes (cooked)	Fiber (G)
Lentils, ½ cup	8.0
Black beans, ½ cup	7.5
Chickpeas, ½ cup	6.0
Kidney beans, ½ cup	5.5
Soy beans (edamame, out of shell), ½ cup	5.0
Lima beans, ½ cup	4.5

Vegetables	Fiber (G)
Artichoke hearts, ½ cup	7.0
Green peas, ½ cup	4.5
Sweet potato, without skin, 1 medium	4.0
Pumpkin, canned, ½ cup	3.5
Potato, baked, with skin, 1 small	3.0
Broccoli, cooked, ½ cup	2.5
Carrot slices, cooked, ½ cup	2.5
Spinach, cooked, ½ cup	2.0
Bell pepper, 1 medium	2.0
Brussels sprouts, cooked, ½ cup	2.0
Green beans, cooked, ½ cup	2.0
Corn, cooked, ½ cup	2.0
Carrot, 1 medium	1.5
Tomato, 1 medium	1.5
Cauliflower, cooked, ½ cup	1.5

Fruits	Fiber (G)
Pear, with skin, 1 medium	5.5
Raspberries, ½ cup	4.0
Blackberries, ½ cup	4.0
Apple, with skin, 1 small	3.5
Orange, 1 medium	3.0
Banana, 1 medium	3.0
Peach, with skin, 1 medium	2.0
Grapefruit, ½	2.0
Blueberries, ½ cup	2.0
Strawberries, ½ cup	1.5

Grains and Cereals	Fiber (G)
Bran flake cereal, ¾ cup	5.5
Whole-wheat English muffin, 1 whole	4.5
Bulgur wheat, cooked, ½ cup	4.0
Popcorn, popped, 3 cups	3.5
Whole-wheat spaghetti, cooked, ½ cup	3.0
Barley, cooked, ½ cup	3.0
Multigrain bread, 1 oz slice	2.0
Oatmeal, cooked, ½ cup	2.0
Brown rice, cooked, ½ cup	2.0

Source: USDA Nutrient Database for Standard Reference, Release 23. www.ars.usda.gov/ba/bhnrc/ndl.

Last week, you learned about vegetables and fruits, two types of whole foods that supply fiber. This week, we turn our attention to other fiber-rich foods: whole grains and legumes.

The "Whole" in Whole Grains

Whole grains are just that: the whole kernel. A kernel of brown rice, oats, wheat, and other grains consists of three separate parts: the protective fiber-rich bran coating, the starchy center of the kernel (called the endosperm), and the nutrient-rich germ. To take advantage of the health and weight benefits associated with whole grains—lower risk of heart disease, stroke, and type 2 diabetes and healthier body weight—you have to eat the entire grain kernel. People who eat the most whole grains (see the Guide to Whole Grains) tend to have lower BMIs and a smaller waist measurement, and they gain less weight during their adult years.

You can use the food package label to help you find whole grains.

- Read the Nutrition Facts panel for fiber information. Whole-grain foods usually have at least 2 grams of fiber per serving. But fiber alone doesn't mean whole grain, so check the ingredient list.

- Buy foods that have whole grains as the first ingredient on the ingredient list—the word "whole" is your tip-off. Whole-wheat flour and whole oats are whole grains; enriched wheat flour isn't.

- Always double-check the ingredient list when you see terms on the package such as "cracked wheat," "multigrain," "stone-ground," and other descriptions of grain. They do not necessarily mean that the food qualifies as a whole grain.

- Check for a whole-grain logo on the front label that identifies foods that count as a full or half-serving of whole grains.

- Learn more about whole grains at www.wholegrainscouncil.org.

Guide to Whole Grains

This chart shows the variety of whole grains to choose from. The many Volumetrics recipes that call for whole grains in side dishes and mixed dishes can get you started. To prepare the whole grains listed in this chart, follow package directions for cooking or cook as you would rice with one part grain and two parts water.

GRAIN	DESCRIPTION	WORKS WELL IN
Amaranth	Tiny kernels with a slightly peppery flavor	Side dishes
Barley	Sold whole or pearled, which cooks faster	Soups, salads, as a hot breakfast cereal
Brown rice; also colored and wild	Available in long=, medium=, and short=grain	Side dishes
Buckwheat	Distinct nutty flavor	Pancake flour, side dishes
Bulgur	Cracked, precooked, dried wheat kernels	Side dishes, salads, combined with ground meat
Corn	Fresh, frozen, popped, or ground	Side dishes, pancakes, quick breads
Millet	Tiny grains with a mild flavor	Side dishes, as a hot breakfast cereal
Oats	Rolled (quick-cooking, instant) or steel-cut	Hot breakfast cereal, quick breads, pancakes
Quinoa	Small round grains with a nutty flavor	Salads, side dishes
Rye	Unlike most grains, has fiber in the endosperm	Breads
Wheat (includes wheat berries, farro, kamut, spelt)	Available whole and as flour	Pasta, side dishes, as a hot breakfast cereal

The Dietary Guidelines recommend eating at least three daily servings of whole-grain products. Eliminating refined grains in our current food environment is hard to do, but you should try to cut back on foods made with them wherever you can and instead choose whole-grain products. You may want to do this gradually to get used to their texture and heartier flavor. If you are like me, you will learn to prefer them. Here are a few tasty suggestions.

- Include at least one whole grain at each meal—a slice of whole-grain bread, a bowl of whole-grain breakfast cereal or hot cereal, a side dish portion of cooked brown rice or whole-wheat pasta. Three meals, three servings, and you've eaten the recommended amount.
- For reluctant eaters, try white whole-wheat flour in breads and recipes. It looks like white flour but is made from a lighter-colored strain of whole wheat.
- Select from the many whole-grain soup, salad, main course, and side dish recipes in this book, including Vegetable Barley Soup (page 203) and Quinoa Tabbouleh Salad (page 289).
- Snack on whole grains—popcorn, brown rice cakes, or your own trail mix of whole-grain cereals—while managing portion size of these higher-CD "dry" whole-grain foods.
- Mix together your own whole-grain combinations to cook on the stove or in the rice cooker and serve as a side dish.
- Wherever you can, replace refined grain foods such as cakes, cookies, snack foods, and desserts that also have added fats, sugars, and calories with whole grains and other low-CD foods.

THE BOTTOM LINE. Science strongly supports the role of whole grains for health and weight management. Include at least three daily servings of whole-grain foods, choosing them in place of, rather than in addition to, refined grain products to avoid adding calories to your day.

Legumes: Another Fiber-Rich Food

I contemplated the best place in this book to discuss legumes (beans and peas). They're both a vegetable and a source of protein, so they deserve mention in each of those sections. But I decided to include them with fiber since they supply more fiber than any other type of food. Half a cup of legumes—kidney beans, black beans, pinto beans, chickpeas, lentils, split peas, and many others—provides about one-quarter of your fiber needs for the day along with numerous vitamins, minerals, and phytonutrients. They're rich in a type of fiber called resistant starch that can help manage blood glucose and cholesterol levels. And when you eat legumes, you'll quickly notice the benefits of their low CD and high fiber content—you're likely to feel quite full.

One of my Penn State colleagues, Dr. Terry Hartman, was inspired to conduct a weight-loss study using legumes when participants commented on how full they were after eating beans. She and her colleagues offered simple food advice to their study participants: eat about 1½ cups of legumes daily and, important, stop eating when you're satiated. The men in her study lost an average of ten pounds over four weeks! They incorporated legumes into their diet in delicious ways, and you can, too.

- Add them to salad, as I've done in Kim's Black Bean and Barley Salad (page 291) and Succotash Salad (page 308).
- Give them a starring role in soups. Red Lentil Soup (page 200) is one of my favorites, and Dr. Hartman's volunteers were particularly fond of black bean soup.
- Use them in chili recipes (pages 284–288) and casseroles to add flavor, texture, and fiber, lower CD, and give you a bigger and more satisfying portion.
- Purée them to enjoy as a dip or salad dressing, or to sneak into pasta sauce or mixed dishes.
- Substitute puréed beans for some of the fat in dessert recipes.

What About Foods and Beverages with Added Fiber?

As you shop the supermarket aisles, you may notice foods with added fiber. Many are formulated to help control blood glucose and blood cholesterol levels. Might they also help people lose weight? The functional fibers added to foods—including alginate, cellulose, guar gum, inulin (chicory root extract), oat fiber, oligosaccharides, pectin, poly-dextrose, and resistant starch—have many of the properties of fiber-rich foods including the ability to absorb water, but scientists do not yet know if they fill you up in the same way that whole foods do.

The best way to increase your fiber intake and maximize the effects of fiber for weight loss is to eat a wide range of fiber-rich foods throughout the day.

- Continue to manage calories by switching to whole-grain breads, pastas, and breakfast cereals and substituting higher-fiber foods for those lower in fiber.
- Eat more slowly and pay attention to fullness. Give fiber a chance to set off fullness signals that start in your mouth and continue in your stomach and intestines. Fiber won't magically melt away pounds, but its actions can help you eat less.
- Increase your intake of fiber-containing foods gradually over several weeks to give your gastrointestinal tract time to adjust.

I've included plenty of grain and legume recipes for you to enjoy. You'll wonder why you haven't been eating this way all along!

Key Points

- Including satisfying portions of protein, in combination with physical activity, helps retain muscle mass.
- Protein in a meal may boost satiety.
- You can enjoy both animal and plant sources of protein, and choosing those with a lower CD gives you a more satisfying portion.
- A diet with plenty of high-fiber foods can help you to feel full.
- Including fiber-containing foods, such as vegetables, fruits, whole grains, and legumes, in your diet can aid weight loss.

Let's Get Physical

Last week's action plan included strategies for fitting exercise into your schedule, including taking ten-minute activity breaks. Here are a few activities that readily fit into a ten-minute time slot.

- Working in the garden pulling weeds or planting
- Dancing to a couple of favorite songs
- Walking 1,000 steps
- Getting up and moving around during commercials
- Doing strengthening exercises for your arms, legs, and core abdominal muscles

Head and Habits

Think back to your last meal—how much attention did you pay to what you ate? If you hadn't been keeping a food record, would you have remembered what and how much you had to eat? This week, I encourage you to be more mindful of what you eat, as a way to get more satisfaction out of your meals. (We'll return to mindfulness in Week 11 when you look at your personal food environment.)

When you eat mindfully, you experience food with all your senses. You slow down so that you can enjoy the way your meal looks, smells, feels, and tastes. Not only does this make food more enjoyable but it gives you the time to recognize and stop eating when you're full. So take your time, minimize distractions by sitting at the table away from the computer and television, and turn your full attention to the food on your plate.

To Do This Week

- ☐ Try at least two different proteins that you usually don't eat, including meatless entrées, legumes, and fish that are highest in healthy fats, including salmon, mackerel, and sardines.
- ☐ Include at least one new whole-grain food this week: whole-grain bread, hot or cold breakfast cereal, pasta, or a side dish made with whole wheat, amaranth, millet, quinoa, or less common wheat varieties.
- ☐ Break for 10 minutes of activity at least once a day.
- ☐ Slow down, pay more attention to meals and snacks, and take the time to eat more mindfully.

Week 7
Managing Fat and Sugar: Strategies for Enhancing Flavor

I watch high-fat foods like salad dressings and bread and butter and skip high-fat appetizers and desserts. But sometimes I just splurge to pacify the urge—and that's all right! An occasional splurge will not make me fat.—Darryl, Pennsylvania

Just before I sat down to write this chapter, my lab had a birthday celebration for one of my graduate students. This is Penn State, so of course we had our famous Creamery ice cream—a perfect combination of sugar and fat. It was delicious and none of us felt guilty about indulging. After all, it is not an everyday occurrence, and we eat lower-CD foods most of the time. You, too, can enjoy such indulgent treats without guilt. Eating for weight management and optimal health is not an all-or-nothing deal. Volumetrics is about fitting a variety of foods into your day, while remembering that some require more moderation than others!

This week I talk about two of the most palatable components of food: fat and sugar. Each by itself makes food taste good, and this can lead to excess calorie intake. The sensory appeal of foods with fat and sugar, sometimes in combination with salt, perks up our appetite. Dr. Adam Drewnowski of the University of Washington explains: "Foods with fat and sugar taste good. We easily can eat too much of them, even when we're not hungry, and they are so pleasurable that they override our systems for putting on the brakes." It's no surprise that when we're trying to lose weight, foods that are high in fat and sugar often are the first to be eliminated.

Banning them, however, is not the answer. Studies, mostly conducted with kids, show that restricting or eliminating foods just makes them more desirable. That's human nature. You won't stick to a diet that forbids your favorite foods. This week I will help you figure out how to manage your intake of fat and sugar without being lured into overeating.

Fitting In Fat

For years, eating too much fat has been thought to be the biggest problem for weight control. Excess dietary fat is stored as body fat more efficiently than other nutrients. But the more powerful relationship between high-fat food and body fat has more to do with its palatability and effects on CD.

- Fat affects the flavor and sensory properties of foods. It gives meat its juiciness, cheese its creaminess, and crackers and cookies their melt-in-your-mouth sensation. High-fat foods are so palatable that we often ignore fullness signals and keep on eating even though we don't need the food or calories.
- High-fat foods tend to have a high CD—they concentrate a lot of calories in a small portion—so they're easy to overeat.

Because it tastes so good and packs in the calories, fat can be a problem for weight management. But our studies show there is a secret weapon against fat. By now you shouldn't be surprised to hear that I recommend including more vegetables and fruits in your diet to offset the effects of fat on intake—water-rich foods decrease the CD even of diets high in fat. When we analyzed national data on what people in America eat, we found that although diets with lots of high-fat foods were associated with higher obesity rates, eating plenty of vegetables and fruits lowered CD and weakened the link between dietary fat and obesity.

THE BOTTOM LINE. Eating palatable high-fat foods can lead to eating more calories than you need, and that can increase body fat. Having a reasonable amount of fat will not make you fat, especially if it's part of a lower-CD diet that includes plenty of vegetables and fruits. The key is to combine sensible portions of fat-containing foods that you enjoy with plenty of lower-CD foods so that the overall CD of your diet is low enough to ensure satisfying portions.

Does Eating Less Fat Shed Pounds?

Reduced-fat diets are not as popular as they once were, but fat reduction is still the core principle of many weight-loss programs. The majority of studies indicate that advising participants to reduce their fat intake promotes weight loss. However, in recent years, several widely publicized large-scale trials have reported little long-term impact of fat-reduction advice on body weight. Part of the problem is that a low-fat diet, like most restrictive diets, is hard to maintain. In studies lasting a year or longer, reported fat intake crept back up toward its level at the beginning of the study. Another problem is that reducing fat intake does not necessarily make a diet lower in calories. For example, people might swap higher-fat chips for fat-free pretzels with a relatively high CD, or higher-fat cookies for a fat-free version with a similar CD. A number of studies show that fat reduction only leads to lower calorie intake if CD is also reduced.

THE BOTTOM LINE. Focus on your total diet, not just fat or another food component, since you can lose weight on any type of diet as long as you limit calories. The Dietary Guidelines recommend that fat should be between 20 and 35 percent of total calories. This broad range gives you plenty of scope to find a level that works for you and makes your foods taste good while not adding unnecessary calories. You will be surprised at how much fat you can cut without affecting a food's appeal—in my lab, we cut fat by 20 to 30 percent without people noticing. No matter what level of fat you choose, you'll be using healthy Volumetrics strategies to eat appropriate amounts of the right kinds of fat.

All Fats Are Not Created Equal

In the early days of low-fat diets, all fats were grouped together. Fat was fat, whether from meat, dairy, nuts, or oils, and there was almost no limit to how low a diet might go. Our bodies need only a small amount of fat—just enough to help absorb vitamins A, D, E, and K, and to make hormones—so even very-low-fat diets can supply enough. But as the health effects of different fats have become better understood, the focus has shifted from the amount of fat in your diet to the type of fat. Here is a guide to choosing beneficial fats.

- Select foods that supply heart-healthy mono- and polyunsaturated fatty acids. Enjoy plant-based oils such as olive oil and canola oil in cooking and on salads, and add nuts, seeds, olives, and avocados for flavor and texture to salads and sandwiches.

- Include foods that supply omega-3 fatty acids—higher-fat fish such as salmon, mackerel, herring, lake trout, and sardines, along with flaxseeds and walnuts. They benefit the heart and vascular system and may have additional positive effects on health.

- Eat less saturated fat, a type of solid fat linked to increased risk of heart disease. Saturated fat is found in meats and dairy products; animal fats such as lard and beef fat; and the foods that contain high-fat animal and dairy products, for example pizza, ice cream, desserts made with butter, and meat or poultry mixed dishes. To limit saturated fat to no more than one-third of the fat in your diet as recommended in the Dietary Guidelines, switch to low-fat or fat-free dairy products, use butter sparingly, choose leaner cuts and sensible portions of meat, eat fewer processed foods, and limit intake of baked and frozen desserts.

- Keep your intake of trans fatty acids as low as possible. Trans fat, a solid fat found mainly as partially hydrogenated vegetable oil in hard-stick margarine, shortening, and some fried foods and baked goods, negatively affects heart health. Be sure to check the calories of foods labeled "trans fat free." Many contain other fats in place of trans fatty acids and have just as many calories.

Even though healthy fats are an important part of a balanced diet, you need to manage their portion size as you would other high-CD food components. Jill, who lost over 200 pounds on Volumetrics, notes that it's easy to succumb to the halo effect around healthy fats. "You might say no to butter but then slather on the guacamole or sauté food in lots of olive oil." The solution is to incorporate fat sensibly, in a way that enhances the flavor of your food.

Nine Ways to Get the Most from a Small Amount of Fat

You can manage fat in many ways—cutting out extra, using less, switching to equally tasty alternatives—to create satisfying low-CD meals that meet your calorie goals:

1. **Decide where fat matters to you.** You might switch to a nonstick pan for sautéing vegetables so that you can have regular dressing on your salad. Having

your breakfast toast without butter would free up fat for 2% milk in your coffee. To indulge in a piece of chocolate after dinner, you might select a leaner cut of beef rather than a higher-fat steak. It's all about managing the amount and type of fat in places where you enjoy it most.

2. **Use the amount that you need for flavor.** Stop for a moment and consider how much fat is necessary. A tablespoon or two of dressing tossed into your salad can add as much flavor as three or four times that amount. A crusty piece of Italian bread needs just a drizzle of olive oil, rather than a puddle. Onions soften and brown deliciously in a teaspoon or so of oil in a nonstick pan; why use more? Look for ways like these to eliminate excessive amounts of fat that add extra calories.

3. **Revamp your cooking.** Preparing foods in ways that require little or no fat enables you to have a bit more fat in other foods. Consider grilling or roasting vegetables (see Roasted Diced Fall Vegetables on page 303) to bring out their natural sweetness. The broiler in your oven comes in handy for grilling a sandwich—there's no need to spread it with butter. Outdoor grilling is a great way to cook foods while allowing fat to drip off. Cook foods in broth to add flavor with little fat. If you don't have nonstick pans and skillets, spray pots and pans with cooking spray for less sticking—and a bonus, quick cleanup!

4. **Bulk up.** Replace high-fat foods with vegetables and fruits, legumes, and whole grains to bring down CD while giving you satisfying amounts of food. Look back at Weeks 5 and 6 for suggestions on incorporating these lower-CD foods into your meals.

5. **Switch to lower-fat alternatives.** If you're like our study participants, you'll be able to switch to reduced-fat and low-fat alternatives and barely notice a difference. Food manufacturers have vastly improved the quality of fat-saving products such as salad dressing, mayonnaise, sour cream, cheese, yogurts, and deli meats. They've even risen to the challenge of getting low-fat cheese to melt well! You may need to try several different brands and varieties to find those that you like best for eating, cooking, and melting.

6. **Keep the creaminess.** Fat enhances the creamy texture of foods. In dishes such as soups and baked goods, you can replace high-fat ingredients with lower-fat

alternatives such as plain regular or Greek-style yogurt, reduced-fat or fat-free sour cream, or puréed potatoes and other puréed vegetables. Be sure to try the three dips on pages 324–328; they're made with lower-CD ingredients that taste creamy and they're served with vegetables to bring down the CD even more.

7. **Flavor up.** In my lab, our study participants don't notice that we've reduced the fat when we bump up flavor with vegetables, spices, and other seasonings. So try these techniques that you'll see used in Volumetrics recipes.

    *   Cook veggies in broth or wine.
    *   Dice high-flavor vegetables such as onion, garlic, celery, and bell pepper and add to stews, soups, and casseroles.
    *   Use lower-CD condiments, including ketchup, mustard, salsa, soy sauce, hot pepper sauce, plain and flavored vinegars, and Worcestershire sauce. If you are concerned about sodium, choose those lower in sodium when available.
    *   Garnish fish or chicken with flavorful toppings of citrus juice or slices, fresh herbs, salsa, or mustard.
    *   Try different combinations of fresh or dried herbs.
    *   Cook rice or pasta in broth or tomato juice, or add herbs to the cooking water.
    *   Add spices and seasonings. As an added bonus, red pepper and other hot spices may help reduce hunger and modestly increase calorie burning.

8. **Enjoy the flavor of lower-fat dishes.** Whether you try the Cornmeal Pancakes with Cinnamon Apples (page 177) or Vegetable Denver Omelet (page 184) for breakfast, the Chicken Salad Sandwich (page 225) or Pesto Pizza with Chicken and Vegetables (page 235) at lunch, or the Volumetrics Spaghetti Bolognese (page 236) or French Beef Stew (page 254) at dinner, you'll quickly see that you can manage fat and calories in a delicious way.

9. **Consider the whole meal.** For a satisfying and nutritionally balanced meal, you should include several different types of foods. If you spend most of your calories on a high-fat food, you won't have much room in your calorie budget to add anything else. As you look through the recipe section of this book, note the difference in portion size in the before-and-after photographs. Many of the

before photos show high-fat packaged or prepared foods, while the after photos feature lower-CD Volumetrics alternatives that are more satisfying and nutritious.

Ultimately, your decisions about fat will make eating more pleasurable while meeting your Volumetrics goals. Since fat often travels with sugar in indulgent foods, you need to consider both when putting together your meals.

You can trim both fat and sugar to lower the CD, increase the size, and boost the nutrition of your meal. The before-and-after breakfast photos show two typical breakfasts, one with foods relatively high in fat and sugar and the other with lower-fat, lower-CD alternatives. By reducing fat and sugar and lowering the CD, you get about 60 percent more food for the calories!

Lots of Fat and Sugar Equals Puny Portions

Fat and sugar can make a big difference, as you can see in these before-and-after breakfasts. The 400-calorie breakfast on the left includes granola, which is surprisingly high in fat and sugar, along with whole milk, and coffee with half-and-half and sugar. The lower-fat, lower-sugar 400-calorie breakfast on the right—bran flakes, fat-free milk, three types of fruit, and coffee with fat-free milk and a sugar substitute—has a lower CD and provides about two-thirds of a pound more food.

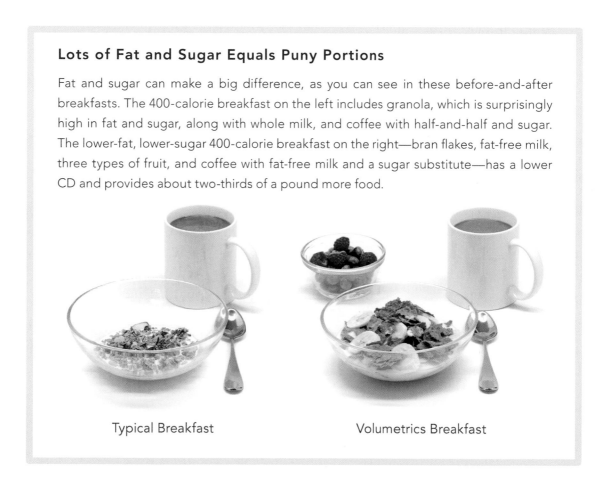

Typical Breakfast   Volumetrics Breakfast

Understanding Your Sweet Tooth

Of all the tastes in our foods, sweetness brings us the most pleasure. Sugar—including sucrose (table sugar), fructose, high-fructose corn syrup, honey, molasses, turbinado sugar, agave syrup, and evaporated cane juice—makes foods and beverages more appealing. It also causes mixed emotions. On one hand, we love sugar because it is so delicious, but on the other, we feel guilty about liking something that is blamed for a variety of illnesses.

Our love of the sweet taste is established even before we are born. This makes sense since breast milk is very sweet. In childhood, sweetness is critical in shaping our food preferences. While our love of supersweet foods declines in our late teen years, most of us don't lose our enjoyment altogether. Many people find that sweet foods taste even better combined with fat and salt. Think kettle corn, chocolate-covered pretzels, and peanut brittle—salt enhances sweetness in a highly appealing way (see Salt and Flavor).

Salt and Flavor

Our bodies need only a small amount of the mineral sodium—salt is our major source—and a diet high in sodium increases the risk of high blood pressure in some people. Breads, pizzas, prepared entrées, processed meats such as cold cuts and hot dogs, and other packaged foods that supply much of our sodium are the types of higher-calorie foods that you should limit, so following Volumetrics can also help you reduce the sodium in your diet. The recipes in the book give you flexibility to reduce the amount of salt in your diet by selecting lower-salt ingredients and adding salt only to taste.

The result of our love for sugar is that we eat way too much. U.S. government surveys estimate that 16 percent of our calories come from added sugars, the equivalent of about twenty teaspoons of sugar in the average diet each day! Can you guess the culprits? We get much of our sugar from sweetened beverages (which you'll learn about in Week 9), desserts, and candy. These high-sugar foods supply calories but few essential nutrients and little dietary fiber. In contrast, foods that have natural sugars—fruits, vegetables, and milk products—are rich in vitamins and minerals. Since sugar intake and obesity rates both have been going up, experts have been questioning whether eating too much sugar might be responsible for the excess pounds.

Does Sugar Make You Fat?
Could Eating Less Help You Lose Weight?

Sugars can cause weight gain if they're adding calories you don't need. That is why government and health initiatives call for children and adults to cut back on added sugars in foods and beverages. In the past, sucrose (ordinary table sugar) was labeled as "pure, white, and deadly" in popular diet books. Now much of this adverse attention is on high fructose corn syrup (HFCS), a widely used sweetener in soft drinks, and its effects on metabolism continue to be studied. Many manufacturers have switched back to sugar (sucrose), but that approach is unlikely to work for managing calories—HFCS and sucrose have similar CD and palatability.

The best approach for weight management and health is to limit foods and beverages with added sugars.

- Look for information on sugars on the label. If at least one sugar is near the top of the ingredient list, then a large proportion of that food's calories come from sugar.
- If a bit of sweetness makes the difference between eating a nutritious food such as oatmeal or plain yogurt and not eating it, go ahead and add a sprinkle. Some recipes, including Juliet's Vegetarian Chili (page 287) and Melissa's Leek Lasagna (page 246), call for a small amount of sugar to enhance flavor.
- Enjoy foods that are naturally sweet and lower in CD, such as fruits, that can satisfy your sweet tooth. Turn fruit into a fancier dessert by drizzling it with liqueur and topping it with a small amount of chopped nuts or grated chocolate. Also try lower-CD fruit desserts such as frozen fruit pops and fruit sorbets that are made with real fruit.

Some people have to keep a close watch on their sugar intake for reasons other than weight. If you have been diagnosed as having prediabetes, diabetes, or insulin resistance, your healthcare providers may suggest that you restrict sugars and use sugar substitutes instead to help control your blood glucose. They also may recommend a low-glycemic-index or low-glycemic-load diet (see box below), which shares many principles with Volumetrics. If you have diabetes, work with your dietitian, diabetes educator, or doctor to create a Volumetrics meal plan that helps you manage your blood glucose.

Glycemic Index, Glycemic Load, and Volumetrics

Glycemic index (GI) and glycemic load (GL)—measures of the effects of carbohydrate-containing foods on blood glucose levels—periodically come into the weight-loss spotlight as tools to help people shed pounds and steady blood glucose after eating. Proponents say that by choosing foods with a low GI instead of those with a higher GI—for example, whole grains rather than processed grains—you can prevent big rises and drops in glucose and insulin. The promised benefits of a low-GI diet include less hunger and reduced storage of body fat.

"The practical value of GI as a tool for selecting foods is limited by the fact that it can vary based on a food's ripeness, other foods eaten in the meal, cooking method, and individual blood glucose responses," notes Dr. Xavier Pi-Sunyer of Columbia University. Low GI also doesn't always favor healthier foods, because other food components such as fat also moderate blood glucose levels. So fatty potato chips have a relatively low GI but high CD, a fat-laden croissant has the same GI as whole-wheat bread, and a chocolate bar has a lower GI than most fruits. While scientists continue to hotly debate the relationship between a low-GI diet and satiety, calorie intake, and weight loss, the evidence is too variable to draw firm conclusions. However, the types of fiber-rich foods recommended in low-GI eating plans—whole grains, legumes, and vegetables—are consistent with Volumetrics principles and are sensible for everyone.

The Place for Sugar Substitutes

Should you consider replacing sugar with one of the many sugar substitutes—aspartame, sucralose, acesulfame K, saccharin, stevia, or neotame? Sugar substitutes, also called intense sweeteners or calorie-free sweeteners, are widely available in foods and as "table-top" sweeteners to offer sweetness without calories or added sugars. While some media reports suggest that sugar substitutes increase hunger and cause people to eat more rather than helping them cut calories, these claims are not supported by research findings.

Sugar substitutes can have a place in your diet for reducing the calories and CD of sweet foods and beverages. They are a tool for eating less sugar, not a green light to eat more of the types of foods that contain them. They should not be used as an excuse to eat other high-calorie foods. Foods labeled sugar-free usually are not calorie-free and many also have a high CD, so read labels before incorporating them into your day. The various intense sweeteners taste slightly different from each other, so if you choose to use them, experiment to see which ones you like best. When using them in recipes, look for brands that specifically can replace sugar in cooking and baking.

Fat and sugar add pleasure to healthy foods and enable us to enjoy small indulgences that can make Volumetrics eating even better. Where and how they can make the biggest impact is for you to decide.

Key Points

- Fat and sugar make food taste good, and that can lead us to eat too much of the foods they're in. Use them in modest amounts while not adding unnecessary calories.
- Foods with a high fat content tend to have a high CD. Pairing fat with low-CD foods such as vegetables and fruits helps offset the effects of fat on calorie intake.
- Decide where to include fat, choosing foods with beneficial mono- and polyunsaturated fats over those with unhealthy saturated and trans fats.
- Portion size is an important consideration for all types of fat, as even healthy fats are high CD.
- Limit foods and beverages with added sugars.

Let's Get Physical

Walking likely has become an important and enjoyable part of your daily routine. Look back at your average daily steps before you began this program. This week, I suggest that you increase the intensity of your walking to burn more calories without having to spend more time exercising.

- If you're walking casually at a slow pace—2 to 3 miles per hour or about 2,000 steps in 20 to 30 minutes—try to cut 5 minutes off the time it takes you to walk 2,000 steps.

- Alternate slow and fast walking.
- Make your stride longer or shorter. Your body will work harder than when you walk at your usual pace.
- Carry light hand weights and move your arms as you walk.
- Walk up and down hills instead of on flat ground.

Head and Habits

People who successfully lose weight talk about the importance of having a support group or support system. We all need people who can cheer for us and help us keep on going. How do you know whom to turn to? Think about connecting in person, over the phone, or online with family members and friends who have conquered or are facing their own weight challenges and will support you in a positive way. They'll have firsthand knowledge of what you're going through. Also consider people who have been particularly supportive of you in the past. Let them know that you're looking for help and tell them how they might help you—by lending an ear, texting or posting words of encouragement, helping you make decisions, distracting you from food, making you laugh. Any type of regular communication and support, whether in person, on the phone, or via email, can reinforce your healthy lifestyle. You could cook and share a meal, swap healthy recipes and tips, go shopping, or take a long walk. Your efforts might even inspire them to make positive changes in their lifestyle!

To Do This Week

- ☐ Look through your food records, particularly those that you kept at the beginning of the program, for sustainable ways to cut out unhealthy fats and added sugars.
- ☐ Talk to a family member or friend about specific ways to help support your weight management efforts.
- ☐ Increase the intensity of your walking by changing your speed, stride, or terrain.

Week 8

To Snack or Not to Snack, That Is the Question

Snacking is the key to controlling my hunger. I include three 100-calorie snacks of fresh fruit each day and always plan ahead when I'm going to be on the road by bringing fruit in a soft cooler. That way, I avoid surprises if I'm ready for a snack and can't find something healthy to eat.—Ric, Florida

You didn't start life eating just three meals a day. As a newborn, you were hungry and ate every couple of hours. During your school years you needed to eat between meals to get enough calories and nutrients. In our adult years, although we organize our day around breakfast, lunch, and dinner, many of us eat between meals or "snack." Could eating more frequently or having snacks between meals help you manage your weight?

How Often Should I Eat?

Many fad diets and articles in the popular press recommend that you change not only what you eat, but how often. Some suggest spreading frequent mini meals across the day, with the promise that they will rev up your metabolism, improve control of blood sugar, reduce hunger, and promote weight loss. This implies that having more meals could help you cut calories. But data from large-scale studies based on reports of what people typically eat show that frequent eating is associated with excess calories rather than with eating less. Several colleagues have reviewed and evaluated the evidence from studies on the effects of the frequency of eating. Here are the takeaway messages.

- Be wary of diets claiming that eating more often during the day will control hunger and melt the pounds away.
- The limited available evidence suggests there is no association between eating frequency and body weight or health, according to a 2009 systematic summary of relevant studies on weight-loss and weight-maintenance interventions.
- Eating *more* than three meals each day has been found to have inconsistent effects on hunger and calorie intake, but eating *fewer* than three meals a day may have negative effects. People who eat just one or two daily meals can feel hungrier and less full than those eating three meals.

How do you decide which eating pattern works best to control your hunger and help you eat healthfully? Should you stick to the three Volumetrics meals you learned about in Week 4, or would eating more frequently be a better strategy? You may find that eating more often is not for you because it tempts you to eat too much. Or you may need to eat every couple of hours to help you avoid the excessive hunger that can lead you to lose control and eat too much food. These individual differences reinforce my suggestion that you have to try different meal patterns to find one that allows you to control your hunger and helps you avoid temptations. Dr. Megan McCrory, at Purdue University, stresses the importance of planning your meals. "Knowing what, when, and how much you're going to eat helps you stay within your calorie goals. You can't just eat more frequently as desired." This is especially true if you increase your eating frequency by adding the types of high-CD convenience foods we typically think of as snacks.

How Snacking Can Add Calories

Snacking definitely is "in." On average, we eat one-and-a-half to two snacks each day, and market aisles are filled with foods created specifically for the occasion. We often choose snack foods based on appeal and availability at the moment rather than on calorie content or nutritional value. But their sensory properties—enhanced by combinations of fat, sugar, and salt—along with their high CD make them easy to overeat.

If you're like people in studies of snacking, you may find that calories from high-CD snack foods (and calorie-rich drinks, which you'll learn about next week) sneak past your body's regulatory systems without triggering appropriate fullness. You won't adjust meal intake enough to compensate for these snack calories and are likely to exceed your daily calorie goals. Even if you do trim back your meals to make room for snack foods, typical snacks tend to be less nutritious, so you may miss out on essential nutrients.

THE BOTTOM LINE. If you decide to eat frequent meals or snack between meals, you need to be consistent and mindful. Try snacking on a similar amount of food at the same time each day to allow your body to adjust to the extra snack calories, allowing you to eat less at meals. Let's look at how Volumetrics strategies can help you manage snacks and ensure balanced nutrition.

CD and Portion Size in Snack Foods

Most traditional snack foods—regular chips, cookies, and other high-fat fare, as well as lower-fat baked chips, reduced-fat crackers, pretzels, and cereal bars—don't contain a lot of water. This means that they fall into Categories 3 and 4, even if they are low in fat or made with "good for you" ingredients such as dried fruit, nuts (see Nuts About Nuts), and whole grains. You don't get much food for the calories.

Nuts About Nuts

Nuts are a popular snack—they're delicious, portable, and filled with protein, fiber, healthier fats, and other nutrients. They have ties to heart health, can be filling, and in studies looking at reports of what people typically eat are not associated with weight gain. But they have a high CD of around 6, so portion size matters. If you include nuts as a snack:

- Measure out your portion rather than eating from the bag or jar.
- Choose nuts in shells to slow down your eating.
- Mix them into lower-CD snack foods such as yogurt, fat-free pudding, or fruit salad.
- Enjoy them in modest amounts that fit your calorie budget.

You also don't get a lot of food in many types of packaged 100-calorie snacks. If you compare several different snack-size packs of chips, crackers, cookies, and candy, you'll see that portions are small because CDs are high. These prepackaged snack foods can make it easier to control the amount you eat when you want a high-CD snack; a study in my lab showed that people ate fewer chips from a smaller bag than from a bigger one. When eating a high-CD 100-calorie snack, be sure to stop at one. Research shows that the small package may send a message that these are okay "diet" foods, leading some dieters to eat more than one.

If you want your snack to help manage your hunger, it should include lower-CD foods. The photo below compares five different snacks to show you what a difference CD can make to your portion.

100-Calorie Snacks : What a Difference Calorie Density Can Make

Each of these snacks supplies 100 calories. You can eat only 16 jelly beans (CD 4.0) or ¼ cup raisins (CD 3.1) because both have a high CD and almost no water. As CD goes down, you get a bigger portion—about a cup of grapes (CD 0.69), close to 2 cups of apple slices (CD 0.53), or almost 4 cups of cherry tomatoes (CD 0.18).

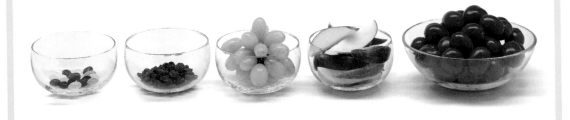

Budgeting Calories for Snacks

Is there an ideal number of calories for a snack? Is it best to include one, two, three, or no daily snacks? The right snacking strategy for you is one that helps you manage your hunger and keep your eating on track within your calorie goals. If you would rather have more calories at meals, try going without snacks or limiting yourself to the lowest-calorie snacks listed in the Snacks and Desserts Modular List (page 365). You also should avoid snacking if it sets off a hard-to-control desire to eat between meals.

Jill, a longtime follower of Volumetrics, finds Volumetrics meals to be so filling that she doesn't need to snack. She also notes that it's hard to have a satisfying meal if she uses up her calorie budget on snacks.

I suggest keeping your total daily snack calories under 200 to leave you with enough calories for meals. The sample menus (pages 156–163) provide about 1,400 calories in meals; if your daily goal is 1,600 calories, you can add 200 calories for snacks or increase the food in your meals. You can use these calories for a single snack or divide them into two snacks—for example, one in the afternoon and one after dinner. By choosing very-low-CD foods, you can have a satisfying snack for less than 100 calories.

Are you trying to limit your snacks to only "healthy" foods? Read labels of snack foods with a healthy-sounding title or ingredients carefully to make sure that the ingredients, calories, portion size, and CD are what you expect. Light ice creams, vegetable chips, fruit roll-ups, and other "healthy" snacks are easy to overeat if you fall into the trap of thinking healthy always means fewer calories.

The Snacks and Desserts Modular List on page 365 can help you choose foods that fit your snack calorie goal. Regardless of which snack strategy you choose, keeping track of what you eat is important.

Snacking Strategies

You can choose your snacks from a wide range of options. If you go for a traditional high-CD snack food such as nuts, chips, or cookies, your portion needs to be small to control calories. Here's how to keep snack calories in check.

FOR MANAGING HUNGER. Planning ahead is important if you know that you'll be really hungry by snack time. Otherwise, it's too easy to be so distracted by your growling stomach that you can't make smart decisions. You might want to eat some low-CD vegetables first to quiet your stomach and then decide on the rest of your snack. Try these filling low-CD snacks:

- Assorted raw veggies with 2 tablespoons low-fat or 1 tablespoon regular dressing
- 6-ounce container of light yogurt with 1 cup sliced strawberries
- A quesadilla made with 1 whole-wheat tortilla (1½ ounces), 2 tablespoons reduced-fat cheese, and 2 tablespoons diced tomato, with ¼ cup salsa for dipping

- 3 lettuce leaves rolled with 3 thin slices (1 ounce total) deli turkey, flavored mustard
- 3 celery stalks stuffed with 3 tablespoons 1% cottage cheese
- A microwaveable cup of broth-based soup

FOR MANAGING TEMPTATION. Snacks help you to manage temptation. If you're particularly vulnerable to overeating at a specific time of day—for example, when you get home from work and are preparing dinner or in the evening when you're watching television—include a snack at that time. Plan ahead for such situations by looking through the Modular Lists for snack ideas and stocking up on low-CD foods to munch on—cut fresh vegetables, chunks of fresh fruit, frozen fruit—to keep from overeating. You also can consider brushing your teeth or chewing gum before snacking. Studies conducted by Professor Marion Hetherington at the University of Leeds found that chewing gum between lunch and a snack reduced feelings of hunger and cravings for salty and sweet foods. "Participants who chewed gum before a snack ate less than those who did not chew gum. It might be that the minty freshness of gum is incompatible with eating a snack or that chewing gum satisfies to some extent the desire for a snack."

FOR YOUR SCHEDULE. Snacks can be well-suited for busy schedules, especially when you plan for your own personal situation.

- If you're on the go, try to bring a snack with you. Pack a small, soft-sided cooler with a light yogurt, half a sandwich, cut vegetables, or a couple of pieces of fruit. You also can bring a portion of nuts, pretzels, or baked chips, but recognize that the high CD means that your portion needs to be small.
- Have a list of six to eight different healthy snacks to rotate through over the course of the week. "It doesn't take a lot of time or planning to make this work," says Megan McCrory.
- Coordinate your snacks with your activity schedule. You may want to have a small snack an hour or so before you work out and another snack after.

FOR BALANCED NUTRITION. Including a snack gives you the opportunity to fill in your day nutritionally. Take a look at the Suggested Food Group Servings guide (page 372) to get an idea of which foods you need to add to your day to make up any food group short-falls. Specifically, the sample Volumetrics meal plans provide about two dairy servings each day, with the expectation that you'll include dairy in your snack. You may also want to have fruits, vegetables, or a whole grain. Here are a few ideas for 100- to 150-calorie snacks that pair dairy with other foods (use the Modular Food Lists to put together additional snacks).

- Broccoli florets with a yogurt dip
- Small apple and a mozzarella cheese stick
- Smoothie made with ½ cup yogurt, half a banana, ½ cup strawberries, and ice
- A yogurt cup and sliced peaches

FOR YOUR FAMILY. What should you do if you have to buy snack foods to pack in lunches or for after-school activities? One strategy is to keep only one or two different snacks around—having a lot of highly appealing snacks in the house can be tempting (you'll learn more about managing variety in Week 11). Consider ways to lessen temptation by storing snack foods in an inconvenient location, and buying individual packs to help manage calories. You also can get your kids accustomed to eating the healthier and more satisfying types of on-the-go snacks that you can enjoy, such as single-serve packs of vegetables or fruit, lower-fat cheese, guacamole, or hummus.

Snacking and its effects on your weight are more about what you eat than about how often. When you create tasty snacks from low-CD, nutrient-rich foods, you reduce between-meal hunger and satisfy the urge to munch while staying within your calorie limit.

Key Points
- Focus more on what you eat than how often you eat.
- Explore different meal and snack patterns to see which best fit your lifestyle and control your hunger levels, using the Am I Hungry? scale before and after meals or snacks.
- Snacks may not be necessary for managing your hunger. You can choose to skip them altogether to free up additional calories for meals.
- Incorporating very-low- and low-CD (Categories 1 and 2) snack foods allows you to have filling portions that fit into your daily calorie budget.

- Higher-CD (Categories 3 and 4) snack foods with low moisture content and combinations of fat, sugar, and salt are highly palatable and easy to overeat. If you choose them at all, manage portion size carefully.
- Strategic snacking should be nutritious, convenient, and effective for managing hunger and temptation. Snacking provides the opportunity to add more vegetables, fruits, and low-fat or fat-free dairy to your day.
- Write down your snacks to help you pay attention and better control what you eat between meals.

Let's Get Physical

Are you sometimes challenged by obstacles to being physically active? Try these strategies for overcoming potential stumbling blocks.

- If you don't have the time, divide exercise into smaller chunks instead of trying to do it all at once.
- If you don't want to miss your favorite show, exercise in front of the TV or at a gym with television sets.
- If you have no energy, exercise anyway; even doing a light cardio workout such as walking can help you feel more energetic and upbeat.
- If you're bored, try different types of activity to find ones that you enjoy, and mix them up to prevent boredom.
- If you're not motivated, find an exercise buddy to help keep you going.

Head and Habits

I hope that you're continuing to keep track of what you eat on paper, on your computer, or using a phone app. Even a few simple notes can help you manage snacking; snackers who record what they eat are better able to keep control of calories. Keeping a food record works so well because it forces you to pay attention to what you choose for a snack. You'll also be better able to keep track of what you've eaten, especially if you are snacking subconsciously while multitasking or nibbling on small amounts of high-CD snacks like a few raisins or pretzels, some cheese, or a small handful of nuts.

If you've drifted away from writing down what you eat, this is a good week to start up again by keeping track just of what you eat between meals. You'll then be better able to tailor your snacks to your schedule, eating habits, and hunger level.

To Do This Week

☐ Monitor hunger and fullness before and after meals and snacks to see which types of snacks have the biggest effect on hunger before the next meal.

☐ Try at least two new Category 1 or Category 2 snacks that fit into your calorie budget.

☐ Keep track of your snacks in your food record.

☐ Come up with at least two strategies for overcoming your obstacles to physical activity.

Week 9
Rethinking What You Drink

Most of us can drink a 20-ounce bottle of regular soda without giving it a second thought. But consider that it's the equivalent of eating 17 teaspoons of sugar! That's why reconsidering your drinks makes so much sense.—Traci Malone, M.H.S., R.D.

A few years ago, I was on a plane next to a father with his overweight young son. He kept his son happy by allowing continuous refills of soda. I don't know what their usual habits were, but it was all I could do to refrain from launching into a full-blown lecture. We get a lot of calories that we don't need from beverages; knowing how to manage their intake is one of the easiest and most sustainable ways to cut calories. People don't realize how quickly drink calories add up—big coffee drinks, for example, often have several hundred calories. This week, you'll learn simple strategies for managing your drink calories.

Filling Up with Water

As you have learned over the past eight weeks, water in foods fills you up without adding calories. You have seen examples of how eating water-rich foods gives you a bigger portion for the same number of calories—and this translates to greater satisfaction. The obvious question is: Can drinking extra water also help you feel full? If you believe what you read in the popular press, the answer appears to be yes. But is it that easy?

Drinking water quenches thirst, but it doesn't satisfy hunger the way water in food does. (See Are You Hungry or Thirsty? on page 107). Four separate studies in my lab showed that drinking up to 16 ounces of water either before or during a meal didn't affect the food intake of young adults. Colleagues at Virginia Tech had similar results with young adults, but found that drinking water before a meal helped older adults feel full and even gave them a small weight-loss boost. How can this be explained? It may be because stomach emptying slows down as we get older, so both liquids and foods stay in the stomach and make us feel full for longer. But for most of us, water that is consumed by itself passes through our stomach quickly and has little impact on satiety.

Are You Hungry or Thirsty?

Dieters are often told that they are eating in response to being thirsty, not hungry. But I am skeptical. Hunger and thirst are triggered in different ways. We get thirsty when our blood volume drops or when the concentration of salt in our blood goes up. Hunger is a signal that the body needs nutrients. When researchers ask people to report how they feel after they have been deprived of either foods or drinks, their answers show that hunger and thirst are sensed differently. Hunger is described as stomach rumblings and growling, while thirst is associated with dry, uncomfortable mouth sensations. Pay attention to what your body is telling you. The next time you need something to relieve a dry mouth, try sipping water or other low-calorie drinks to satisfy the urge, instead of turning to food.

What about the commonly held belief that drinking water helps burn off calories? Research findings have been inconsistent, but any effect that water may have is unlikely to be big enough to have much impact on weight loss. Even though drinking water doesn't effortlessly melt away the pounds, you still need adequate amounts for overall health.

Water: How Much Do You Need?

Humans aren't like camels. Our bodies can't store water, so we need to replenish fluids every day. If I were to ask you how much water you should drink, your likely answer might be the widely publicized eight glasses a day. Surprisingly, this number is not scientifically proven, and current advice is not nearly so specific. The 2010 Dietary Guidelines stress that people who are healthy usually take in plenty of water so long as they have regular access to water and other beverages. For most of us, drinking water with meals and when we are thirsty provides the water we need.

If you really want a number to guide you, the Institute of Medicine suggests that daily totals of nine cups of water for women and thirteen cups for men are adequate to meet bodily needs. All the water you drink counts, and so does the water in the foods you eat—food contributes about 20 percent of the average person's daily water intake. Because your Volumetrics diet is filled with water-rich foods (see Percentage of Water in Foods), the percentage of water coming from the foods you eat probably is even higher.

Your water needs can vary widely with your physical activity and the temperature of your environment. Be sure to drink plenty of water and other beverages and eat water-rich foods when you're active or in a hot climate, in order to replace the fluids your body is losing through perspiration and respiration.

Percentage of Water in Foods

FOOD	WATER CONTENT (%)	FOOD	WATER CONTENT (%)
Vegetables and fruits	80–95	Pasta, cooked	60–65
Soups	80–95	Meats	45–65
Hot cereal	80–85	Cheese	35–55
Yogurt, low-fat fruit-flavored	75	Bread	35–40
		Nuts	2–5
Egg, boiled	75	Crackers and chips	2–3
Fish and seafood	60–85	Oil	0

Source: USDA National Nutrient Database for Standard Reference, Release 23, Water Content of Selected Foods per Common Measure, 2010

Choosing Beverages Wisely

While simply drinking water won't fill you up, it plays an important role in your diet by quenching your thirst and satisfying your need for liquid . . . and it's calorie-free. Compare that to the numerous calorie-containing beverages—soft drinks, fancy and flavored coffee drinks, bottled tea, flavored waters—that are so much a part of our lives. Both children and adults get an average of about 400 calories per day from beverages with added sugars!

In the past few years, soft drinks have often been labeled as the number one culprit in the obesity epidemic. It is true that soft drink intake and rates of obesity have increased at the same time. However, the types of controlled studies needed to establish a clear relationship between sugar-sweetened beverages and body weight have not been conducted. The available data suggest that cutting back on soda helps overweight people manage their weight. And it is clear that no one needs extra calories from nutrient-poor beverages. Sadly, adolescents now consume more soda than any other beverage including milk!

THE BOTTOM LINE. Many people drink high-calorie beverages when they're thirsty. Soft drinks don't work as well as water to satisfy thirst and do little to satisfy hunger. So even though you might drink a fair number of calories, you're likely to eat just as much food. That's why the biggest benefit to drinking water when managing your weight is that it will help you escape this beverage calorie trap. Check out the Beverages Modular List (page 370) to see how quickly beverage calories can add up. If you decide to drink some of your calories, choose nutrient-rich beverages lower in CD, such as fat-free milk, 100% vegetable juice, or a small portion of 100% fruit juice.

The availability of many tasty lower- and zero-calorie beverage options makes this one of the easiest places in your diet to make sustainable changes.

- *Bottled waters:* Plain mineral water and seltzer are calorie-free, but watch out for flavored varieties that have added sugars. To create your own flavor, make a spritzer with a splash of orange juice, grapefruit juice, cranberry juice, or tropical juice.
- *Milk:* Milk is important for calcium, protein, vitamin D, and other nutrients. Try to gradually move down to fat-free milk, because it has the lowest CD and calories. If you prefer other types of milk, you'll need to adjust your food choices to compensate for the additional calories.
- *Diet sodas:* Diet sodas as an alternative to regular soda can save a lot of calories and lower the CD of your beverages. You still need to watch what you eat and avoid making up the calories with more food.
- *Coffee:* Coffee on its own or sweetened with a low-calorie sweetener has almost no calories, and a splash of fat-free milk adds just a few more.

- *Iced tea:* Skip the bottled or canned varieties that are loaded with sugar and calories. Instead, look for unsweetened brands, or make your own with a small amount of sugar or other sweetener and add flavor with lemon or lime wedges or a sprig of mint.

What if you're really in the mood for a more indulgent coffee drink? You still can have a treat while making changes that lower calories and CD. Order the smallest size. Request that your drink be made with fat-free or lower-fat milk, along with light or sugar-free syrup. Skip the whipped cream, or taste just a spoonful and remove the rest. For sweetness, use a low-calorie sweetener or just a small amount of sugar.

THE BOTTOM LINE. Water and fat-free milk are your best choices. Skip drinks with added sugars that contribute calories without nutrients. (See Think Your Drink).

Think Your Drink

Each of the beverages in this photo provides 100 calories: whole milk, orange juice, cola, and fat-free milk. Make the switch from whole milk to fat-free milk and you can drink almost twice as much for the same number of calories. The CD and calories of orange juice and cola are similar, but orange juice is preferable because it is more nutritious.

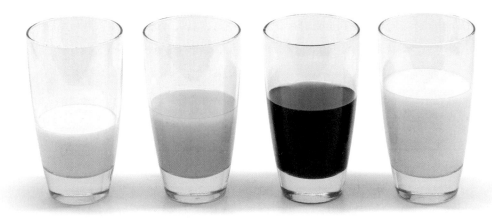

Whole milk (5.3 oz)   Orange juice (6.8 oz)   Regular cola (8 oz)   Fat-free milk (9.3 oz)

Alcohol and Volumetrics

You may be asking: Do I have to stop drinking my favorite alcoholic beverages to lose weight? The answer is no. Moderate drinking is consistent with weight management and can have health benefits for many adults. But you need to make wise choices. Consider:

- Alcohol is calorie-dense, with 7 calories per gram compared to 4 for carbohydrate or protein. An ounce of 80 proof alcohol contains 70 calories, and mixed drinks often contain more.
- Calories from alcoholic beverages don't satisfy hunger; instead, they add to the calories you're getting from food.
- Alcohol consumed both before and during a meal primes your appetite and can increase calorie intake.

Calories from alcohol have the potential to be particularly fattening if consumed along with high-fat foods. When you add alcohol to a high-fat, high-calorie meal, your body burns less dietary fat and stores more excess calories as body fat. If drinking a beer means you are likely to reach for chips, chicken wings, pizza, or other high-fat, high-CD foods, work toward breaking this pattern to keep calories under control.

Another reason to plan what and how much you are going to eat is that alcohol is likely to break down your resolve to manage your calories. After the first drink, all bets may be off, especially if you are enjoying yourself with friends and family and not paying attention. If you want to include alcohol in your diet, develop new habits that help you avoid eating excess calories. You may want to drink only with lower-CD meals, rather than between meals with high-CD snacks. Research shows that a glass of wine or a beer consumed along with your evening meal is unlikely to increase total calories. For example, if you have a glass of wine or beer with a dinner of soup, lean steak, green vegetables, and fruit salad for dessert, you're likely to stay within your calorie goals. Alcohol doesn't have to affect your weight, as long as you keep the rest of your diet consistent with Volumetrics.

THE BOTTOM LINE Keep alcohol to a minimum, and when you do drink, consume it with a low-CD food or meal to reduce the chances of overeating.

In summary, your body needs water, so drinking throughout the day is essential. What's not essential is getting a lot of calories from beverages, particularly those that supply calories with few or no nutrients. By drinking primarily water, you can quench your thirst without adding unnecessary calories to your day.

Key Points

- Limiting intake of caloric beverages is a relatively easy and sustainable strategy to cut unwanted calories.
- While for most of us drinking water doesn't enhance fullness, it quenches thirst and helps meet the body's need for fluids without adding calories.
- Water should be the beverage of choice, along with fat-free milk to meet nutrition recommendations.
- Alcoholic beverages add calories and can stimulate the appetite. If you choose to include alcohol in your Volumetrics diet, consume it with a meal or with very-low- or low-CD Category 1 and 2 foods.

Let's Get Physical

Even if you've chosen to do other types of physical activity, I encourage you to walk every day. Think about walking in the same way that you think of other aspects of your daily routine—brushing your teeth, taking a shower, getting dressed. Walking is a given. Your decisions involve where and for how long you're going to walk.

Mix up your routine for variety and to help you meet your daily step goal. Hop on a treadmill at home or in a fitness center. Set the TV to your favorite show to make time go by quickly. Find out if your local mall opens early for walkers; you can window-shop without spending money!

Head and Habits

Do you find that certain situations trigger eating even though you're not hungry? It may be a tempting food ad on television that sends you back into the kitchen shortly after dinner. You might instinctively grab a snack to eat every time you sit in front of your computer. The office candy bowl or treats brought in by coworkers may be your weakness. Being around certain friends and family members could derail your healthy habits.

You might drink juice or regular soda at a party because they're available. Here are a few suggestions for handling eating triggers.

- Become more aware of what sets off your eating, so that you can prepare mentally ahead of time.
- Make a conscious effort to avoid the trigger—get up and walk around during food commercials, don't eat while you're at the computer, stay away from office treats.
- Limit or eliminate trigger foods and drinks like candy, desserts, snack foods, soda, and beverages with alcohol.
- Make plans with friends and family members that don't involve eating and drinking.

To Do This Week

- ☐ Buy a sports bottle or travel container and fill it with water. Keep it with you to ensure you turn to water to quench your thirst over the course of the day.
- ☐ Look through your food records and develop a plan to eliminate drinks with added sugars.
- ☐ Decide how you are going to manage alcohol calories and how they fit with your calorie goals.

Week 10
Eating Away from Home

Your restaurant plate should resemble your plate at home, with half vegetables and the remaining half split between protein and grain. There are a lot of ways that you can do this by changing the size of your entrée, ordering vegetable side dishes, or even making a meal from all side dishes. It is most important to be mindful of your choices.—Emily Fonnesbeck, R.D.

When I was a kid, eating out was something we did once in a while and mainly for special occasions. Now surveys show that we spend about half of our food dollars on meals and snacks purchased and eaten away from home. Sometimes it is a necessity—we are on the road—and other times it's a great way to relax and spend time with friends and family. But many people find eating out to be the most difficult part of weight management.

Restaurants know what sells: big portions of indulgent, calorie-dense foods. The result is that people who eat out frequently eat more calories and tend to be heavier than people who have most of their meals at home. That is why I've devoted this week to helping you make choices when eating away from home that are both enjoyable and consistent with the principles of Volumetrics.

Portion Size and the Restaurant Plate

Have you noticed that restaurant portions have grown before your eyes in recent years? My colleagues Drs. Marion Nestle and Lisa Young at New York University found that portions are up to five times as large as they were thirty to forty years ago! It is not unusual for a pasta bowl to hold a pound of pasta and meatballs. Steakhouses brag about their 12- to 16-ounce steaks. Sandwiches in chain restaurants often start at 700 calories and easily can top 1,000 calories. That's a lot of calories compared to your daily budget!

How does a chef decide how much food to put on your plate? My colleagues and I were curious about whether chefs understand appropriate portion sizes. Of the 300 chefs we surveyed, about three-quarters thought they serve regular-size portions. But the portions of pasta and meat they reported serving were up to eight times larger than the standards the government recommends. When it came to vegetables, on average, the chefs reported dishing up barely half a cup, which is not nearly enough. It turns out that most chefs don't think about calories when they plate up your meal, and over half say that it is your responsibility to know how much to eat rather than their job to serve the right amount.

Calorie Density in a Restaurant

Calorie density is an important consideration when ordering a restaurant meal, but here's the challenge: often you can't tell which ingredients the chef used to make your dish, or how your dish was prepared, by just reading the restaurant menu. So the CD is hard to figure out.

Suppose you go out with a group of friends to a Chinese restaurant and order your favorite dish, chicken with broccoli. If calorie information is not listed on the menu, can you tell whether your dish is low or high in calories? The chef may have chosen high-fat pieces of meat, used a heavy hand with oil during stir-frying and in the sauce, and skimped on broccoli, so calories and CD would be on the high side. On the other hand, if the chef prepared your dish with lower-CD ingredients such as skinless chicken breast fillet, a large portion of broccoli, just a small amount of oil along with broth for cooking and a light sauce, you could get a bigger portion for the calories, or eat a satisfying amount for fewer calories. The example in the chart CD Comparisons in a Chinese Meal (page 116) shows how CD can vary in a typical Chinese restaurant dish. That is why knowing how to order is so important.

CD Comparisons in a Chinese Meal

Calories and CD can vary a lot, depending on the ingredients in a healthy-sounding dish like chicken and broccoli. You can enjoy a portion that is twice as large and has less than two-thirds the calories when lower-CD ingredients are used.

HIGHER-CD CHICKEN AND BROCCOLI			LOWER-CD CHICKEN AND BROCCOLI		
Food	Grams	Calories	Food	Grams	Calories
½ cup fried chicken thigh chunks	85	225	½ cup stir-fried chicken breast	70	115
¼ cup stir-fried broccoli	40	10	1 cup stir-fried broccoli	155	45
1 tbsp peanut oil	15	120	1 tsp peanut oil	5	40
Stir-fry sauce	30	15	Stir-fry sauce	30	15
CD = 2.2 cal/g Serving = ¾ cup	170	370	CD = 0.83 cal/g Serving = 1½ cups	260	215

Take Action: Plan Ahead

One of the best ways to manage your restaurant meal is to prepare ahead of time. You'll be better able to control your hunger and order a satisfying amount of food with a little advance planning.

- Have a low-CD snack beforehand to cut your hunger so that you can be just as satisfied with smaller restaurant portions, particularly of higher-CD foods. Remember that this strategy could backfire if you order and indulge in a first course at the restaurant anyway.
- Come up with your own "go-to" dish that you can order almost anywhere. Easy options include grilled chicken or a large house salad with dressing on

the side, a turkey breast sandwich with mustard and plenty of lettuce and tomato, or grilled salmon with a couple of vegetable side dishes.

- Pick a restaurant that has plenty of lower-CD options on the menu. Check out the menu on the restaurant's website, read diner reviews on food and restaurant sites, and call the restaurant in advance to find out if it can accommodate your particular requests.

Navigating the Restaurant Menu

Did you know that experts in the field of menu engineering manipulate the restaurant menu to entice you to order certain dishes? I was surprised to learn how much thought goes into where and how foods appear on the menu. Items that the restaurant wants you to buy appear in the middle of the menu, at the top or bottom of a list of foods, or high-lighted in a box. Photos and evocative descriptive language stimulate diners to order those dishes. An expensive item at the top of a list is there to make the dishes that follow look more affordable. And be careful if prices are listed without a dollar sign—for example, 16. rather than $16. People tend to spend more when the dollar sign is missing.

Restaurants also use a health "halo" to help them sell food. People tend to buy more and consume more calories from chains with healthier options on the menu. If a dish has a healthy name or ingredient list, you're likely to think it's lower in calories. Often it's not! Now that a growing number of restaurants list calories on their menu, picking foods that fit into your eating plan is easier. But you still need to order wisely—the calories in your dish could be very different from the calories on the menu. Here's how.

- The calories refer to the primary dish—for example, a salad or soup—but not extras like dressing, croutons, or bread that are served with it.
- The listing of calories and other nutrition information on the menu does not include condiments such as mayonnaise, sauce, or cheese.
- The calories listed are for a single portion of the entire dish, for example, one slice of a personal size pizza, but people typically eat the whole thing.

Becoming an informed menu reader helps you be more knowledgeable about what you're ordering and know which questions to ask for personalizing your meal.

The Importance of Speaking Up

Do you ever feel too nervous to ask questions in a restaurant? It is perfectly normal to want to avoid making waves, especially when you are dining with others. But keep in mind that restaurants are in business to serve you and that you deserve to have foods prepared the way you like, when possible. The website of the National Restaurant Association, www .restaurant.org, encourages diners not to be afraid to ask for special low-calorie or low-fat preparation of a menu item. So speak up when you need information that can help you order a lower-CD meal. (See page 119 for Ten Questions You Shouldn't Be Afraid to Ask.)

Course-by-Course Strategies for Volumetrics Eating

Over the past several weeks, you've been putting together your meals in ways that help fill you up while managing calories—building breakfast around Category 1 and 2 foods, filling up first with a big, low-CD appetizer at lunch and dinner, incorporating vegetables and fruits, and including foods with healthy fats strategically. These same strategies apply when you're eating out, and they can make the difference between a Volumetrics meal and one that is too high in calories.

BREAKFAST. Do you grab a quick breakfast at the local coffee shop, food truck, or fast-food chain on your way to work? Restaurants and fast-food outlets have expanded their breakfast menus into more healthful choices such as yogurt parfaits, oatmeal, fruit platters, and grilled sandwiches filled with egg whites and vegetables. When I can, I try to mix and match three different types of foods on the menu: whole-grain bread or cereal, fruit, and a fat-free or low-fat dairy product. Here are a few suggestions.

- Whole-grain or high-fiber cereal, berries, and fat-free milk
- Oatmeal, diced fruit salad, and fat-free milk to drink
- Whole-wheat toast, fruit, and plain yogurt
- Bran muffin, melon half, and fat-free milk to drink
- One pancake, berries, and plain yogurt

THE BREAD BASKET. Request whole-grain breads and rolls when available and manage portion size. I like to pick out a favorite and then put the basket at the other end of the table or ask the waiter to take it away so that I am not tempted to eat more.

Ten Questions You Shouldn't Be Afraid to Ask

1. **How is this dish prepared and which ingredients are used?** Ask if the dish can be prepared in a healthful way—for example, grilled with a small amount of butter or oil instead of pan-fried. Find out if high-fat, high-calorie, or high-CD ingredients can be reduced or eliminated. If the answer is no, get suggestions for alternative dishes.

2. **Which soups are made with broth rather than cream?** Common broth-based soups on restaurant menus include chicken noodle, minestrone, vegetable, and beef barley.

3. **What are my salad dressing options?** Many restaurants offer both lower-fat and regular dressings. Ask for dressing on the side and dab it on lightly with your fork to control calories. Or lightly dress your salad with vinegar and olive oil.

4. **Is this dish available in a smaller portion?** Pastas in particular may be available in both appetizer and entrée portions. An appetizer portion of many options is often large enough to have as your main course.

5. **What vegetables can I order or have in place of the side dish that comes with my meal?** Select veggie dishes that are not swimming in oil or sauce, or request them steamed. Asian restaurants are particularly good at making flavorful steamed vegetable dishes.

6. **Can I split this dish with someone at my table?** Check the menu for a splitting charge so that you are not surprised when the bill comes. If the charge seems unreasonable, order the dish and bring home half.

7. **Can we order this for the table, with plenty of spoons/forks?** This is an easy way to enjoy a taste or two without the calories of the whole dish.

8. **Can I have this dish without cheese/sour cream/gravy/sauce/butter on top?** If your waiter says no—the dish already is prepared or the chef refuses to serve the dish without—ask for recommendations for popular dishes that may be lighter.

9. **Could I have fat-free or another milk instead of cream for my coffee?** This is a common request that is easy to satisfy.

10. **Can I take the rest of this home?** Doggy bags are the answer to too much food—once I took home enough food for three additional dinners from one Mexican dish! You can even act in advance—ask to have your meal split and wrapped to take home before it is brought to the table.

SALADS AND SALAD BARS. As you know, my lab staff and I have done a lot of research on salads, and our research has shown that having a large, low-CD salad as either your first or main course will help you feel full and eat fewer calories. But salad bars can be calorie minefields. Sure, there are plenty of greens, but usually there are all kinds of mayonnaise-covered pastas and other high-CD healthy pretenders. Look at all the available foods before you fill your plate, to decide which and how many foods you want. Then use the salad-building strategies that you learned in Week 5.

APPETIZERS. You can find plenty of lower-CD picks on the appetizers menu. Best bets include steamed shellfish, shrimp cocktail, melon with prosciutto, vegetables that have been grilled without a lot of oil, or a fresh vegetable platter. Appetizers at family and burger restaurants tend to be fried; if you have a craving for onion rings, mozzarella sticks, fried zucchini, or other classic appetizer menu fare, order the smallest portion, share with everyone at the table, and leave some food on the plate. This is not the type of food you want to bring home! As with all appetizers, I suggest that you keep your appetizer portion to 150 calories or less (see the Modular Food Lists on pages 357–371 for ideas).

MAIN COURSES. Ask questions before you decide on a main course. Find out if a dish can be grilled or broiled and served with little or no sauce, or with sauce on the side. Chicken cooked with the skin on is fine—the skin helps keep in moisture—as long as you remove it before eating. Order your pizza with less cheese and extra veggies. Choose dishes with low-CD buzz words and be cautious if you see or hear high-CD hot button phrases in the name or description of a dish (see page 121).

SIDES. A menu's side dish section can be filled with options for lowering the CD of your meal. Ask how vegetables are prepared—steamed, stir-fried, and grilled vegetables tend to have the lowest CD. I don't often see whole grain choices on the menu so I have learned to ask for brown rice instead of white rice. If my dish comes with buttery mashed potatoes, I request a baked potato instead, with salsa or a small amount of butter or sour cream on the side. You can make the choice that is best for you—either less potato with an indulgence of butter or sour cream or a larger portion of potato if you cut down on higher-fat toppings. Use the Condiments and Spreads Modular List (page 369) to compare the CDs of various toppings.

LOW-CD BUZZ WORDS	HIGH-CD HOT BUTTONS
Baked	Basted
Broiled	Béarnaise (butter, egg yolks)
Grilled	Butter sauce
Lightly sautéed	Crispy
Poached	Cream/Creamed/Cream sauce
Roasted	Cheese/Fromage
Steamed	Gratin (butter, crumbs)
Stir-fried	Hollandaise (butter, egg yolks)
	Scalloped (cream, cheese, crumbs)
	Stuffed

Ordering in Ethnic Restaurants

Ethnic cuisines are fun to explore and can fit well into a Volumetrics eating style. Here are some choices and swaps to lower the CD of your meal.

AT A CHINESE RESTAURANT

- Order dishes with chicken breast strips instead of chicken thigh pieces and with meat that is not breaded and fried.
- Mix a dish of steamed vegetables into your main course.
- Ask for brown rice rather than white or fried rice.

AT AN ITALIAN RESTAURANT

- Ask for an appetizer-size portion of pasta as a main course.
- Select extra vegetable side dishes, preferably steamed, for sharing family style.
- Look for red sauce dishes with *marinara*, *cacciatore*, or *pomodoro* in their name.

AT A MEXICAN RESTAURANT

- Order corn tortillas—they're smaller, and some are whole grain—instead of flour tortillas.
- Request a small portion of one higher-fat topping—guacamole, sour cream, or cheese—and ask for the others to be left off your dish.
- Use salsa as a salad dressing and topping.

AT A STEAKHOUSE

- Order leaner steaks—sirloin, strip steak, filet mignon—rather than higher-fat prime rib and T-bone.
- Select the smallest portion of meat—remember that the recommended serving size is about 3 ounces cooked—and bring home any extra.
- Go for a baked potato with a pat of butter and a tablespoon of sour cream instead of home- or french-fried, scalloped, au gratin, or mashed potatoes.

AT A SANDWICH SHOP

- Order the smallest size or half a sandwich, paired with a small broth-based soup.
- Hold the dressing, mayonnaise, and spreads, and ask for mustard or barbecue sauce instead.
- Pile on the vegetables.

AT A FAST-FOOD RESTAURANT

- Order the salad main course topped with grilled rather than "crispy" chicken, beef, or fish, and use as little of the dressing packet as you can without compromising taste.
- Switch to the smallest size single patty or a veggie patty, with a thin slice of cheese if you like, plus extra lettuce and tomato. Skip the mayo and "special" sauce.
- Consider having a yogurt parfait for breakfast rather than a breakfast dish that has a high CD.

Smart Eating on the Road

Traveling for several days? Even just one day on the road can be hard on your diet. You lose a lot of control over when you eat, what you eat, and how your meals are prepared over the course of the day. It is easy to feel grumpy and out of sorts when your daily food routine is upended. Here are some of the strategies that help me stay on track when I travel to meetings and conferences.

I stock a small cooler for car trips that overlap a meal. Breakfast might include yogurt, maybe a hard-cooked egg, and fresh fruit, along with a small muffin or roll. For lunch or dinner, I bring either a sandwich with hummus and vegetables (see page 229), or fixings for a picnic sandwich if the weather is nice. The cooler has fresh vegetables and fruit for snacking and frozen gel packs to keep everything cool.

At the airport, I pick up food in the terminal. The options on planes are limited and usually high in CD, so don't wait to find food until you are in the air and hungry. If you are going to take the food on the plane, be kind to your fellow passengers and choose ones that are not too fragrant—no fish or onions.

When I arrive at a hotel, I ask if they have a refrigerator I can use, or if they can provide one. I then search out the closest grocery store and stock the refrigerator with a few healthy foods, especially so I can have an inexpensive, healthy in-room breakfast. If you are at a breakfast meeting, seek out cereal with low-fat milk, or a high-fiber muffin, and pass up high-CD pastries. Choose fresh fruit over juice.

Make sure you get enough dairy. One option is to order a latte, cappuccino, or café au lait made with fat-free milk. Have yogurt from the breakfast buffet, order yogurt from the restaurant menu, or pick a carton up at a mini mart.

Eating away from home has become a big part of our everyday eating, rather than something we do only once in a while. That is why your restaurant food decisions are so important for managing your weight and nutrition. You still can enjoy indulgences on occasion, and do so without feeling guilty.

Key Points

- Restaurant portions are generous and most chefs don't consider calories when dishing up meals. You'll need to manage the amount you eat to keep calories in check.

- A chef's decisions about ingredients and cooking methods can make the difference between a high- and lower-CD dish. Ask questions and modify your order to help lower the CD of your meal.
- Plan ahead by filling up first on a low-CD appetizer, looking at the restaurant menu in advance, and selecting restaurants with lower-CD options.
- Remind yourself that you don't have to treat every meal as if it is the last one you will ever eat—share, take food home, or just leave some on the plate.

Let's Get Physical

Experts agree on the benefits of physical activity, but myths still abound. You may be wondering about whether these are true.

Myth: Exercise makes you tired.
Reality: People often feel energized and less stressed after physical activity.

Myth: If you can't reach 10,000 daily steps, don't bother.
Reality: Any amount of walking is better than not walking at all. Increase steps at your own pace.

Myth: It takes too much exercise to lose weight.
Reality: It is true that it is easier to overeat than it is to burn off excess calories. But when it comes to weight management, every bit of exercise helps—remember, small changes add up. Exercise provides other important benefits, including better physical and emotional health.

Myth: If I don't feel it, it isn't working.
Reality: Your muscles should feel like they've been moving, but physical activity shouldn't hurt.

Head and Habits

Many of us spend more waking hours at work than anywhere else. That is why it is important to adapt your work routine to support your weight management efforts.

- Plan your meals. Bring breakfast with you if you don't have time to eat at home. Pack a lunch to eat at work—Volumetrics leftovers, a salad or sandwich, soup, or a portion-controlled frozen entrée. Store your lunch in an insulated bag with freezer packs if refrigerator space isn't available.

- Seek out healthy choices in the company cafeteria or your favorite local spot. You don't have to avoid eating out and miss the opportunity to bond with coworkers and find out what's going on. Identify a few different meal options that can fit into your eating plan—for example, an entrée salad, a lean deli meat sandwich on wheat bread, or a bowl of chili.

- Manage temptation. Bring fresh veggies for a midafternoon snack to help you resist office goodies. Use Volumetrics strategies for filling your plate at office parties. Change your path to and from your office so that you don't pass by the vending machines.

- Take a few activity breaks over the course of the work day. Try to spend a portion of your lunch hour outside or walking around inside the building. Encourage coworkers to join you if that will make your break more enjoyable.

To Do This Week

- ☐ Think of questions to ask about the menu at your favorite restaurant.
- ☐ Review restaurant menus online and check calorie counts to help you decide what to order.
- ☐ Try at least one strategy for lowering the CD of a meal eaten away from home.
- ☐ Add steps this week if you're not yet at 10,000 steps per day.

Week 11
Your Personal Environment

When your environment is filled with tempting foods, controlling your eating can be a challenge. Since being overweight has much more to do with your appetite than your metabolism, you may find that it's easier, and ultimately more effective, to change your physical food environment than to change the way you respond to food.—Michael Lowe, Ph.D.

For the past ten weeks, we have been working together on the fundamentals and benefits of making healthier food choices and increasing physical activity. I hope you are pleased with the results—feeling better and weighing less. Now it's time to start looking ahead toward the maintenance phase of your personal plan, which I will cover next week. This week I am giving you a head start by showing you how to structure your food environment so that it encourages you to stick with your Ultimate Volumetrics Diet and lifestyle.

We live in an environment that surrounds us with opportunities to overeat. Huge portions of calorie-dense foods are not just in grocery stores and restaurants but almost everywhere we go—gas stations, bookstores, and even home improvement shops. It's no secret that these foods are designed to tempt us and appeal to our love for sugar, salt, and fat. They also seem like good value since they provide lots of calories for the dollar. But they are not a good value if they cause you to overeat.

Your personal eating environment is not just about the types of foods you buy. It also involves the foods you keep around at home and at work, the way you eat them, and the people you eat them with. How do we keep temptation at bay? This week I am going to tell you about a number of strategies that can be used to structure your personal environment so that it works with you rather than undermining your best intentions. But first, let's explore your personal vulnerability to delicious foods.

The Power of Food

We are not known as a species with a lot of willpower. Most of us succumb to the lure of indulgent high-CD foods when we are tired, stressed, or feel we need a treat or deserve a reward, or just because the food is there. So far, the types of self-control you have been learning and practicing should be helping you stay on course. But to be successful at managing your weight long term, you need to structure your food environment so that it's less conducive to overeating. Dr. Michael Lowe of Drexel University suggests making specific changes to the foods available in the places where most of your eating takes place—your home, workplace, and even your car.

Dr. Lowe and his colleagues developed a self-test to evaluate how strongly you are affected by the availability of tasty foods in your immediate environment where you spend most of your time. Take the short Power of Food quiz (page 128) to find out more about your personal vulnerability to delicious foods.

THE BOTTOM LINE. For many of us, changing our food environment is necessary for supporting our weight-loss efforts. Changes can be extensive or quite simple, as long as they're effective and permanent. Dr. James Hill of the University of Colorado suggests that small changes in the right direction can make your environment work with rather than against your weight management goals. One place to start is with managing variety—that is, the number and types of different foods you keep around.

Make Variety Your Ally

Humans are omnivores. We need to eat a varied diet to ensure that we get the nutrients our bodies require. And variety in our diet is truly the spice of life—can you imagine how boring it would be to eat the same few foods over and over? But the type of dietary variety in your environment matters. If you surround yourself with lots of calorie-dense foods, you are bound to eat more calories than you need.

Much of my earlier work looked at how the variety of foods offered in a meal affects the amount of food people eat. Consider these results.

Power of Food

Indicate the extent to which you agree that the following items describe you. Use this 1–5 scale for your responses.

1   don't agree at all
2   agree a little
3   agree somewhat
4   agree
5   strongly agree

___

- ☐ If I see or smell a food I like, I get a powerful urge to have some.
- ☐ When I'm around a fattening food I love, it's hard to stop myself from at least tasting it.
- ☐ When I know a delicious food is available, I can't help myself from thinking about having some.
- ☐ I love the taste of certain foods so much that I can't avoid eating them even if they're bad for me.

Add up your four scores; the total will be between 4 and 20. The higher your score, the more important it is for you to make permanent changes in your "personal food environment" to reduce food temptations and help you control your weight.

4–8: Change in food environment may not be necessary
9–12: Some changes in food environment are recommended
13–20: Major changes in food environment are recommended

- When we fed students four very different foods, they ate 60 percent more than when they received just one of the foods, even if it was their favorite.
- People who were served sandwiches with four different fillings ate one-third more than when they were served sandwiches that had the one filling they liked best.
- Just varying the shape of pasta increased intake. People ate 15 percent more pasta when served three different shapes than when they were offered only one shape.

We tire of the taste of individual foods as we eat them, a response called sensory-specific satiety. During a meal that includes a variety of foods, the foods we have not yet eaten still seem pleasant and appealing, particularly those that have very different tastes, textures, shapes, and aromas from those we have already eaten. We switch without realizing it from one food to another as each food declines in pleasantness. Sensory-specific satiety helps ensure we get the variety of nutrients we need, and explains why we still have room for dessert even when we already feel full. The salty and savory tastes of the foods we have been eating are less pleasant, but sweet foods still are desirable so we keep on eating.

How can sensory-specific satiety and variety be used to positively influence intake? The answer is not to just cut variety out of your meals and in your home. Restricting variety may help you eat less in the short run, but eventually the desire for variety will win because it is so fundamental. You can make variety work for you by stocking your personal environment with an appealing selection of lower-CD Category 1 and 2 foods. This helps ensure that when you are planning a meal or dealing with the "munchies," rather than turning to high-CD food you will find lower-CD foods that you want to eat. A study conducted at Tufts University shows that this strategic approach to variety is consistent with weight loss: people who eat a greater variety of vegetables weigh less than those who eat a variety of more calorie-dense foods. What are some ways to use variety to help you eat a Volumetrics diet?

- At home and at work, surround yourself with a wide selection of Category 1 and 2 foods you enjoy—apples, carrots, soups, yogurts, or one of your favorite Volumetrics recipes—in place of a stash of calorie-dense cookies, candies, and chips. That way, when one food becomes less appealing as you're eating it, you can switch to another one that fits into your eating plan.

- Add flavor. Stock your kitchen with a variety of condiments, such as ketchup, mustard, or low-fat dressing, to make low-CD foods even tastier and help you resist higher-CD options.
- Vary colors, textures, and shapes of veggies and fruits.
- Limit the different types of Category 3 and 4 snack foods you buy so that you're not driven by their variety to sample them all.

Managing variety is an important aspect of your Volumetrics food environment. A related but different challenge is keeping control of the types and amounts of trigger foods you have around.

Handle Trigger Foods

The top reasons people give for choosing foods are good taste and convenience. It's important not to sacrifice taste. But by now you should have a clear idea of your trigger foods—those you can't resist, and that are hard to stop eating once you start. You will need to come up with personal strategies and firm rules to help you control how much you eat of these foods. Here are a few suggestions to try; choose the ones that work better for you.

- Avoid temptation altogether and ban trigger foods from your personal food environment. This works for some people, but studies show that restricting access to high-CD foods can backfire, making them even more tempting and desirable. Dr. Lowe suggests that strong trigger foods be eliminated from your home environment and eaten only away from home.
- Keep small amounts around as treats. Snack-size candy, now available year-round, is good for portion control as long as you can stop after eating just one or two.
- Figure out if these foods can still be a part of your life . . . in moderation. There's no need for a sense of panic and urgency about eating them, since they are not going to disappear from the marketplace. You can buy them whenever you want. So take a step back, think about whether they might trigger overeating, and consider the calories before you buy or bite in.

- Substitute a lower-CD alternative—for example, a frozen fruit pop—for a higher-CD trigger food such as full-fat ice cream.
- Crowd out trigger foods by surrounding yourself with lots of your favorite low-CD foods. Your long-term goal is to make these foods your default, the ones you automatically turn to when you have the urge to eat something.
- Chew gum or brush your teeth to give your taste buds a calorie-free flavor hit and distract you from eating.

Ultimately you need to be reassured that your favorite foods are not going to disappear from your life. You are in charge, so don't let them derail your resolve to manage your weight.

Get Your Family On Board

Despite your best efforts, it may be impossible to banish all higher-CD trigger foods because family members or housemates might not be willing to give up their stash of favorites. Since having the support of family members can help you be more successful, try to find a solution that satisfies everyone.

- Minimize temptation by keeping one or two treats in the house that family members like but you don't.
- Stock up on lower-CD foods and create lower-CD dishes from the recipes in this book or from electronic sources at your fingertips.
- Be a role model. By watching you, your kids will learn healthful habits, including eating vegetables and fruits (Week 5), how to fill their plate (Week 4), when to stop eating, having water or fat-free milk with most meals (Week 9), and other Volumetrics practices.
- Try the stealth approach! Don't tell your family that the meals are healthy, and consider hiding vegetables or fruit in your recipes. As you learned in Week 5, this not only significantly increases intake of these foods but it also helps cut calories.

Make Convenience Work for You

I mentioned that people also choose foods for convenience. Food companies are doing their part to make foods much more convenient, with single-serve portions of soup, pre-portioned frozen meals, individually packaged snacks, and other food products. Be sure to add a Volumetrics twist to convenience.

- Keep appealing Category 1 and 2 foods at hand. Stock up on prepared soups, low-fat yogurt, frozen meals, hummus, and your favorite veggies and fruits. Read labels for portion size and calorie information and compare products to find those with the lower CD.
- Make your own single-serving meals with leftovers. Many of my Volumetrics recipes are delicious the next day or suitable for freezing and reheating.
- Cook big batches of foods and divide into individual portions—it takes just a few minutes more.
- Label and date all food that goes into the freezer to help you keep track of what you have on hand.
- Use the sample menus (page 156–163) as a guide for incorporating convenience foods into your meals.
- Exercise caution when buying portion-controlled bags of chips, cookies, and candy, and energy bars. If you fill your home and office with these easy, high-CD options, they are likely to lure you into eating too much because they are not very satisfying for the calories.

Good planning makes convenience possible in a low-CD environment. Create a menu to cover several days and make a shopping list. People who go to the market with a shopping list usually stay on track, and they also save money by avoiding items not on the list and wasting less food. Consider buying smaller packages, especially of higher-CD foods, rather than stocking up at the warehouse store. Whatever you do, make sure you don't shop for groceries when you are hungry. Hunger increases the probability that you will fill your cart with more high-CD foods than you planned or wanted.

Reset Your Table

Your food environment is about more than food. It also encompasses the physical aspects of eating, including the plates you use for meals and snacks, the bowls you serve from, and even where you place foods in your fridge and cupboards. Could fixes as simple as downsizing your plates and utensils or repositioning your fruit bowl really help you to manage how much you eat? Absolutely yes, says Dr. Brian Wansink of Cornell University, who suggests using these strategies to support your weight-loss efforts. Here is sampling of his suggestions.

- Use smaller bowls or plates. They are a good reminder of the appropriate amount of food to eat, and you are likely to serve yourself less because a smaller bowl or plate fills up faster.
- Drink from tall, narrow glasses rather than short, wide ones. These create a visual illusion of holding more liquid so you will pour yourself a smaller amount.
- Place healthy, low-CD foods in easily accessible spots in the kitchen, such as at eye level at the front of the refrigerator or in a prominent bowl on the counter. Wash, peel, and cut them ahead of time so that they're ready to be eaten. Do the opposite for high-CD foods: put them out of sight and out of your way by freezing, wrapping, or positioning them behind other foods to make them less convenient and accessible.

My take on such environmental "engineering" is that it is a simple, positive approach to reinforce healthy eating habits. But don't count on these measures to automatically cut calories. When we gave nondieters smaller plates at a buffet, they went back to fill their plates more often and ended up eating as much as they did with big plates. They were not paying attention and didn't use the plate size to guide their portions.

THE BOTTOM LINE. You have to play an active part in controlling what you eat. If you decide to use physical tools such as plate and glass size or the placement of foods in your environment to nudge you toward eating less, do it mindfully. Use them to focus your attention and design an environment that directs you to healthy, low-CD options. Remember that when you're following Volumetrics, you will be filling your plate with lots of Category 1 veggies and fruits, so focus more on what you put on your plate than its size.

Do I Remember Eating That?

If I hadn't asked you to keep a daily food record, would you remember what you ate yesterday? Were you doing anything else—watching TV, checking email, working, texting, talking on the phone—while eating a meal or snack? If you don't pay attention to what you eat, you're likely to lose track and eat more. You don't want to end up like the two men with amnesia who were tested at the University of Pennsylvania. When they were served a meal, they ate it. A few minutes later, they were served a second meal, and they ate that, too. Because they had no memory of their meals, they just kept on eating. If you habitually eat in front of the TV or computer, you, too, may not remember what you ate, and that puts you at risk of eating too much. Distractions like playing computer games or watching TV interfere with the memory of eating, and this translates to greater intake when food is next available.

Distraction is not the only problem with too much screen time. TV viewing is associated with increased intake of high-CD foods such as snacks and pizza that are easy to grab and balance on our laps or the arm of the couch. Also, TV ads are designed to get us thinking about food. Studies show that people who spend the most hours in front of network TV with commercials eat the most fast food, especially at dinner. Speaking of dinner, it is now commonplace for families to eat dinner while watching TV. Not a good idea. Children who watch TV during dinner have a poorer diet quality, with fewer fruits and veggies and more soda, than those who don't watch.

In addition to TV time, many of us spend hours in front of a computer screen. Computer time is so pervasive in our daily lives that Dr. James Levine of the University Hospitals Case Medical Center in Cleveland designed a treadmill desk so that people can be active while working at their computer. While that isn't practical for most of us, you can try these strategies to help you turn your attention back to your meals and cut back on screen time.

- Eat at a table, not in front of a screen.
- Take your time and savor your food. This advice has been standard in weight-management clinics for years—it helps you experience, enjoy, and remember what you eat.
- Continue to keep your daily food journal. You learned when you began this program that food and activity diaries are associated with successful weight

management. Enhancing your memory of what you have eaten reduces intake later in the day.

- Reduce screen time. Adults in the United States watch an average of four hours of TV a day, and screen time is probably even higher now with all of our portable electronics such as smartphones and tablets. If you can't cut back, position the screen so that you can be active while watching. Or get up from the chair and take "activity" breaks.

- Remove the bedroom TV. A bedroom TV has been found to increase the chances that children are overweight. The same is likely true for adults—one study found they watch an average of 5.4 hours a day with a bedroom TV and 3.6 hours without one.

THE BOTTOM LINE. Family meals should be a time to build relationships and set a healthy eating example for children. And the more time we spend in front of our computers or TVs, the less time we spend on physical activity in our day.

The Company You Keep and the Food You Eat

A few years ago, headlines proclaimed that you can "catch" obesity from your friends and family. A study of social networks of over 12,000 men and women found that if someone has a friend who starts gaining weight, their chances of putting on extra pounds go up by 57 percent. Spouses affected each other's weight, and so did adult brothers or sisters. People of the same sex had a greater influence on one another than those of the opposite sex. The good news from this study is that thinness also was contagious. If your friends and relatives successfully lose weight, your chances of success increase.

The mechanism is thought to be social contagion. When your friend or partner gets heavier, you ramp up your idea of what constitutes a normal weight and you may be less vigilant about your weight. Friends also influence how much you eat. Studies from my lab and the labs of colleagues show that we eat more when we are with friends and family than when dining alone or with strangers, and that many of the excess calories come from high-CD foods such as desserts. Eating is an intensely social activity and our eating companions drive our food choices and consumption without our realizing it.

Many of our decisions about how much to eat are made before we even serve ourselves. We are influenced by what seems to be appropriate or the "social norm" among the people we eat with. Women in particular tend to look to others to guide their eating, and a woman's eating provides a way for her to present herself positively in social situations. Women adapt to the situation, choosing dainty portions and making healthy choices when that's the image they want to project, or being indulgent if that seems like the appropriate way to get the party going.

The answer to managing these social effects is not to ditch your friends and family or eat alone. You need them as a support network. These tips may help you overcome the influence of others and help protect you from "catching" obesity.

- Be proactive. Suggest restaurants with healthy options you can enjoy. Offer to bring a dish that happens to be low-CD to a party.
- Take the lead and order or fill your plate first at a social gathering. See if your companions follow suit with healthier choices!
- Pay attention. If you're distracted when eating with family and friends, you're apt to order more, put additional food on your plate, and eat bigger portions.
- Share. This is a tip I especially like. For me, sharing dessert is a perfect ending to a meal. Research shows that such sharing reduces intake.

Managing your weight has more to do with your physical and social environment than with your self-control. "If you are vulnerable to the power of delicious foods, you're more likely to be affected by the tempting high-CD foods in the places where you spend the most time," says Dr. Lowe. "If you struggle with your weight, your willpower and commitment will help but are no match for the lure of living amidst lots of highly tempting foods. That is why it is so important to permanently change your food environment if you want to permanently control your eating."

Key Points
- Engineer your food environment to help you resist the power of food and reinforce positive eating habits and physical activity.

- Use variety strategically to fill your environment with lower-CD foods that you enjoy eating and that will help you resist high-CD temptations.
- Find your own personal strategy for keeping favorite high-CD foods in your life.
- Build a social support network that reinforces your healthy habits; be the leader, not the follower.

Let's Get Physical

Just as you're making changes to your food and eating environment, you can make changes to your environment that may make it easier for you to keep up your activity routine.

- Make sure you have comfortable exercise clothing and shoes that you enjoy wearing.
- Lay out your exercise clothing the night before so it's ready to go when you are.
- Update your music player with your favorite upbeat tunes and make sure your headphones are in good working order.
- Prepare your postexercise snack or meal ahead of time.
- Keep the computer off until after you've finished your physical activity.

Head and Habits

In Week 4, you learned how small changes in your diet and exercise routines add up to a noticeable difference. The same holds true for your environment. While it may be tempting to completely overhaul your kitchen and environment all at once, that approach is too drastic. Making changes gradually over several weeks allows you to adjust and helps you determine which specific actions work best for managing the temptations in your environment. You might divide the changes into the following categories:

- Food package size
- Variety of foods in your cupboards and refrigerator
- Placement of low- and high-CD foods in your cupboards and refrigerator
- Types of condiments and seasonings

- Availability of trigger foods
- Cooking ahead and freezing
- Mindfulness during meals

To Do This Week

- ☐ Make at least two changes to your personal food environment.
- ☐ Decide on a promising strategy to manage trigger foods and try it.
- ☐ Change your environment to be more conducive to activity.

Week 12
Maintaining Your Volumetrics Lifestyle

The odds of keeping pounds off for good are much more encouraging than we've been led to believe, and it's in your power to take charge of your lifestyle in a way that makes it happen.—Anne M. Fletcher, M.S., R.D.

Volumetrics is about helping you find patterns of eating and activity that you can live with long term. Lots of people who have followed Volumetrics tell me what a revelation it has been. They find they can eat plenty of food while managing calories. While I hope you have found sustainable habits, everything I know shows that maintenance is difficult but doable. That's why this week I am going to help you develop a plan to continue with the healthy habits you have learned over the past eleven weeks.

Many of the strategies I suggest are those used by "successful losers." The National Weight Control Registry (www.nwcr.ws) tracks more than 5,000 participants who have lost at least thirty pounds and maintained a thirty-pound loss for one year or more. Through interviews and questionnaires, the Registry research team studies how successful losers keep the weight off. This week I will share with you observations from the Registry, along with findings from other researchers and stories from followers of Volumetrics that show lasting weight loss is possible!

The first step is to revisit the goals you set at the beginning of this program and adjust them to fit where you are today and where you want to be in the future.

Getting Ready to Move Forward

Twelve weeks ago, you set personal goals for your weight, daily calories, and activity. How did you do? If you are satisfied with what you accomplished and the amount that you lost, this is the week to map out your course for maintenance. The box For Additional Weight Loss outlines next steps if you are not yet at your goal.

For Additional Weight Loss

- Set a new weight-loss goal of 5 to 10 percent of your current weight.
- Cut out 100 to 200 calories per day if your rate of loss has slowed or stalled; a slimmer body burns fewer calories.
- Increase your daily activity goal.
- Continue to follow the Volumetrics strategies that have worked for you and reevaluate your progress in several weeks.

The Ultimate Volumetrics Diet gives you the opportunity to explore different approaches for managing your eating and your weight. Dr. Chris Sciamanna, a physician and researcher at Penn State Hershey Medical Center who compares successful weight-loss strategies to those found beneficial for weight maintenance, stresses the importance of this process: "At the beginning of any program, you try out lots of new things, each of which may or may not help. Both weight loss and maintenance require that you think about what is working and what is not, and continue those strategies that help you." I encourage you to go back through the book and flag your most helpful strategies and tips; pick the ones that you can sustain so they will support you in keeping off what you lost. Let's look first at your diet and then consider the place for activity, self-monitoring, emotions, your environment, and habits for maintaining your loss.

Choosing Your Maintenance Diet

What do you think is the most important factor for maintaining your weight? Anne Fletcher studied the habits of successful weight maintainers when writing *Thin for Life* and *Eating Thin for Life*. When she asked them how they think they're different from the many people who gain back lost weight, they told her that they finally realized they couldn't go back to their old eating habits. They changed their perspective from being "on" or "off" a diet to eating in a way that would help manage their weight long term. Many of the Volumetrics strategies you've been using are ones used by long-term "losers" from the Registry, "masters" interviewed by Anne Fletcher, and respondents in Dr. Sciamanna's research.

- Continue to enjoy satisfying, low-CD meals and snacks that include plenty of vegetables and fruits, whole grains, legumes, lean protein, and low-fat and fat-free dairy products. Eating foods with a low CD has helped successful losers maintain weight loss and avoid weight gain over time.
- Include fat strategically to help you manage your calories. Registry members say they maintain their weight by following a lower-fat diet. They specifically mention incorporating lean cuts of meat and other lower-fat protein foods, as well as using lower-fat dressings, sauces, and dairy products as alternatives to those that have more fat. Dr. James Hill, a cofounder of the Registry, explains that controlling fat is necessary for maintenance because fat is so calorie-dense, and eating too much can lead to weight regain.
- Cut added sugar, especially in beverages. Registry participants report incorporating sugar-modified foods and calorie-free soft drinks into their diet.
- Manage your portions, using your toolkit from Week 3. Even though you may be comfortable with your diet, weighing and measuring high-CD foods once a week or so can help prevent portion size "inflation."

As you look back through this book to find your personal food strategies, you can feel proud of the number of changes you made to the way you eat. I encourage you to make a photocopy of the Summary of the Ultimate Volumetrics Diet Principles (page 142) to keep handy as a reminder.

As you've learned and experienced, Volumetrics enables you to manage your calories with satisfying amounts of food. The photos on page 143 bring the Volumetrics message home by comparing two 1,600-calorie meal plans, one with high-CD foods and the other with low-CD choices, including dishes made from the recipes in this book. The Volumetrics day gives you three times the weight of food!

Summary of *the* Ultimate Volumetrics Diet Principles

Volumetrics is based on healthy eating principles. When following these recommendations, find an eating pattern that is both enjoyable and sustainable.

FOODS	RECOMMENDATIONS
Portions	Appropriately sized portions will help you eat the amount of food that meets your daily calorie goal. • Fill your plate with satisfying portions of very-low-CD Category 1 and low-CD Category 2 foods. • Choose medium-CD Category 3 foods less frequently and in smaller portions. • Limit portions of high-CD Category 4 foods.
Water-rich foods	Water-rich foods give you satisfying portions that will help you feel full with fewer calories. • Eat more fruits and vegetables, with little to no added sugar or fat. • Have a large broth-based soup or salad at the start of a meal. • Substitute vegetables for higher-CD ingredients in stews, casseroles, pizzas, sandwiches, and rice and pasta dishes.
Fiber-rich foods	Fiber can help you to feel full. Rather than eating refined carbohydrates: • Switch to whole grains like whole-wheat bread, whole-grain cereals or brown rice. • Add more beans (legumes) to your diet.
Lower-fat foods	Fat is high in CD. Reducing intake of unhealthy fats is good nutritionally and can help control calories. • Include foods with healthy fats. • Choose low-fat animal products such as dairy and meats. • Substitute lower-fat foods for those high in fat. • Bake, steam, grill, or broil instead of frying. • Learn how to use small amounts of fat strategically to ensure you enjoy your food.
Lean protein foods	Low-CD lean protein choices help maintain muscle mass, provide essential nutrients, and are satisfying. • Include fish, poultry without skin, lean meats, eggs, legumes, and tofu. • Select dairy products that are low in fat or fat-free.
Low-calorie beverages	Beverage calories can add up quickly, so: • Remember, water is your best choice. • Limit your intake of sugary drinks and alcoholic beverages.

Same Calories, Three Times More Food

Both these meal plans contain 1,600 calories! The top photo shows typical high-CD foods that a person might eat over a day: a cinnamon bun, a burger with fries, fettuccine Alfredo and garlic bread, chips and dip, and a regular cola. The low-CD foods in the bottom photo were selected based on the principles of Volumetrics, with plenty of water- and fiber-rich vegetables and fruits, and moderate amounts of fat. You could eat a Berry Parfait (page 186), toast, melon, and a glass of milk for breakfast; a Rainbow Chef's Salad (page 216), The Volumetrics Soup (page 196), a whole-wheat English muffin, and fat-free pudding for lunch; and a dinner with an appetizer of Crudités with Cilantro-Lime Ranch Dip (page 317), followed by Chicken and Zucchini Skewers with Peanut Dipping Sauce (page 281), rice pilaf, a mixed green salad, and peach slices for dessert, plus as much as you want of my favorite beverage, water. Which would you rather eat for managing your weight?

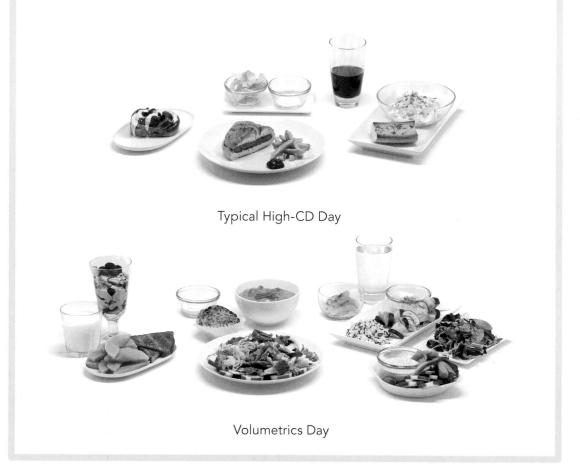

Typical High-CD Day

Volumetrics Day

What are your personal success strategies? Look back at your notes on the food, activity, behavior, and other strategies that helped you meet your goals each week. Write down those that worked best on the Weight Maintenance Worksheet and update the worksheet as you discover new strategies and behaviors that can be incorporated into your game plan for keeping your weight on track.

Weight Maintenance Worksheet

Weight_____   Daily Calorie Goal_____
Daily activity goal (in minutes or steps)_____

My favorite food strategies

_____

_____

_____

_____

My favorite activities

_____

_____

_____

_____

Ways I get support

_____

_____

_____

Mindset, attitudes, and behaviors that help me

_____

_____

Maintaining Daily Activity

Ric, a successful longtime follower of Volumetrics, says that physical activity is a must for maintaining his weight. "I make exercise part of my morning routine. It makes maintenance so much easier, and helps blow off steam."

At the beginning of this program, I suggested that you work toward an activity goal of 10,000 daily steps. If this goal was not realistic for you, I hope that you were inspired to increase your daily activity to a comfortable level. Even low levels of physical activity improve your health, help you feel more energetic, boost feelings of well-being, and reduce stress. Importantly, being active reinforces your commitment to a healthy lifestyle for maintaining your weight loss.

Whether you are highly active or get just modest amounts of activity, experts agree that exercise is essential.

- Keep up your activity level and follow a consistent routine. National Weight Control Registry participants who exercise most often are more successful at maintaining their weight loss. Dr. Sciamanna's research on weight loss and maintenance success factors shows that "while people try different types of exercises for losing weight, they settle into a routine with activities they like best in order to keep up their loss."
- If you can, add more steps to your walking program and pick up the pace, especially if you find it hard to maintain your new weight. Registry participants say that much of their physical activity is moderate to vigorous rather than leisurely.
- Data from the Registry show that you should be physically active whenever possible—turn off the TV and get away from the computer screen. Your body doesn't burn many calories when you're sitting, so cutting down on sedentary time is important.
- List your favorite activities on the Weight Maintenance Worksheet.
- Continue to record your daily activity.

Keeping Track

Maintaining a record of your eating and activity is one of the most important ways to improve your chances of success. I want to remind you that your food records don't have to be detailed. Writing things down makes you pay attention to what you're doing. You don't have to keep precise measurements of your daily diet and exercise unless you want to or feel you need to.

Here's another success factor: getting on the scale. Registry participants say that they weigh themselves often, even daily, to keep motivated and allow themselves to make small adjustments to keep their weight steady. It's better to catch and reverse a gain of one or two pounds than to be surprised by an extra five or ten pounds because you weren't monitoring your weight.

What should you do if your weight gradually goes up and gets "stuck" at a higher number than you like? Checking your records can help you spot possible causes.

- Think about and note problem situations that may have resulted in extra calories or less activity, along with strategies for handling them differently the next time (see the Solutions Worksheet on page 147).
- Consider going back to the weight-loss plan you followed earlier in the program to get rid of extra pounds. Then return to maintenance, knowing that you'll need to take fast action if the scale starts moving up again.
- Be diligent about keeping track of your diet and activity and checking to see if they are in sync with your goals.
- Think about whether emotional ups and downs may have affected your eating.

Solutions Worksheet

Life is full of tempting and challenging situations that call for creative solutions for staying on track. Write down those that have derailed you in the past and ways to handle them differently. Then keep track of new situations and solutions as they arise.

Problem Situation	New Approach
Example: Mom serves big dessert portions	*Serve myself a smaller piece*
_____	_____
_____	_____
_____	_____
_____	_____
_____	_____
_____	_____

Separating Emotions from Food

Food and emotions often go hand in hand. I know I often feel the urge to comfort myself with food after a stressful day. But this type of eating can be hard to control. Ric sums it up.

Emotional eating was a challenge, especially after a bad day at work. Eating my favorite sweet treats would knock me off track for weeks. Now I'll munch on a big bowl with of strawberries, blackberries, and blueberries—just as sweet and way more filling—while relaxing with a great book. Most important, I won't let one emotion-driven, poorly chosen meal turn into a month of lousy eating.

Anne Fletcher reinforces the importance of not turning to food during tough times. "Food can comfort and soothe you temporarily but it won't make your problems go away. Put your efforts toward constructive problem solving and stay in control of your eating to avoid adding stress to an already stressful situation." Include on the Weight

Maintenance Worksheet the types of support that gave you strength over the past eleven weeks. If you find that you are continuing to eat for psychological or emotional reasons and Volumetrics has not helped, consider switching to a behavioral program that is more targeted toward your specific needs.

Managing Your Environment

As you learned last week, changing your personal food environment can help you control the power food has over the way you eat. One way you can do this is by being the gatekeeper and making sure the foods in your home fit with your goals.

Reorganize your kitchen to support your Volumetrics diet. Darryl, who started Volumetrics in November 2008 and has maintained a loss of fifty pounds, changed his food environment by giving his kitchen a makeover.

> I stocked the cabinet with only better food choices so that anything in there is a good pick. That way, I don't have to think much about what to eat. I also moved foods to different locations. Now fresh fruit is out in the open on the counter or in the fridge and tempting foods are in the back section of the cabinet so that I don't see them.

You can control the selection and storage of foods in your home, but it is impossible to remove all tempting foods from your environment. So give yourself permission to indulge on occasion. An important part of weight maintenance is fitting in occasional treats while continuing to eat according to Volumetrics principles. A one-time indulgence does not have to become a habit.

Reinforcing New Habits

A habit is an established pattern that you repeat without much thought. Over the past eleven weeks, you've been trying out different Volumetrics strategies, and the ones that have become habits can help you maintain your weight. An important part of maintenance is to continue developing new habits to support your Volumetrics lifestyle.

Darryl got into the habit of keeping himself busy.

I needed to find ways to avoid sitting around thinking about and reaching for food out of boredom. Now one of my habits is to get up off the couch, turn off the TV, and walk the dog. I go places and do things, anything to distract myself from the boredom that leads me to overeat.

Here's another habit that can help you maintain a healthy weight: a good night's sleep. A growing number of studies show that people who don't get enough sleep are more likely to be overweight. You may find that heeding the advice in Week 11 to cut down on television time, particularly when you're in bed at night, also could improve your sleep.

Staying Motivated

What a great feeling to step on the scale and see that the number has gone down! When you're losing weight, watching the pounds come off is a strong motivator for keeping up your efforts. Once you reach your goal weight, the number on the scale stays fairly steady, so it's important to find other forms of motivation to give you the reinforcement you need to keep going.

When successful weight maintainers were asked how they keep their weight in check, they mentioned several strategies for staying motivated.

- Reward yourself for sticking to your program. Rewards can be small and simple—a manicure or pedicure, an afternoon with friends, a trip to the ballpark, a new scarf or belt—as long as they make you feel good and help keep you going.
- Think about how much progress you've made. Keep a running list of everything that has changed for the better—you have more energy; you wear a smaller clothing size; your stamina has improved; you sleep better—to remind you of where you were and how far you've come so far. (See My Successes on page 150.)
- Remind yourself of your healthy weight goal.

- Keep in mind the benefits of maintaining a healthy weight. What reminders might work? Sabrina, who participated in her employer's Volumetrics weight loss program, says that "regular exercise is important because it reminds me that I am working to improve my health, and that helps me make better food choices." You can feel good knowing that by keeping up your diet as well as your activity routine, you're improving your health and well-being.

My Successes

You were successful in large and small ways while losing weight. Remind yourself of those successes and of how much has changed for the better.

My weight-loss program is successful because today I am able to:

Example: Wear clothing that is two sizes smaller _____

Example: Play catch with my kids _____

_____

_____

_____

_____

There will be times when life hits you hard and distracts you from your healthy lifestyle. Your weight and health move to the back burner as you feel yourself slipping into old habits. But wait! You need to reignite your motivation. Regaining weight and eating poorly will just make you feel worse. You'll be better able to deal with life's stresses if you're eating right, getting activity, and making your health a priority. When life seems to be spinning out of control, two things you do have control over are food and activity. Your personal support system—friends, family members, coping strategies, mindset—can help you put your problems in perspective and remind you of the importance of taking care of yourself by taking care of your weight. While testimonials are not proof that a diet works for everyone, the experience of Jill O'Nan (see A Volumetrics Success Story, page 151) can help you move forward on your own personal journey for lifelong weight loss.

A Volumetrics Success Story

Jill O'Nan, a professional writer who lost 220 pounds using Volumetrics, offered to share her story about the challenges she is overcoming in maintaining her weight.

When I finally reached my goal weight, I was extremely proud of myself, but I knew an even bigger challenge lay ahead. Lots of people lose weight only to gain most or all of it back again. Long-term maintenance can be a minefield for chronic overeaters who struggle with weight control.

Yet I felt better prepared than most to make a successful transition. It had taken me four years to reach my goal weight, and during that time I schooled myself on healthy living. I learned to make satisfying meals by following the recipes in the first two *Volumetrics* books. I shopped for fresh, nutrient-rich produce, meat, bread, and eggs at the local farmers' market. I exercised regularly at my gym and did nearly all my errands on foot or by bike. Maintenance to me meant continuing the active lifestyle I had come to love.

For five years I maintained my weight loss fairly easily. Although my weight fluctuated from time to time—particularly around the holidays—I always resumed my healthy habits and shed excess pounds before they became permanent. After nine years of successful weight loss and maintenance on Volumetrics, I believed my battles with food were over forever.

Then things changed. I became ill and wasn't able to exercise. By the time I recovered, I had regained several pounds. A new job required me to work long hours at my computer, and my more sedentary lifestyle made it difficult to burn calories. But it was the stress of purchasing and then moving into a new home that proved to be my real undoing. Unexpected problems with my kitchen made it difficult to prepare food, so I turned to fast food. My focus was no longer health and nutrition. If I had a stressful day, I felt entitled to eat a bag of potato chips for dinner and a pint of ice cream for dessert.

Fortunately, my meltdown didn't last long. Within a couple of months, with the support of many kind friends, I began pulling myself back together. I joined a new gym and started working out regularly again. I hired a contractor to fix the kitchen so I could cook healthy meals at home again. I said good-bye to fast-food restaurants and went back to the farmers' market again.

Every day I chip away at the twenty-five pounds I gained, and little by little it is coming off. To keep myself going when progress is slow, I celebrate small victories along the way. This month the scale didn't move much, but I made it to the top of the hill on one of my favorite hiking trails. My legs felt stronger and my breath came easier than the last time I climbed it. Successes like this reassure me that by eating healthfully and exercising regularly, I will get back to my healthy weight in the near future.

Look at the many ways that you've changed your behaviors and attitudes to help manage your weight. *You* made your new healthy lifestyle happen with your dedicated efforts to eat, move, think, and act in a different way. These conscious efforts to alter your behaviors in meaningful ways will help you to be successful in a world filled with temptations to eat more, indulge often, and add convenience.

Successful losers say that keeping weight off becomes easier over time as weight management strategies become habits and don't require as much forethought and effort. You have what it takes to support new habits: realistic goals, a toolkit of new strategies, skills for spotting and solving problems without turning to food, and a strong support system. Keep coming back to your Volumetrics diet to remind yourself of the tips, strategies, support, and delicious foods that helped you reach this milestone.

Your new weight is a reminder of your most important goals: to enjoy good health, have a positive attitude about yourself, and sustain the energy to do the things that you like and need to do to live a fulfilling life. Be proud of what you've accomplished and what you can and will go on to do!

Your Personal Ultimate Volumetrics Diet Plan

The primary purpose of this sample menu plan is to guide you toward the amounts and types of foods to eat at your personal calorie level. Each day's menu provides 1,400 calories divided into three meals.

400 calories for breakfast
500 calories for lunch
500 calories for dinner

To match your calorie goal, hunger and fullness levels, and lifestyle, you can increase portions and add snacks. You also may need to adjust your calories up or down if you're losing weight too slowly or quickly.

Many of the meals are based on the recipes in this book, while others include easy dishes to make at home or order when eating out. A few meals contain frozen entrées and fast-food menu items to show you that you can adapt the meal plan to your lifestyle. I encourage you to mix and match meals, even interchanging a lunch for a dinner and vice versa, and to repeat a meal the next day to use up leftovers.

My goal is for you to learn how to incorporate Volumetrics eating habits into your lifestyle and to create an eating plan that's right for you. Use these meal plans for several weeks as a guide to the amounts and types of foods to eat. You can then move away from the focus on calories and concentrate instead on making nutritious food choices for enjoyable, satisfying meals.

Using the Modular Lists

To give you even more flexibility, I organized common foods into "modular" lists, on pages 357–371. You can use these lists to create meals with combinations of foods that you like best by substituting foods and dishes with similar calorie counts. For example, you might prefer chunky chicken soup to butternut squash soup—each has 90 calories per cup—or select the 90-calorie Baby Arugula Salad (page 210) instead. You also can refer to the lists for picking out snacks and adding foods to your meals. Meal and Snack Strategies by Calorie Level offers guidance for adjusting your diet to your calorie goal.

Meal and Snack Strategies by Calorie Level

CALORIE LEVEL	STRATEGY
1,400 calories	Use the menu plan for meals. If you want to add a 100- to 200-calorie snack, reduce meal calories by the number of calories in your snack.
1,600 calories	In addition to the foods in the meal plan, either increase your lunch and dinner from 500 to 600 calories by adding a 100-calorie dish at each meal, or add 200 calories in snacks.
1,800 calories	In addition to the foods in the meal plan, add 200 calories in snacks and increase lunch and dinner to 600 calories by adding foods or increasing portion sizes.
2,000 calories	In addition to the foods in the meal plan, add 200 calories in snacks. Also, increase your breakfast from 400 to 500 calories and increase your lunch and dinner to 650 calories by adding foods or increasing portion sizes.
Greater than 2,000 calories	If you need more calories, don't keep adding snacks. Instead, increase portion sizes for breakfast, lunch, and dinner. Main meals contain more protein and more nutrients than most snacks, so this is a healthier approach.

What about beverages? You'll notice that with the exception of fat-free milk, meals do not include beverages. As discussed in Week 9, beverage calories add up quickly. The calories you drink, including sugar and milk or cream in your coffee or tea, need to be subtracted from your meal or snack calories. I recommend water as your main beverage, or other noncaloric drinks if you enjoy them, so that you can have your calories available for food.

Milk, along with other dairy products such as yogurt and cheese, is an excellent source of protein and calcium. The Dietary Guidelines recommend three daily servings of milk or dairy products. Many of the meals in the menu plan include one serving; depending on your meal selection, you will need to incorporate one or two additional servings into your snacks or meal. See the Modular Food Lists on pages 357–371 for calorie and CD information on milk, yogurt, and cheese. Talk to your doctor about taking calcium supplements if you can't consistently fit three calcium-rich foods into your menu plan. Additionally, I recommend taking a daily multivitamin and multimineral supplement, especially if you are at the 1400- or 1600-calorie level. Meeting all of your nutrient recommendations from food alone is difficult at that level.

A Lifetime of Healthy Eating

The Ultimate Volumetrics Diet is a healthy eating plan for life. Here are a few more tips.

- Because Volumetrics meals use everyday foods, not special "diet" products, they're appropriate for sharing with a spouse, a friend, or family members. Your weight-loss efforts can result in healthier, more satisfying meals for everyone!
- At any meal or snack, you can eat more vegetables (except high-CD vegetable dishes with butter, oil, or high-fat sauce) while only slightly increasing your calorie intake.
- Don't worry about counting portions or calories exactly, especially of very-low-CD Category 1 foods and low-CD foods at the lower end of Category 2. The plan is designed to maintain the appropriate calorie levels, but you don't have to measure everything perfectly for it to work.

The Ultimate Volumetrics Diet plan is designed to help you fill up on fewer calories and lose weight without feeling deprived. More important, I want to show you that healthy eating can be enjoyable!

Week 1 Meal Plan

	Monday	Tuesday	Wednesday
Breakfast (400 calories)	2 whole-wheat waffles with 1 tbsp maple syrup, 1 small sliced banana (295 calories)	2 *Apple Oatmeal Muffins* (230 calories)	*Berry Parfait* (265 calories)
	1 cup fat-free milk (80 calories)	1 cup blueberries (85 calories)	½ whole-wheat English muffin with 2 tsp peanut butter (125 calories)
		1 cup fat-free milk (80 calories)	
Lunch (500 calories)	*Mixed Greens with Strawberries, Pears, and Walnuts* (105 calories)	1 frozen entrée of your choice (300 calories)	15 baby carrots with ¼ cup hummus (155 calories)
	2 slices whole-wheat bread with 2 oz turkey breast, 1 oz light cheese, mustard, and veggies of choice (325 calories)	6 oz light yogurt (80 calories)	1 bean and cheese burrito (260 calories)
	1 orange (70 calories)	1 cup grapes (110 calories)	1 medium apple (95 calories)
Dinner (500 calories)	*Asian Salmon in a Packet* (315 calories)	*Chili-Rubbed Steak Salad on a Deconstructed Guacamole Salad* (270 calories)	*Chilled Cucumber and Summer Vegetable Soup* (135 calories)
	½ cup brown rice (110 calories)	1 small (1¼ oz) whole-wheat tortilla (75 calories)	½ cup pasta sauce with 3 oz lean ground beef, ½ cup whole-wheat pasta (320 calories)
	1 cup raspberries (65 calories)	½ cup low-fat frozen yogurt with 5 banana slices and 5 sliced strawberries (160 calories)	1 cup cantaloupe (60 calories)

Thursday	Friday	Saturday	Sunday
1¼ cup bran flakes with ⅔ cup sliced banana, 2 tsp chopped walnuts, ½ cup fat-free milk (320 calories)	½ cup rolled oats cooked with 1 cup fat-free milk (230 calories)	*Light as a Feather Pancakes with Berry Sauce* (310 calories)	*Greek Frittata* (220 calories)
½ cup fresh blueberries (40 calories)	1 cup cut-up fruit (80 calories)	1 cup fat-free milk (80 calories)	1 slice whole-wheat toast with 1 tsp whipped butter (90 calories)
½ cup fat-free milk (40 calories)	6 oz light yogurt (80 calories)		1 cup fat-free milk (80 calories)
Caribbean Bean and Squash Soup (340 calories)	1 sandwich on a small whole-wheat sub roll with 3 oz ham, 1 slice cheese, mustard, veggies of choice (370 calories)	*Salade Niçoise* (270 calories)	1 frozen veggie pizza (360 calories)
1 medium whole-wheat roll with 1 tsp whipped butter (115 calories)	½ cup deli three bean salad (90 calories)	1 whole-wheat English muffin (135 calories)	6 oz nonfat plain Greek-style yogurt with 1 cup sliced strawberries (145 calories)
2 plums (60 calories)	½ cup raspberries (30 calories)	6 oz light yogurt (80 calories)	
Korean-Style Steak Fajitas (205 calories)	1 small garden salad with 2 tbsp light Italian dressing (60 calories)	3 oz grilled tilapia (110 calories)	*Crudités with Cilantro-Lime Dressing* (75 calories)
½ cup brown rice (110 calories)	*Pesto Pizza with Chicken and Vegetables* (300 calories)	½ cup rice pilaf (140 calories)	3 oz grilled pork chop with ½ cup mashed potatoes (305 calories)
1 cup steamed broccoli (55 calories)	1 slice angel food cake with 1 cup sliced strawberries, 1 tbsp light whipped topping (135 calories)	½ cup steamed sugar snap peas (35 calories)	1 cup grilled asparagus with 1 tsp whipped butter (60 calories)
6 oz light yogurt with 1 sliced peach (140 calories)		1 medium baked apple with cinnamon and 1 tsp brown sugar, topped with ⅓ cup light ice cream (200 calories)	½ cup raspberries (30 calories)

Week 2 Meal Plan

	Monday	Tuesday	Wednesday
Breakfast (400 calories)	1 hard-cooked egg (80 calories)	*Greek Apple Parfait* (260 calories)	2 slices whole-grain toast with 2 tsp whipped butter (180 calories)
	1 cup spoon-size shredded wheat cereal with 1 cup strawberries, 2 tbsp sliced almonds (235 calories)	1 medium (2 oz) bran muffin (145 calories)	½ cup low-fat cottage cheese with 1 sliced peach (140 calories)
	1 cup fat-free milk (80 calories)		1 cup fat-free milk (80 calories)
Lunch (500 calories)	1 fast-food green salad with grated cheese, 2 tbsp light Italian dressing (130 calories)	1 cup raw bell pepper strips with 2 tbsp light Italian dressing (75 calories)	1 cup cherry tomatoes (25 calories)
	1 regular cheeseburger (305 calories)	*Juliet's Vegetarian Chili* (375 calories)	1 frozen entrée of your choice (300 calories)
	6 oz light yogurt (80 calories)	½ cup raspberries (30 calories)	1 medium whole-wheat roll (95 calories)
			1 medium apple (95 calories)
Dinner (500 calories)	1 cup raw veggies with 2 tbsp light ranch dressing (95 calories)	3 oz BBQ chicken breast (165 calories)	1 small garden salad with 2 tbsp light Italian dressing (60 calories)
	3 oz grilled haddock, snapper, or other white-flesh fish (145 calories)	*Succotash Salad* (125 calories)	2 oz ground turkey in ½ cup tomato-based pasta sauce on ½ cup whole-wheat fusilli with 2 tbsp grated parmesan cheese (395 calories)
	1 medium baked potato with 1 tsp whipped butter, 1 tbsp grated Parmesan (215 calories)	1 medium baked sweet potato (105 calories)	1 orange (70 calories)
	1 cup sautéed spinach (45 calories)	6 oz light yogurt (80 calories)	

Thursday	Friday	Saturday	Sunday
2 scrambled eggs with 1 chopped tomato, 2 tbsp guacamole (290 calories)	1 whole-wheat English muffin with 1 tbsp peanut butter (230 calories)	*Pumpkin Cranberry Bread* (145 calories)	*Vegetable Denver Omelet* (160 calories)
1 corn tortilla (55 calories)	1 small sliced banana (90 calories)	6 oz nonfat plain Greek-style yogurt with ½ cup blueberries, 2 tbsp low fat granola, 1 tbsp walnuts (270 calories)	1 small (2 oz) whole-wheat bagel with 2 tbsp light cream cheese (215 calories)
1 cup fat-free milk (80 calories)	1 cup fat-free milk (80 calories)		½ cup cantaloupe (30 calories)
Rainbow Chef's Salad (230 calories)	1 cup minestrone soup (80 calories)	1 veggie burger patty on a whole-wheat bun with ½ oz reduced-fat cheese, ketchup, lettuce, tomato, roasted pepper strips (295 calories)	3 oz grilled chicken on a bed of lettuce with 1 oz cheese, 2 tbsp light Italian dressing (270 calories)
1 medium whole-wheat roll (95 calories)	*Hummus and Veggie Sandwich* (290 calories)	1 carrot and 1 celery stalk, cut into strips (30 calories)	1 slice whole-wheat bread (70 calories)
2 cups cut-up fruit (175 calories)	½ cup grapes (55 calories)	⅓ cup deli three-bean salad (60 calories)	6 oz light yogurt (80 calories)
	6 oz light yogurt (80 calories)	*Red, Black, and Blue Berry Medley* (115 calories)	1 cup pineapple chunks (80 calories)
South-of-France Ratatouille with 2 thin slices French bread (150 calories)	*Pork Stir-Fry with Asian Cabbage and Red Peppers* (345 calories)	*Tomato and Mozzarella Mini Sticks* (95 calories)	½ avocado, sliced, drizzled with lemon juice (115 calories)
3 oz grilled chicken breast (140 calories)	1 medium pear (105 calories)	3 oz grilled sirloin steak with ½ cup grilled mushrooms (175 calories)	3 oz grilled salmon (175 calories)
½ cup egg noodles with 1 tsp whipped butter (125 calories)	2 fortune cookies (60 calories)	1 medium baked potato with 1 tbsp light sour cream (180 calories)	½ cup microwaveable brown rice (110 calories)
1 cup steamed carrots (60 calories)		1 cup steamed broccoli (55 calories)	1 cup sautéed spinach with garlic (70 calories)

Week 3 Meal Plan

	Monday	Tuesday	Wednesday
Breakfast (400 calories)	2 cups corn flakes with ½ sliced, small banana and 1 cup fat-free milk (330 calories)	2 slices whole-grain toast with 2 tsp whipped butter (180 calories)	1 whole-wheat English muffin with 1 oz reduced-fat cream cheese, tomato slices (220 calories)
	1 cup blueberries (85 calories)	½ cup low-fat cottage cheese with 1 cup sliced strawberries (140 calories)	1 medium apple (95 calories)
		1 cup fat-free milk (80 calories)	1 cup fat-free milk (80 calories)
Lunch (500 calories)	1 small garden salad with 2 tbsp light Italian dressing (60 calories)	1 sandwich on a small whole-wheat sub roll with 2 oz turkey, 1 slice cheese, mustard, lettuce, tomato (335 calories)	*Red Lentil Soup* (150 calories)
	Chicken Salad Sandwich (400 calories)	*Asian Sesame Slaw* (60 calories)	1 frozen entrée of your choice (300 calories)
	1 clementine (35 calories)	6 oz light yogurt (80 calories)	½ cup blueberries (40 calories)
		½ cup raspberries (30 calories)	
Dinner (500 calories)	½ oz fresh mozzarella cheese with 2 tomato slices, basil, balsamic vinegar (45 calories)	1 cup wonton soup (70 calories)	1 small garden salad with 2 tbsp light Italian dressing (60 calories)
	Pasta Bolognese (330 calories)	4 oz stir-fried tofu (90 calories)	*Melissa's Leek Lasagna* (425 calories)
	1 cup steamed green beans (45 calories)	*Vegetable Fried Rice* (210 calories)	
	1 cup honeydew (60 calories)	½ cup low-fat frozen yogurt (110 calories)	

Thursday	Friday	Saturday	Sunday
Peach Melba Parfait (310 calories)	2 packets instant oatmeal with 1⅓ cups fat-free milk, 2 tbsp dried cranberries, 1 tbsp chopped walnuts (405 calories)	*Fajita Breakfast Burrito* (390 calories)	*Cornmeal Pancakes with Cinnamon Apples* (330 calories)
1 slice whole-grain toast (70 calories)			1 cup fat-free milk (80 calories)
15 baby carrots with ¼ cup hummus (155 calories)	1 cup black bean soup (115 calories)	1 cup broccoli florets with 2 tbsp light ranch dressing, 10 olives (120 calories)	*The Volumetrics Soup* (130 calories)
Tuna Salad Sandwich (350 calories)	3 oz lean burger patty on a whole-wheat bun with lettuce, tomato, ketchup, extra veggies (320 calories)	*Very Veggie Pizza* (360 calories)	2 cups lettuce plus veggies of choice, 3 oz grilled lean steak, 2 tbsp light Italian dressing (225 calories)
	2 clementines (70 calories)	½ cup watermelon (25 calories)	1 medium whole-wheat roll (95 calories)
			½ cup grapes (55 calories)
Turkey Piccata with Broccoli (230 calories)	1 cup butternut squash soup (90 calories)	*Orange Chicken* (290 calories)	1 cup red pepper strips with ¼ cup salsa, 2 tbsp guacamole (80 calories)
½ cup brown rice (110 calories)	3 oz grilled salmon with 1 small baked potato (305 calories)	½ cup brown rice (110 calories)	*Enchilada Casserole* (265 calories)
1 small pear with 1 oz reduced-fat cheese (165 calories)	½ cup steamed carrots (30 calories)	1 cup steamed green beans (45 calories)	1 slice angel food cake with 1 cup sliced peaches, 1 tbsp whipped topping (140 calories)
	6 oz light yogurt (80 calories)	1 cup sliced strawberries with 2 tbsp whipped topping (70 calories)	

Week 4 Meal Plan

	Monday	Tuesday	Wednesday
Breakfast (400 calories)	1 cup oat flakes with ⅔ cup fat-free milk, 2 tbsp raisins, 1 tbsp sliced almonds (280 calories)	6 oz Greek 0% fat plain yogurt with 1 cup pineapple chunks, ¼ cup low-fat granola (265 calories)	1 whole-wheat English muffin with 1 tbsp peanut butter (230 calories)
	1 cup fresh fruit salad (100 calories)	1 medium (2 oz) bran muffin (145 calories)	1 medium apple (95 calories)
			1 cup fat-free milk (80 calories)
Lunch (500 calories)	2 cups vegetable beef soup (240 calories)	2 cups lettuce plus veggies of choice, ¼ cup kidney beans, ¼ cup garbanzo beans, ¼ cup grated reduced-fat cheese, 2 tbsp light Italian dressing (280 calories)	*Chicken Tortilla Soup* (320 calories)
	½ sandwich with 1 slice whole-wheat bread, 1½ oz roast beef, lettuce, tomato, mustard (175 calories)	*Chocolate Chip Zucchini Squares* (200 calories)	Medium whole-wheat roll (95 calories)
	2 cups watermelon (90 calories)		6 oz light yogurt (80 calories)
Dinner (500 calories)	¼ cup hummus with 1 small whole-wheat pita, 15 baby carrots (230 calories)	*White Turkey Chili* (440 calories)	1 small garden salad with ¼ cup kidney beans, 2 tbsp light Italian dressing (115 calories)
	Grilled skewers with 3 oz shrimp, pepper pieces, zucchini rounds, onion wedges (165 calories)	½ cup grapes (55 calories)	3 oz grilled chicken breast (140 calories)
	Lemony New Potato Salad (125 calories)		*Cauliflower Rice* (135 calories)
			1 cup cherries (95 calories)

Thursday	Friday	Saturday	Sunday
2 oz whole-wheat bagel with 2 tbsp light cream cheese (215 calories)	6 oz 0% fat plain Greek yogurt with ½ cup blueberries, 2 tbsp low-fat granola, 1 tbsp chopped walnuts (270 calories)	*Blueberry Lemon Bread* with 1 tbsp light cream cheese (200 calories)	*Cherry-Vanilla French Toast* (385 calories)
2 grapefruit halves with 1 tsp honey (100 calories)	1 slice whole-wheat toast with 1 tsp whipped butter, 1 tsp jam (110 calories)	1 cup fresh fruit salad (100 calories)	½ cup fat-free milk (40 calories)
1 cup fat-free milk (80 calories)		1 cup fat-free milk (80 calories)	
Classic Spinach Salad (80 calories)	2 cups lettuce plus veggies of choice, 3 oz canned tuna, 1 oz reduced-fat cheese, 2 tbsp light ranch dressing (285 calories)	*Baked Potato with Black Bean and Pepper Salsa* (325 calories)	1 cup raw veggies with 2 tbsp light ranch dressing (95 calories)
1 sandwich on a small whole-wheat sub roll with 2 oz grilled chicken breast, lettuce, tomato, mustard, veggies of choice (280 calories)	1 whole-wheat pita (75 calories)	⅓ cup low-fat frozen yogurt (75 calories)	*Chili con Carne* (415 calories)
6 oz nonfat plain Greek-style yogurt with 1 cup sliced strawberries (145 calories)	1 sugar-free pudding cup with 1 medium orange (120 calories)	1 cup cherries (95 calories)	
1 cup vegetable beef soup (120 calories)	*Grilled Chicken and Zucchini Skewers with Peanut Dipping Sauce* (245 calories)	1 cup onion soup (55 calories)	*Creamy Broccoli-Feta Salad* (125 calories)
3 oz grilled lamb chop (170 calories)	½ cup brown rice (110 calories)	1 2-oz wheat tortilla topped with ½ cup fat-free refried beans, shredded lettuce, chopped tomato, salsa, 2 tbsp shredded reduced-fat cheese, ¼ sliced avocado (300 calories)	3 oz roasted turkey breast with ½ cup sautéed mushrooms (140 calories)
1 medium baked potato with salsa and yogurt (180 calories)	1 cup shredded cabbage topped with rice vinegar (20 calories)	1 oz piece of dark chocolate (170 calories)	1 medium baked sweet potato (105 calories)
½ cup steamed snow peas (35 calories)	2 cups watermelon (90 calories)		1 medium pear (95 calories)

Ultimate Volumetrics Recipes

Your Volumetrics Recipes

Are you ready to start cooking? You can choose from the 105 delicious Volumetrics recipes in this book or use them as inspiration for creating your own signature dishes. You'll find several types of breakfast dishes, a variety of sandwiches, soups, and salads, main dish favorites, grain and vegetable side dishes, and desserts. And what would life be without celebrations? I also give you a choice of recipes suitable for parties. When you're feeding your family, there is no need to prepare Volumetrics recipes just for yourself—most recipes and meals are suitable for everyone in your family!

About the Recipes

Each grouping of recipes includes features to help you incorporate the Volumetrics approach into your kitchen.

- A **before-and-after photo** compares single servings of a classic dish and the Volumetrics version. For example, regular coleslaw is compared to Asian Sesame Slaw; 3 tablespoons of regular coleslaw or 1 cup of Asian Sesame Slaw each has about 60 calories.
- Curious about how we increased portions and lowered the calories? Check out the **comparison box** under the before-and-after photos. You can use these strategies as a starting point for modifying your favorite recipes.
- For each category I've included a **gorgeous photo** of one of the recipes to show you how appealing healthy eating can be.

- Each recipe lists the suggested **number of servings**—usually four, although some recipes serve more—and the approximate **size of a single serving.**

- Ingredient quantities are listed in **household measures** and **corresponding gram weights** from measurements made during the recipe development process. The kitchen scale I recommended that you use for learning about appropriate portions is also a handy tool for measuring the weight of ingredients when cooking. When you use the scale, you won't have to worry about how tightly to pack the measuring cup or whether the ingredient in your measuring spoon should be rounded or flat.

    Although I am listing gram amounts for recipe ingredients, I don't want you to obsess over exact measurements unless you are baking. If a recipe calls for a whole can or package, add the whole thing rather than weighing the contents. Weights can vary from manufacturer to manufacturer and from can to can. When you're shopping for vegetables and fruits, pick those that are about the size specified in the recipe. Keep in mind that vegetables and fruits differ in size and weight; for example, a medium onion weighed anywhere between 110 to 145 grams in the tested recipes.

- Each recipe includes **nutrition information per serving** for calories, macronutrients, and CD. If the recipe gives a choice of ingredients, the first ingredient was the one used to calculate the nutrition information. CD was calculated from the weight of the finished dish. This weight often is different from the total weight of the ingredients. Other factors that affect the final weight include the trimming of vegetables and fruits, draining of canned ingredients, and loss of water during cooking. Calories, macronutrients, and CD listed at the end of each recipe have been rounded.

- **Special icons** indicate which recipes are suitable for leftovers, freezer-friendly, or appropriate for vegetarians. Vegetarian recipes conform to the standards of a lacto-ovo vegetarian diet and may include dairy products or eggs.

When Planning Your Menus

The sample menus (pages 156–163) give you a running start on incorporating recipes, prepared foods, and simple food combinations in a way that supports your Volumetrics way of eating. Long term, your meals and menus will reflect your own food tastes, budget, and schedule. One of my favorite time and cost savers is leftovers. I enjoy preparing extra food I can pack in single-serve containers, label, and refrigerate or freeze. That way, if time is tight, I'm in a rush, or my schedule changes, I know that I have access to a healthy meal that will take just minutes to heat up in the microwave. Most of the recipes can be doubled or tripled to allow for leftovers or feed more people.

Stocking Your Volumetrics Kitchen

Stock your kitchen wisely and it will be one of the best tools for supporting your Volumetrics diet. This includes having a ready supply of the types of lower-CD foods and staples you need to prepare healthy meals. To start, make a master list of the staple food items you want to have on hand, including nonperishable canned and packaged foods, baking supplies, and seasonings. Use this list to keep track of items as you run out so that you can replace them on your next trip to the market. Then consider the meals and recipes you want to make in the coming week. Which ingredients do you have on hand and what do you need to buy? As you write your shopping list for staples, include items for dressing up and lowering the CD of mealtime favorites.

- *For sandwiches:* jarred and canned vegetables such as water-packed artichoke hearts, roasted red peppers, pickles, flavored mustards
- *For soups:* beans packaged in cans or bags; reduced-sodium chicken, beef, and vegetable broths; frozen vegetables; canned tomato products; whole grains such as brown rice and pearled barley; spices and seasonings
- *For salads:* canned beans, canned fish, healthy fats such as olive oil and olives, nuts to sprinkle as a topping, vinegars, dressings or dressing ingredients
- *For mixed dishes:* lean meat and poultry to divide into portions and freeze, beans packaged in cans or bags, whole-wheat pasta, brown rice, frozen vegetables, spices and seasonings

At the Supermarket

I enjoy grocery shopping—it gives me a chance to remind myself of the huge variety we have available! I go to the market when it's not too crowded, and I try to eat beforehand—I find that when I'm hungry, high-CD foods are too hard to resist buying. A shopping list is a must, but I allow myself wiggle room to buy low-CD foods and seasonal vegetables and fruits that are inexpensive or on sale. But don't let a sale lure you into purchasing high-CD foods! To manage my grocery bill, I consider supermarket-brand staples, especially canned beans, canned tomatoes, and frozen vegetables. I also switch to frozen vegetables and fruits when they're on sale, or when fresh is out of season or of low quality. This aisle-by-aisle guide can help direct you when you're shopping for your Volumetrics meals.

Produce aisle

- Stock up on vegetables and fruits that keep well such as onions, shallots, garlic, celery, potatoes, winter squash, carrots, cabbage, apples, and citrus.
- For the best flavor, shop for veggies and fruits that are in season. Your market may also carry produce from local farms.

Bread aisle

- Choose whole-grain versions of bread, buns, bagels, pita, English muffins, and tortillas.
- Choose brands of bread, pita, tortillas, wraps, and buns with the lowest CD, and check how the calories per slice fit into your meal plan.
- Look for thin-sliced breads or buy a loaf and slice it thin at home.
- Limit breads made from refined grains, as well as higher-fat breads such as biscuits, croissants, cheese bread, focaccia, garlic bread, and bread brushed with oil.

Grains aisle

- Shop for different types of whole-grain rice, including long-grain brown rice, brown basmati rice, red rice, and wild rice.
- Choose from the growing variety of whole-wheat and whole-grain pastas— whole grain should be listed as the first ingredient.
- Buy at least one less-common whole grain such as quinoa, barley, or bulgur wheat. Store whole grains in the refrigerator or freezer to help keep them fresh; their natural oils turn rancid over time at room temperature.

Meat, poultry, and fish cases

- When possible, shop for weights that are easy to split into 4-ounce uncooked portions—for example, 1 pound (4 portions), 1½ pounds (6 portions) or 2 pounds (8 portions). When you get home, divide them into single servings and wrap, label, and freeze extras.

- Always buy lean meat (the five leanest beef cuts are eye round, sirloin tip, top round, bottom round, and top sirloin) and trim visible fat before cooking. If lean ground beef, pork, or poultry is not readily available, ask if the meat department can grind a lean cut for you.

- Pay attention to package weight and number of pieces when buying chicken breast fillets. A single fillet can range from about 3 ounces to half a pound, depending on size and thickness.

- If you prefer chicken parts, purchase either skin-on or skinned, but remove skin after cooking and before serving.

- When buying deli meats, request lean and thinly sliced.

- Include both light- and darker-flesh fish. Lighter fish have a lower CD, while those with a darker color provide healthy fats.

Dairy case

- Select low-fat or fat-free milk and yogurt and reduced-fat and low-fat cheeses. Fat-free cheeses may not deliver the same flavor or texture as cheese with a small amount of fat. Shop for light or reduced-fat sour cream—or fat-free, if you prefer—as an alternative to regular.

- Purchase strongly flavored cheeses—cheddar, Swiss, Parmesan, Asiago, feta, blue, Gruyère—that can be grated or crumbled and added in small amounts to enhance a dish.

- Buy low-fat cottage cheese for salads and part-skim ricotta cheese to use in pasta dishes.

Canned and frozen food aisles

- Include lower-salt canned vegetables and fruits canned in water or juice along with frozen vegetables, berries, and fruit mixtures.

- Shop for a variety of canned and dried legumes, including dried lentils and split peas for soups.
- Choose the variety of veggie burgers that you like best—soy and mushroom burgers can resemble ground beef, while all-vegetable patties have a different look and texture. Consider meatless crumbles, sausages, and other meatless products in the freezer case.
- Compare the CD and calories of different brands and types of ice cream and frozen yogurt. Regular (nongourmet) ice cream and frozen yogurt can have similar CDs and calories.

Condiments and spices aisles

- Go for high-flavor, low-CD condiments such as flavored mustards, hot peppers, relishes, horseradish, capers, olives, and pickles.
- Choose healthy oils with neutral flavors such as canola for cooking and baking and oils with distinct flavors—olive, walnut, sesame, hazelnut—for salads. Peanut oil is particularly suited for stir-frying because it can tolerate high cooking temperatures, but canola oil also works.
- Stock up on plain and flavored vinegars for salads, including white and regular balsamic, cider, champagne, and tarragon. You can keep vinegars in the cupboard or refrigerator for months.
- Purchase an assortment of dry spices to create your own combinations for adding to mixed dishes or rubbing onto meat, poultry, fish, and veggies.

Save Time or Save Money?

Would you rather save time or money? Each of these ingredient pairs offers you a choice between convenience and cost.

SAVE TIME	SAVE MONEY
Precut vegetables in bags or from the salad bar	Seasonal whole vegetables
Frozen vegetables in steamer bags	Create your own combos and microwave
Sliced mushrooms	Buy whole mushrooms and slice
Bagged coleslaw mix	Cabbage shredded at home
Bagged broccoli slaw mix	Peel and cut broccoli stalks at home
Shredded carrots	Shred at home with a grater or food processor
Canned pumpkin	Roast and purée fresh pumpkin or winter squash
Peeled, cut butternut squash cubes	Whole butternut squash
Frozen puréed or cubed winter squash	Whole squash
Frozen corn kernels	Seasonal corn on the cob
Jarred minced garlic	Garlic heads
Single-serving fresh herb packets	Large bunches or plants
Canned beans	Beans packaged in bags
Prepared tomato-based sauce	Sauce from canned tomatoes, seasoning
Heat-and-eat packets of cooked rice	Cook rice in advance and refrigerate or freeze
Bottled sauces	Prepare from a recipe
Seasoning blends	Individual spices and seasonings
Precut meat, poultry	Family pack to cut at home

SAVE TIME	SAVE MONEY
Trimmed, marinated meat and poultry	Trim and marinate at home
Grilled chicken breast fillets at the deli counter	Grill skinless, boneless fillets in a grill pan, under the broiler, or on an outdoor grill
Grated cheese	Grate by hand or in a food processor
Egg whites in a carton	Whole eggs, separated
Hard-cooked eggs	Cook and peel eggs at home
Packaged hummus	Hummus from a recipe
General time savers: frozen cut vegetables, quicker-cooking whole grains, bottled lemon and lime juice	General money savers: Onions in place of leeks or shallots, canned tomato products, generic or store brand, larger package size, sale items

Modifying Your Favorite Recipes

Once you're comfortable with the Volumetrics meal strategies, you're ready to branch out into modifying your favorite recipes. Here are some strategies you can try to lower CD without sacrificing taste.

- How can I add more vegetables and fruit?
- Where can I add water and water-rich ingredients?
- Can I switch to whole grains?
- Which lower-fat cooking method can I use?
- Can I substitute a lower-fat ingredient for one higher in fat?
- Where can I reduce the sugar?

I suggest using the Sample Menus on pages 156–163 to show you how to incorporate Volumetrics recipes into your meals. You can browse through the recipes and pick the ones that appeal most to you. You have 105 delicious dishes to choose from!

BREAKFAST
Pancakes and French Toast

Cherry-Vanilla French Toast

This feels like a luxurious breakfast, but the fat-free ricotta cheese and fat-free milk help lower the CD. I prefer whole-grain bread to 100 percent whole wheat—it absorbs the egg mixture better. If you like, you can assemble this the night before and put it in the refrigerator until the morning.

Makes 4 servings (320g each), 1 French toast "sandwich" plus ½ cup cherries each

 Vegetarian

FRENCH TOAST

1 cup (248g) fat-free ricotta cheese

1½ tablespoons (20g) sugar

2½ teaspoons (2g) pure vanilla extract

8 slices (208g) whole-grain bread

2 large (100g) eggs

3 large (99g) egg whites

1 cup (244g) fat-free milk

2 teaspoons (5g) ground cinnamon

SAUCE

One 1-pound (448g) bag frozen dark cherries

1 teaspoon (3g) cornstarch

1 teaspoon (4g) sugar

1. Spray an 8-inch square baking pan with cooking spray.
2. Combine the ricotta, 1½ teaspoons of the sugar, and ½ teaspoon of the vanilla in a small bowl. Spread onto 4 slices of bread and top each with a second slice of bread. Place the four "sandwiches" in the pan.
3. Whisk together the eggs, egg whites, milk, the remaining sugar and vanilla, and the cinnamon. Pour over the tops of the sandwiches and let soak for several minutes until the liquid is absorbed.

4. Meanwhile, preheat the oven to 350°F.

5. Bake the French toast, uncovered, for 40 minutes or until the bread is lightly browned and the egg mixture is fully cooked; a knife inserted into the center will come out clean.

6. While the French toast is baking, toss the cherries with the cornstarch and sugar in a medium microwaveable bowl. Microwave at 1-minute intervals, gently stirring between intervals, until the cherries are soft and the liquid is bubbling and thickened, about 5 minutes. Serve the cherries on top of the French toast.

Nutritional Information per Serving
Calories 385 • CD 1.2 • Carbohydrate 62g • Fat 5g • Protein 24g • Fiber 7g

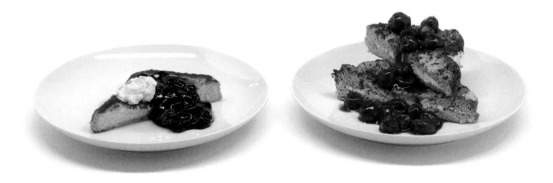

Traditional	How we lowered the CD	Volumetrics
French toast with butter, fruit sauce, and syrup	• Substituted extra egg whites for some of the yolks • Switched to fat-free milk • Replaced thick blueberry topping with fruit • Omitted butter and syrup	Cherry-Vanilla French Toast

Cornmeal Pancakes with Cinnamon Apples

It's easy to turn any packaged muffin mix into pancake batter, lowering CD by using fat-free milk and less butter or oil. I find the apple topping to be really satisfying in combination with these pancakes.

Makes 6 servings (235g each), 3 pancakes with ¾ cup cinnamon apples each

 Vegetarian

PANCAKES

One 8 to 8.5-ounce (225 to 240g) package corn muffin mix

1 cup (244g) fat-free milk

2 large (100g) eggs

1 tablespoon (14g) butter, melted

SAUCE

6 medium apples (700g), cored and sliced (do not peel)

2 tablespoons (16g) cornstarch

2 tablespoons (26g) sugar

2 teaspoons (5g) ground cinnamon

1. Stir together the muffin mix, milk, eggs, and butter in a medium bowl until well blended. It is okay if the batter has a few small lumps. Allow it to sit for 5 minutes.

2. Heat a nonstick griddle or large skillet on the stove over medium-low heat. Place 2 tablespoons of batter on the griddle for each pancake, leaving space for the pancakes to spread without touching each other, and cooking several at a time, depending on the size of the pan. Flip the pancakes with a spatula when the bubbles on the top begin to pop and the bottom appears dry. Cook for 1 or 2 minutes more, until the bottom is lightly browned.

3. Meanwhile, toss the apple slices with 1 cup water, the cornstarch, sugar, and cinnamon in a large microwaveable bowl. Microwave at 1-minute intervals, gently stirring between intervals, until the slices are soft and the liquid is bubbling and thickened, about 8 minutes.

Nutritional Information per Serving
Calories 330 • CD 1.4 • Carbohydrate 58g • Fat 9g • Protein 9g • Fiber 6g

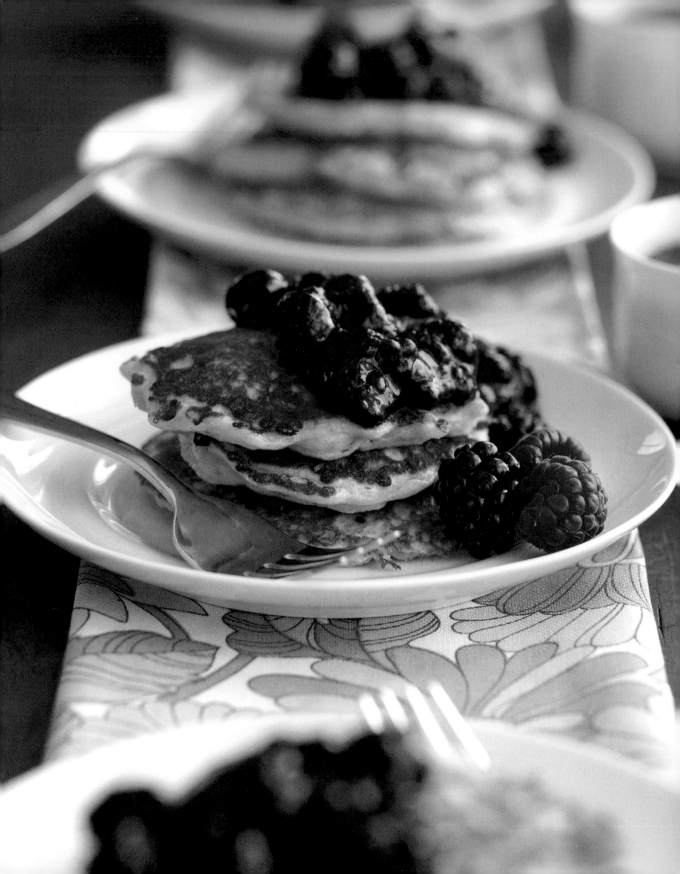

Light as a Feather Pancakes with Berry Sauce

I like the light and delicate texture of these cottage cheese pancakes, and they have a lower CD than the traditional ricotta cheese version. When I want an even fluffier pancake, I separate the eggs, combine the yolks with the cottage cheese, beat the whites separately, and then fold the whites into the yolk mixture.

Makes 4 servings (240g each), 3 pancakes with ⅓ cup fruit sauce each

 Vegetarian

PANCAKES

½ cup (60g) white whole-wheat flour

2 tablespoons (16g) cornstarch

2 tablespoons (26g) sugar

1½ teaspoons (4g) baking powder

¼ teaspoon (1g) table salt

1¼ cups (226g) 1% fat cottage cheese

3 large (150g) eggs

1 tablespoon (15g) melted butter or oil

SAUCE

3 cups (450g) frozen or fresh mixed berries, strawberries, or blueberries

1 tablespoon (8g) cornstarch

1 tablespoon (13g) sugar

1. Stir together the flour, cornstarch, sugar, baking powder, and salt in a large bowl. Whisk together the cottage cheese, eggs, and butter in a small bowl. Add to the flour mixture and stir to combine. It is okay for the batter to have a few small lumps.

2. Heat a nonstick griddle or large skillet on the stove over medium-low heat. Place 2 tablespoons of batter on the griddle for each pancake, leaving space for the pancakes to spread without touching each other. Flip the pancakes with a spatula when the bubbles on the top begin to pop and the bottom is dry. Cook for 1 or 2 minutes more, until the bottom is lightly browned.

3. Meanwhile, toss the berries with the cornstarch and sugar in a medium microwaveable bowl. Microwave at 1-minute intervals, gently stirring between intervals, until the berries are soft and the liquid is bubbling and thickened, about 5 minutes.

Nutritional Information per Serving
Calories 310 • CD 1.3 • Carbohydrate 43g • Fat 9g • Protein 16g • Fiber 4g

Eggs

Fajita Breakfast Burrito

The peppers and onion strips are what give this burrito its fajita flavor. Pick your favorite red or green salsa with the level of spiciness that you like.

Makes 4 servings (260g each), 1 burrito each

 Vegetarian

2 medium (238g) yellow, orange, or red bell peppers, seeded and chopped

1 medium (115g) red onion, peeled and chopped

8 large (400g) eggs

⅓ cup (37g) grated reduced-fat cheddar or Monterey Jack cheese

Salt and freshly ground black pepper to taste

Four (172g) 7-inch whole-wheat tortillas

¼ cup (62g) reduced-fat sour cream

1 (150g) avocado, split, pitted, peeled, and sliced

¼ cup (66g) salsa

1. Spray a large skillet with cooking spray and place over medium heat. Cook the peppers and onion, stirring occasionally, until soft, about 5 minutes. Transfer the mixture to a bowl.

2. Whisk the eggs in a separate medium bowl. Spray the skillet again with cooking spray. Scramble in the skillet over medium heat until fully cooked. Stir in the peppers and onion mixture and cheese, and season with salt and pepper to taste. Remove from the heat.

3. Spread each whole-wheat tortilla with 1 tablespoon of the sour cream down the center and top with one-quarter of the avocado slices. Place one-quarter of the egg mixture on each tortilla, fold over the side edges, and roll into a burrito. Top each with 1 tablespoon of salsa.

Nutritional Information per Serving
Calories 390 • CD 1.5 • Carbohydrate 33g • Fat 20g • Protein 20g • Fiber 6g

VARIATION: Replacing the eggs with egg substitute can reduce CD more. Use 2 cups egg substitute in place of 8 eggs.

Nutritional Information per Serving with egg substitute
Calories 310 • CD 1.1 • Carbohydrate 34g • Fat 10g • Protein 20g • Fiber 6g

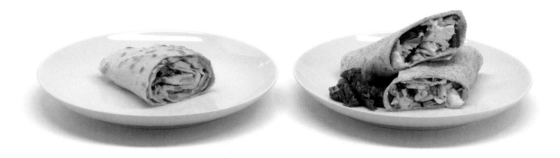

Traditional	How we lowered the CD	Volumetrics
Breakfast burrito	• Filled the burrito with lots of vegetables instead of breakfast meat • Used reduced-fat cheese • Switched to a smaller whole-wheat tortilla	Fajita Breakfast Burrito

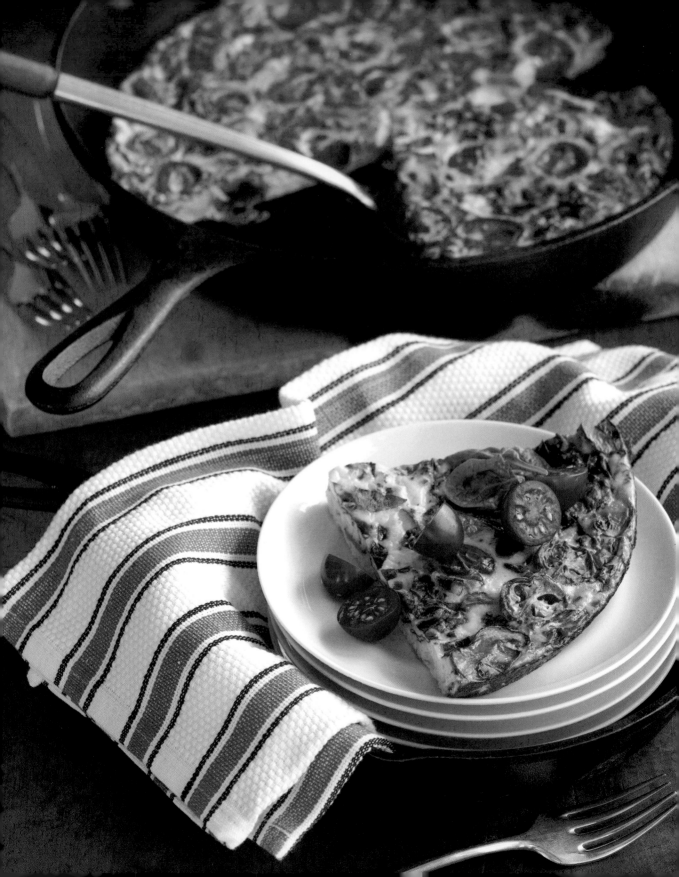

Greek Frittata

This reminds me of mornings out at a Greek diner, but without the unnecessary fat. For additional Greek flavor, garnish with finely chopped fresh oregano or basil.

Makes 4 servings (200g each), 4-inch wedge or square each

 Vegetarian

1 cup (96g) sliced mushrooms

1½ cups (45g) shredded, fresh baby spinach (one-quarter of a 6-ounce bag) (see note)

8 large (400g) eggs

½ cup (122g) fat-free milk

½ cup (100g) diced tomato, or grape tomatoes, cut in half

¾ cup (102g) crumbled reduced-fat feta cheese

1. Preheat the oven to 350°F. Spray a 9-inch cast-iron skillet or glass baking dish with cooking spray.

2. Heat a large nonstick skillet over medium heat. Spray with cooking spray. Cook the mushrooms for 5 minutes, stirring occasionally, until they start to release their liquid. Stir in the spinach and cook for 1 minute. Remove from the heat.

3. Whisk together the eggs and milk in a large bowl. Add the mushroom-spinach mixture, tomatoes, and cheese.

4. Pour the egg mixture in the prepared skillet. Bake for 35 to 45 minutes, until the eggs are firm and a knife inserted into the center comes out clean. Cool for 5 minutes before cutting.

NOTE: To shred leaves, stack them on a cutting board and thinly slice crosswise.

Nutritional Information per Serving
Calories 220 • CD 1.1 • Carbohydrate 6g • Fat 14g • Protein 21g • Fiber 1g

VARIATION: Replacing the eggs with egg substitute can reduce CD more. Use 2 cups egg substitute in place of 8 eggs.

Nutritional Information per Serving with egg substitute
Calories 135 • CD 0.62 • Carbohydrate 7g • Fat 4g • Protein 20g • Fiber 1g

Vegetable Denver Omelet

I make this meatless version of a coffee shop classic with smoked cheese in place of the more traditional ham. Poblano peppers are mildly spicy; switch to a green bell pepper for less heat or to an Anaheim chile for more. Using an egg substitute will lower calories and CD.

Makes 4 servings (145g each), ½ omelet each

 Vegetarian

2 teaspoons (8g) olive oil

1 medium (145g) red onion, peeled and finely chopped

1 small (31g) poblano pepper, seeded and finely chopped

5 ounces (142g) fresh button mushrooms, sliced

4 large (200g) eggs

4 large (132g) egg whites

¼ cup (61g) fat-free milk

¼ cup (28g) grated smoked gouda or cheddar cheese (1 ounce)

1. Heat the oil in a large nonstick skillet over medium heat. Add the onion and pepper and cook, stirring occasionally, until soft, about 5 minutes.

2. Add the mushrooms and cook, stirring occasionally, until the mushrooms give up their liquid and are soft, about 7 minutes. Transfer the vegetables from the skillet to a plate or bowl and set aside.

3. Wipe the skillet clean with a paper towel, spray with cooking spray, and heat over medium-low heat. Whisk together the eggs, egg whites, and milk in a medium bowl. Pour half of the egg mixture into the skillet and swirl the skillet to evenly distribute the eggs. As the eggs cook, use a spatula to gently lift the edges of the omelet and allow the uncooked egg to flow underneath. When the bottom of the omelet is just firm, place half the vegetables onto one side of the omelet, top with 2 tablespoons of the cheese, and using the spatula, gently fold the uncovered half over the filling. Cook for 30 seconds or until the cheese softens. Transfer to a plate and cut in half.

4. Repeat step 3 with the remaining ingredients.

Nutritional Information per Serving
Calories 160 • CD 1.1 • Carbohydrate 6g • Fat 9g • Protein 14g • Fiber 1g

VARIATION: Replacing the eggs with egg substitute can reduce CD more. Use 1½ cups egg substitute in place of the 4 eggs and 4 whites.

Nutritional Information per Serving with egg substitute
Calories 115 • CD 0.62 • Carbohydrate 6g • Fat 3g • Protein 13g • Fiber 1g

Parfaits

Berry Parfait

This parfait makes a colorful and tasty breakfast or dessert. I get creative with variations on this dish, especially when berries are in season.

Makes 4 servings (370g each), 2 cups each

 Vegetarian

1 quart (900g) light blueberry yogurt (see note)

½ cup (41g) low-fat granola

2 cups (288g) sliced fresh strawberries

2 cups (246g) raspberries

Place ¾ cup yogurt in each of four tall glasses. Top each with 1 tablespoon granola and ½ cup strawberries. Repeat with another layer of ½ cup yogurt and ½ cup raspberries. Top each with 1 tablespoon granola.

NOTE: Light yogurt is fat-free and sweetened with sugar substitutes.

Nutritional Information per Serving
Calories 265 • CD 0.72 • Carbohydrate 54g • Fat 3g • Protein 10g • Fiber 9g

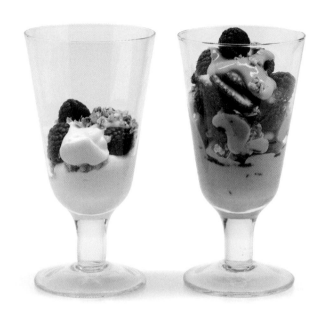

Traditional	How we lowered the CD	Volumetrics
Yogurt parfait with granola	• Switched from regular yogurt with honey to light yogurt • Used low-fat granola instead of regular and reduced the portion • Added more fresh fruit	Berry Parfait

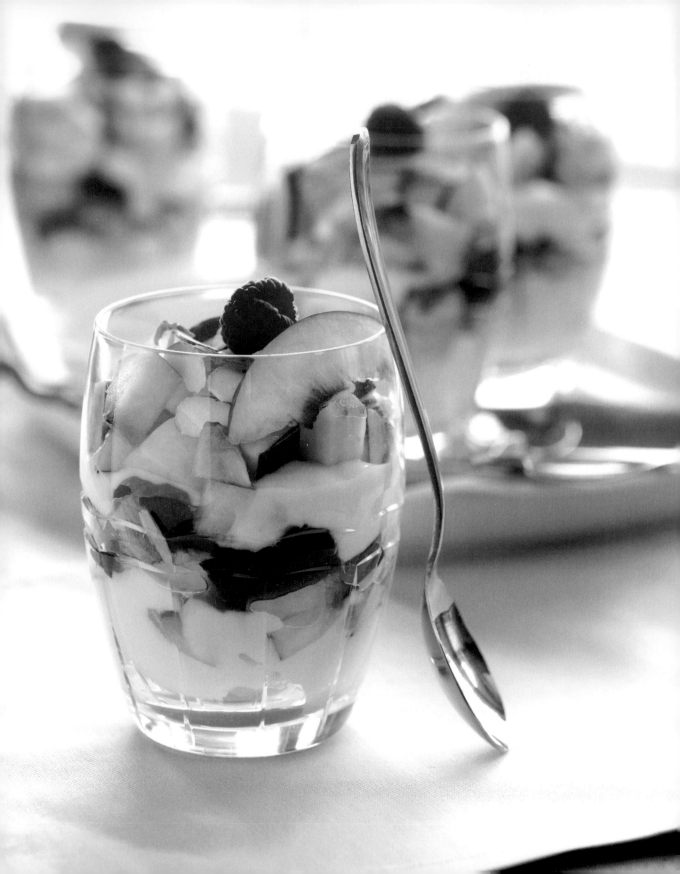

Peach Melba Parfait

I love the flavor and crunch of sliced almonds in this parfait. When I want something a little less sweet, I switch to plain yogurt instead of vanilla.

Makes 4 servings (310g each), 1½ cups each

 Vegetarian

3 cups (744g) light vanilla yogurt (see note)

3 cups (390g) chopped fresh or thawed frozen peach slices

½ cup (50g) sliced almonds (about 1½ ounces)

¼ cup (68g) reduced-sugar raspberry preserves or all-fruit spread

Place ⅓ cup yogurt in each of four tall glasses. Top each with ⅓ cup chopped peaches, 1 tablespoon almonds, and 1½ teaspoons preserves. Repeat once to use up all the ingredients.

NOTE: Light yogurt is fat-free and sweetened with sugar substitutes.

Nutritional Information per Serving
Calories 310 • CD 1.0 • Carbohydrate 45g • Fat 10g • Protein 11g • Fiber 3g

Greek Apple Parfait

Plain Greek-style yogurt is thicker and less tangy than traditional plain yogurt. I used the nonfat variety and it still seems rich and creamy. Low-fat granola saves a few calories over regular granola.

Makes 4 servings (300g each), 1¾ cups each

 Vegetarian

3 cups (744g) nonfat plain Greek-style yogurt

3 medium (390g) apples, cored and diced (about 3 cups)

1 cup (80g) low-fat granola

½ teaspoon (1g) ground cinnamon

Place a generous ⅓ cup yogurt in each of four tall glasses. Top each with ⅓ cup chopped apples and 2 tablespoons granola. Repeat once to use up the ingredients. Sprinkle the top of each parfait with cinnamon.

Nutritional Information per Serving
Calories 260 • CD 0.87 • Carbohydrate 43g • Fat 2g • Protein 20g • Fiber 4g

Muffins and Breads

Apple Oatmeal Muffins

Chopped apple gives this muffin flavor and texture while lowering CD. A large peach, nectarine, pear, or plum can take the place of the apple.

Makes 18 servings (50g each), 1 muffin each

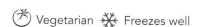 Vegetarian ❄ Freezes well

1½ cups (120g) quick-cooking oats
1 cup (120g) whole-wheat flour
¼ cup (50g) granulated sugar
¼ cup (55g) packed light brown sugar
1½ teaspoons (7g) baking soda
1 teaspoon (2g) ground cinnamon
½ teaspoon (3g) table salt

1 cup (244g) low-fat buttermilk
¼ cup (56g) canola oil
1 teaspoon (4g) pure vanilla extract
1 large (50g) egg, lightly beaten
2 medium (276g) or 1 large apple, peeled, cored, and chopped

1. Preheat the oven to 375°F. Spray three 6-cup muffin pans with cooking spray.
2. Stir together the oats, flour, granulated and brown sugars, baking soda, cinnamon, and salt in a large bowl. Push the mixture to the sides of the bowl to make a well in the center.
3. In a small bowl, combine the buttermilk, oil, vanilla, and egg. Pour into the well in the flour mixture and stir just until all the flour is moist.
4. Gently fold the apple into the batter.
5. Spoon the batter into the prepared muffin pans, filling each cup about three-quarters full.
6. Bake for 20 minutes, or until the muffins spring back when lightly touched in center. Remove the muffins from the pan immediately and place on a wire rack to cool.

Nutritional Information per Serving

Calories 115 • CD 2.3 • Carbohydrate 18g • Fat 4g • Protein 3g • Fiber 2g

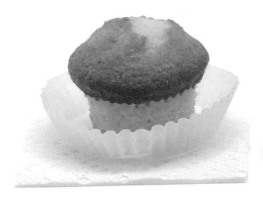 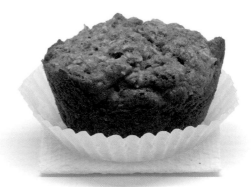

Traditional	How we lowered the CD	Volumetrics
Corn muffin	• Added oats • Decreased sugar • Decreased oil • Added fruit	Apple Oatmeal Muffin

Pumpkin Cranberry Bread

I add lots of pumpkin to make a moist and lower-CD bread. Buy and freeze an extra bag or two of cranberries in the fall or check the freezer case of your market for frozen berries year round.

Makes 24 servings (80g each), about 2-inch square each

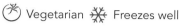 Vegetarian ❄ Freezes well

One 29-ounce (822g) can pumpkin

1½ cups (300g) granulated sugar

¼ cup (56g) vegetable oil

2 teaspoons (8g) pure vanilla extract

4 large (200g) eggs

3 cups (360g) whole-wheat flour

2 teaspoons (9g) baking soda

½ teaspoon (1g) baking powder

1 teaspoon (4g) table salt

2 teaspoons (5g) ground cinnamon

1½ teaspoons (3g) ground nutmeg

1½ cups (165g) fresh or frozen cranberries (see note)

1. Preheat the oven to 350°F. Spray a glass 9 by 13-inch baking pan with cooking spray.

2. Stir together the pumpkin, sugar, oil, vanilla, and eggs in a large bowl. Stir in the flour, baking soda, baking powder, salt, cinnamon, and nutmeg. Gently fold in the cranberries.

3. Place the batter into the prepared pan and bake for 55 minutes or until the top is dry and a toothpick inserted into the center of the bread comes out clean. Put the pan on a wire rack to cool for 5 minutes, then turn out the loaf onto the rack to cool to room temperature before slicing.

NOTE: Leave the cranberries frozen to prevent them from becoming watery.

Nutritional Information per Serving
Calories 150 • CD 1.9 • Carbohydrate 27g • Fat 4g • Protein 3g • Fiber 3g

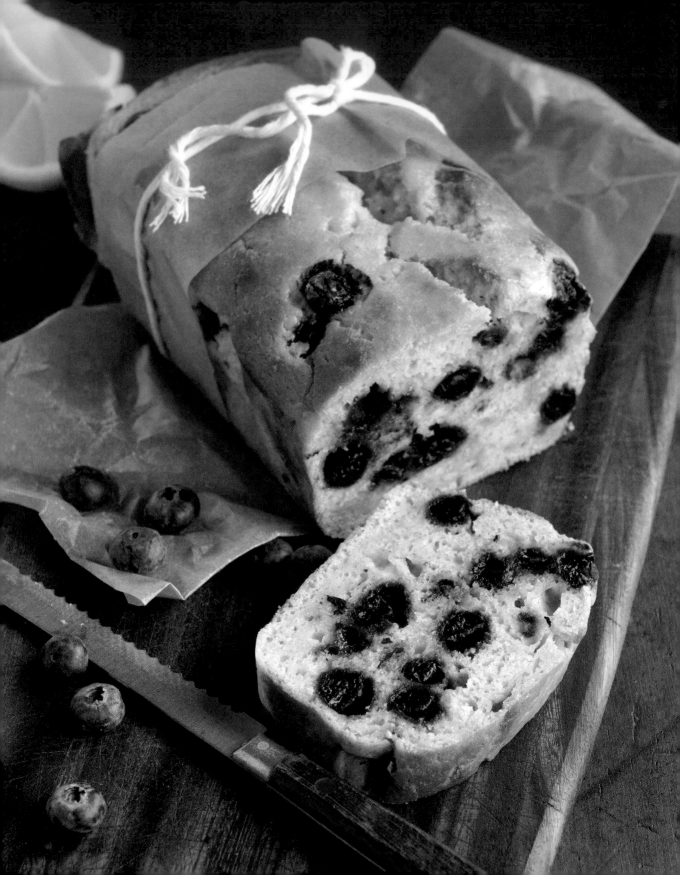

Blueberry Lemon Breakfast Loaf

I use light lemon yogurt in this recipe to add moisture and flavor while lowering CD. White whole-wheat flour has the nutrition and fiber benefits of traditional whole-wheat flour without the darker color.

Makes 12 servings (90g each), ¾-inch slice each

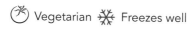 Vegetarian ❄ Freezes well

1 cup (125g) all-purpose flour

1 cup (120g) white whole-wheat flour

2 teaspoons (5g) baking powder

½ teaspoon (3g) table salt

¾ cup (150g) sugar

¼ cup (63g) egg substitute

2 tablespoons (28g) melted butter

One 6-ounce (170g) carton light lemon yogurt

½ cup (122g) low-fat buttermilk

1 tablespoon (15g) lemon juice

1 teaspoon (2g) grated lemon peel (optional)

1 teaspoon (4g) lemon or pure vanilla extract

2 cups (310g) frozen or fresh blueberries (see note)

1. Preheat the oven to 375°F. Spray a 9 by 5-inch loaf pan with cooking spray.

2. Stir together the flours, baking powder, and salt in a large bowl. Whisk together the sugar, egg substitute, butter, yogurt, buttermilk, lemon juice, lemon peel, if using, and extract in a medium bowl. Gently fold the sugar-egg mixture into the flour mixture just until completely combined. Gently fold in the blueberries.

3. Pour the batter into the prepared pan and bake for 55 minutes, or until the top is lightly browned and a toothpick inserted into the center of the loaf comes out clean. Put the pan on a wire rack to cool for 5 minutes, then turn out the loaf onto the rack to cool to room temperature before slicing.

NOTE: Do not thaw frozen berries, or they will turn the batter blue.

Nutritional Information per Serving
Calories 170 • CD 1.9 • Carbohydrate 33g • Fat 3g • Protein 4g • Fiber 2g

SOUPS AND SALADS
First Course Soups

The Volumetrics Soup

This is a soup that was used in a study in my lab. We served it as a first course and found it was so filling that people ate 20 percent less for lunch.

Makes 4 servings (390g each), about 2 cups each

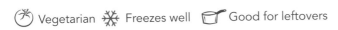 Vegetarian ❄ Freezes well ⊐ Good for leftovers

1½ cups (155g) peeled, cubed white potato (1-inch cubes)

One 32-ounce (946g) carton or can vegetable or reduced-sodium chicken broth

2 cups (312g) frozen broccoli florets

2 cups (248g) frozen cauliflower florets

¾ cup (110g) frozen carrot slices

1½ tablespoons (21g) butter

Salt and freshly ground black pepper to taste

1. Boil the potato in water for 15 minutes. Drain. Combine the cooked potato, broth, broccoli, cauliflower, carrot, and butter in a large pot and simmer over medium heat, covered, for 20 minutes.

2. Purée until the soup is fairly smooth but with a few small chunks of vegetables. Use a stick or immersion blender right in the pot, or purée it in batches in a countertop blender. Season to taste with salt and pepper.

Nutritional Information per Serving
Calories 130 • CD 0.33 • Carbohydrate 18g • Fat 4g • Protein 4g • Fiber 5g

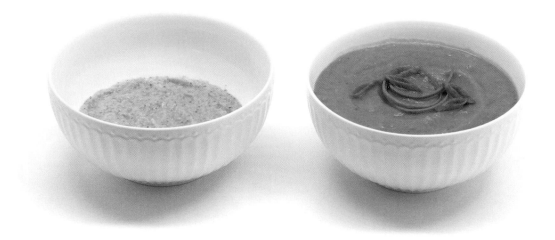

Traditional	How we lowered the CD	Volumetrics
Broccoli soup	• Used potato rather than milk and cheese for creaminess • Increased vegetables	The Volumetrics Soup

Chilled Cucumber and Summer Vegetable Soup

Cold soup is a refreshing treat in warm weather. For more color contrast in the garnish, I leave the peel on the cucumber. Try different combinations of seasonal vegetables, including summer squash, peppers, peas, or green beans. Chop the basil immediately before serving to keep color bright.

Makes 4 servings (305g each), about 1 cup soup plus ½ cup chopped vegetables each

 Vegetarian

SOUP

1 medium (290g) seedless English cucumber (about 11 ounces), peeled and sliced

2 cups (454g) nonfat plain Greek-style yogurt

1 small (3g) garlic clove, peeled and coarsely chopped

½ teaspoon (3g) table salt

¼ teaspoon (1g) ground white pepper

GARNISH

16 (272g) grape tomatoes, cut in quarters

1 (180g) small regular cucumber, finely diced

½ cup (65g) fresh corn kernels (from 1 ear) or frozen corn, thawed

2 (30g) green onions (scallions), white and light green parts only, sliced into thin rounds

1 tablespoon (15g) white balsamic vinegar

Salt and ground white pepper to taste

1 tablespoon (14g) extra virgin olive oil

¼ cup (10g) chopped fresh basil leaves

1. Purée the sliced cucumber, yogurt, garlic, salt, and pepper in a food processor or blender until smooth. Refrigerate for at least 20 minutes.

2. Meanwhile, combine the tomatoes, diced cucumber, corn, green onions, and vinegar in a medium bowl. Season with salt and pepper.

3. Divide the soup into four bowls. Top each with one-quarter of the vegetable garnish. Stir together the oil and basil in a small bowl and divide among the four bowls.

Nutritional Information per Serving
Calories 135 • CD 0.44 • Carbohydrate 14g • Fat 4g • Protein 12g • Fiber 2g

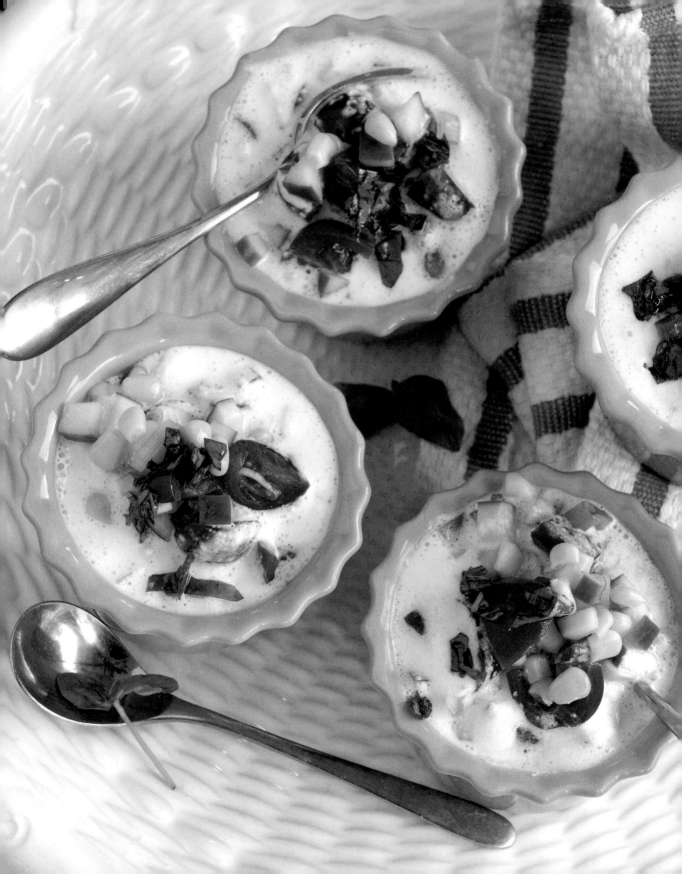

Red Lentil Soup

This standard of mine has become a favorite of my daughter Juliet's family. The flavor of red lentils is milder and less earthy than the better-known brown lentils. With cooking, they break down into a thick and creamy base that pairs well with tart and savory seasonings. This recipe evokes the flavors of Lebanese cuisine. Pictured on page 63.

Makes 8 servings (250g each), about 1 cup each

 Vegetarian Freezes well Good for leftovers

SOUP
2 tablespoons (28g) olive oil

1 large (200g) onion, peeled and finely chopped

2 (6g) garlic cloves, peeled and finely chopped

One 32-ounce (946g) carton or can vegetable or reduced-sodium chicken broth

One 8-ounce (227g) can tomato sauce

¾ cup (144g) dried red lentils

1 medium (100g) carrot, peeled and finely chopped

One 10-ounce (280g) package frozen squash

1 tablespoon (7g) ground cumin

⅛ teaspoon (1g) cayenne pepper

Juice of ½ lemon (40g)

Salt and freshly ground black pepper to taste

GARNISH
¼ cup (61g) nonfat plain yogurt or fat-free sour cream

¼ cup (4g) chopped fresh cilantro

1. Heat the olive oil in a medium pot over medium heat. Add the onion and garlic and cook, stirring occasionally, until soft, about 5 minutes. Add the broth, tomato sauce, lentils, carrot, squash, cumin, and cayenne. Increase the heat to bring to a boil, then reduce to medium-low. Cover and simmer until lentils are soft, about 25 minutes.

2. Stir in the lemon juice and season with salt and pepper.

3. Serve as is or purée in the pot with a stick or immersion blender if you prefer a smooth consistency, adding water if the soup is too thick. Garnish each bowl with a tablespoon each of yogurt and cilantro.

Nutritional Information per Serving
Calories 150 • CD 0.60 • Carbohydrate 22g • Fat 4g • Protein 8g • Fiber 4g

Main Course Soups

Caribbean Bean and Squash Soup

Light coconut milk gives this soup its creamy texture and distinct tropical flavor, but with about one-third the CD of regular coconut milk. Any type of bean or combination of beans can be used in this recipe; rinse well to lower the sodium. To give the soup a creamier consistency, purée until smooth, or substitute frozen squash or canned pumpkin.

Makes 6 servings (505g each), 2 cups each

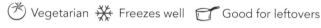 Vegetarian ❄ Freezes well 🥘 Good for leftovers

- 1 tablespoon (14g) canola or vegetable oil
- 1 large (200g) onion, peeled and finely chopped
- 1 (3g) garlic clove, peeled and finely chopped
- One 32-ounce (946g) carton or can of vegetable or reduced-sodium chicken broth
- Three 15.5-ounce (1,320g) cans white beans, drained and rinsed well
- 1 pound (454g) peeled butternut squash or other winter squash, cut into 1-inch cubes

- One 13.5-ounce (405g) can light coconut milk
- One 14.5-ounce (411g) can plain diced tomatoes
- 1 tablespoon (7g) ground cumin
- 2 teaspoons (5g) ground coriander
- 2 teaspoons (3g) dried oregano
- Salt and freshly ground black pepper to taste
- ½ lime, cut into 6 wedges
- Caribbean hot sauce to taste (optional)
- ¼ cup finely chopped cilantro (optional)

1. Heat the oil in a medium pot over medium heat. Add the onion and garlic and cook, stirring occasionally, for 5 minutes or until soft. Add the broth, beans, squash, coconut milk, tomatoes, cumin, coriander, and oregano. Bring to a boil, then reduce the heat and simmer the soup uncovered for 30 minutes. Stir in salt and pepper to taste.

2. Ladle into bowls and serve with a lime wedge and hot sauce and cilantro if desired.

Nutritional Information per Serving
Calories 340 • CD 0.67 • Carbohydrate 54g • Fat 8g • Protein 16g • Fiber 12g

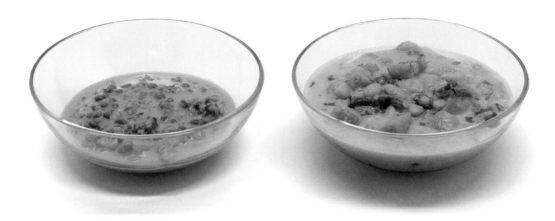

Traditional	How we lowered the CD	Volumetrics
Southern creamy bean soup	• Used broth and light coconut milk instead of half-and-half • Added vegetables • Eliminated high-fat meats	Caribbean Bean and Squash Soup

Vegetable Barley Soup

Kim, my administrative assistant, introduced me to this family favorite. It is hearty, tasty, and best of all, can be made with staple ingredients. Make extra to keep in the freezer for a quick meal.

Makes 8 servings (400g each), about 1½ cups each

🍅 Vegetarian   ❄ Freezes well   🍲 Good for leftovers

1 tablespoon (14g) canola oil

1 cup (160g) chopped onion

1 cup (122g) chopped carrots

1 cup (101g) sliced celery

1 (3g) garlic clove, chopped

One 32-ounce (946g) carton or can vegetable broth

One 28-ounce (794g) can crushed tomatoes

One 15.5-ounce (439g) can black beans, rinsed and drained

One 8-ounce (227g) can tomato sauce

1 cup (200g) pearl barley, rinsed

1 tablespoon (5g) dried basil

½ teaspoon (1g) freshly ground black pepper

One 10-ounce (284g) package frozen chopped spinach

½ ounce (14g) Parmesan cheese, for garnish (see note)

1. Heat the oil in soup pot over medium heat. Add the onion, carrots, celery, and garlic and cook for 5 minutes.

2. Add the broth, tomatoes, beans, tomato sauce, barley, basil, 1 cup water, and the pepper. Bring to a boil, reduce the heat, cover, and simmer for 15 minutes.

3. Add the frozen spinach, cover, and simmer for 10 minutes or until the spinach is completely thawed and heated. Stir occasionally to break up and distribute the spinach.

4. Ladle into bowls and garnish each bowl with a generous teaspoon of Parmesan.

NOTE: ½ ounce Parmesan equals about ¼ cup freshly grated cheese or 2 tablespoons packaged grated cheese.

Nutritional Information per Serving
Calories 225 • CD 0.56 • Carbohydrate 38g • Fat 3g • Protein 10g • Fiber 9g

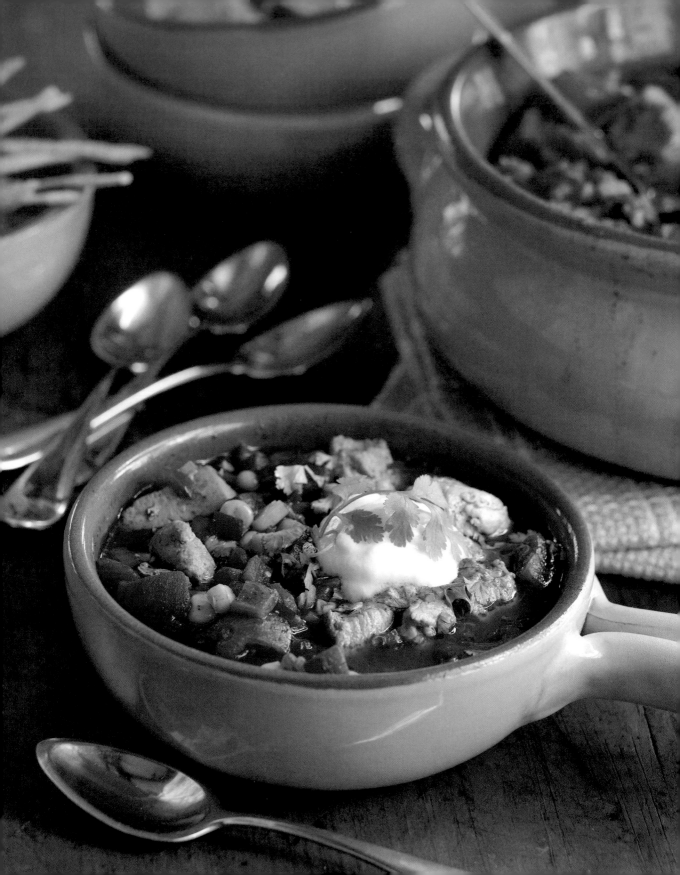

Chicken Tortilla Soup

I make a meal of this hearty quick and easy soup on weeknights. The amount of heat is up to you, depending on the type of salsa and canned tomatoes you select. Add extra broth or water if you prefer a thinner consistency; this also will lower the CD. Leftover turkey or lean grilled steak works well as a substitute for the chicken.

Makes 4 servings (550g each), 2 cups each

👐 Good for leftovers

SOUP

1 tablespoon (14g) olive oil

1 medium (145g) onion, peeled and finely chopped

2 medium (238g) red bell peppers, seeded and finely chopped

1 (3g) garlic clove, peeled and finely chopped

1 cup (264g) mild or medium salsa

Two 14.5-ounce (822g) cans reduced-sodium chicken broth

One 14.5-ounce (411g) can plain or seasoned fire-roasted diced tomatoes

2 cups (280g) diced cooked chicken breast

1 cup (130g) fresh or frozen corn kernels

1 tablespoon (8g) chili powder

Salt and freshly ground black pepper to taste

Juice of ½ lime (22g) (optional)

GARNISH

½ cup (122g) nonfat plain yogurt or fat-free sour cream

1 ounce (28g) baked tortilla chips (about 18), crumbled

4 sprigs (8g) fresh cilantro

1. Heat the oil in a medium pot over medium heat. Add the onion, red pepper, and garlic and cook, stirring occasionally, for 5 minutes, or until soft. Add the salsa, broth, tomatoes, chicken, corn, and chili powder. Bring to a boil, then reduce the heat and simmer the soup partially covered for 15 minutes.

2. Add the salt and pepper to taste and lime juice if desired.

3. Ladle into bowls and garnish each with 2 tablespoons each of yogurt and tortilla chip crumbles, and 1 sprig cilantro.

Nutritional Information per Serving
Calories 320 • CD 0.58 • Carbohydrate 36g • Fat 7g • Protein 31g • Fiber 7g

First Course Green Salads

Classic Spinach Salad

With baby spinach readily available in supermarkets, I enjoy this nutrient-rich salad year-round. The red onion and bell pepper slices add flavor and color contrast.

Makes 4 servings (150g), 1¼ cups each

 Vegetarian

Half a 6-ounce (170g) bag baby spinach (about 4 cups)

8 ounces (226g) sliced button mushrooms

1 small (115g) red onion, peeled and thinly sliced

1 medium (119g) orange or red bell pepper, seeded and thinly sliced

1 (50g) hard-cooked egg, peeled and chopped

3 tablespoons (45g) red wine vinegar

1 tablespoon (14g) olive oil

2 teaspoons (10g) Dijon mustard

Dash of liquid smoke (optional)

Salt and freshly ground black pepper to taste

1. Toss together the spinach, mushrooms, onion, orange pepper, and egg in a large salad bowl.

2. Whisk together the vinegar, oil, mustard, and liquid smoke, if using, in a small bowl. Season with salt and pepper. Pour over the salad and toss.

Nutritional Information per Serving

Calories 85 • CD 0.57 • Carbohydrate 6g • Fat 5g • Protein 5g • Fiber 2g

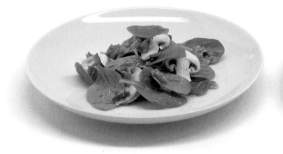 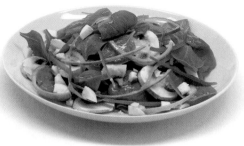

Traditional	How we lowered the CD	Volumetrics
Traditional spinach salad	• Made a lower-fat dressing without bacon • Added more vegetables	Classic Spinach Salad

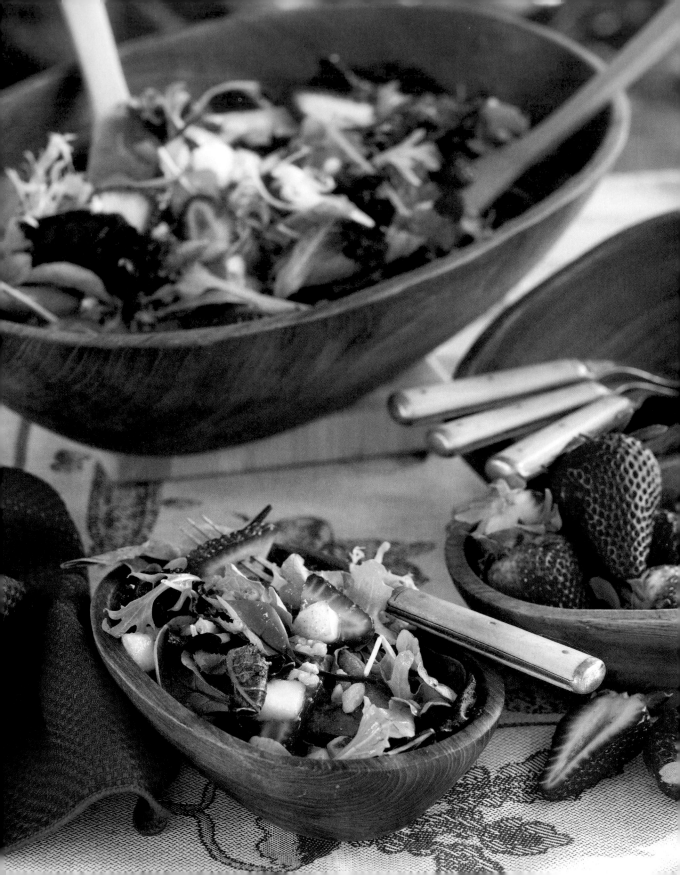

Mixed Greens with Strawberries, Pears, and Walnuts

I make the dressing for this pretty salad with orange juice and a small amount of flavorful oil. Look for the most colorful assortment of salad greens that you can find, or create your own with a combination of baby lettuce, radicchio, and fresh herbs.

Makes 4 servings (200g each), 1½ cups each

 Vegetarian

4 cups (220g) spring salad mix
(8 ounces)

1 pint (288g) strawberries, stemmed
and sliced

1 medium (178g) pear, cored and
chopped

2 tablespoons (15g) chopped walnuts

3 tablespoons (45g) champagne
vinegar

3 tablespoons (47g) orange juice

1 tablespoon (14g) walnut or olive oil

1 teaspoon (5g) Dijon mustard

Salt and freshly ground black pepper
to taste (optional)

1. Gently toss together the salad mix, strawberries, pear, and walnuts in a large salad bowl.
2. Whisk together the vinegar, orange juice, oil, and mustard in a small bowl. Pour over the salad and toss gently to avoid crushing the fruit. Season with salt and pepper, if desired, and toss again gently.

Nutritional Information per Serving
Calories 105 • CD 0.53 • Carbohydrate 17g • Fat 4g • Protein 2g • Fiber 4g

Baby Arugula Salad

I love the flavor of baby arugula, with its peppery overtones. To enjoy this salad year-round, switch to fresh orange slices or canned Mandarin oranges when fresh clementines are not available. Pictured on page xvii.

Makes 4 servings (155g each), 1½ cups each

🍅 Vegetarian

4 cups (80g) baby arugula (3 ounces)

1 small (175g) fennel bulb, sliced, fronds reserved

1 small (119g) red bell pepper, seeded and chopped

3 (222g) clementines, peeled and divided into sections

3 tablespoons (45g) white wine vinegar

1 tablespoon (14g) olive oil

2 teaspoons (10g) honey mustard

Salt and freshly ground black pepper to taste

1. Toss together the arugula, fennel, red pepper, and clementines in a large salad bowl.
2. Whisk together the vinegar, oil, mustard, and salt and pepper in a small bowl. Pour over the salad and toss. Garnish with the reserved fennel fronds.

Nutritional Information per Serving
Calories 90 • CD 0.58 • Carbohydrate 14g • Fat 4g • Protein 2g • Fiber 3g

Vegetable Salads

Asian Sesame Slaw

You can put together this recipe in minutes using packaged coleslaw mix, or take a bit more time to shred your own. For a quick and easy change, I make it with broccoli slaw mix in place of the cabbage. Substitute 2 teaspoons each sugar and soy sauce if you don't have hoisin sauce.

Makes 4 servings (130g each), about 1 cup each

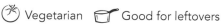 Vegetarian Good for leftovers

4 cups (280g) packaged coleslaw mix

1 large (150g) red bell pepper, seeded and diced (about 1 cup)

¼ cup (60g) rice wine vinegar

1 teaspoon (4g) granulated sugar

1 tablespoon (16g) hoisin sauce

1 tablespoon (9g) sesame seeds

½ teaspoon (2g) sesame oil

Combine all ingredients in a large bowl. Toss well to coat vegetables with sauce. Cover and refrigerate for at least 30 minutes.

Nutritional Information per Serving
Calories 60 • CD 0.46 • Carbohydrate 9g • Fat 2g • Protein 3g • Fiber 3g

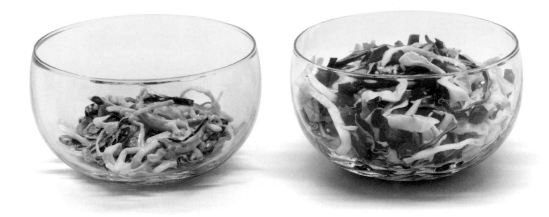

Traditional	How we lowered the CD	Volumetrics
Coleslaw	• Replaced mayonnaise with a low-fat Asian dressing • Added more vegetables	Asian Sesame Slaw

Spicy Lentil Salad

The ginger and cumin provide light Indian overtones to this warm and hearty side salad. Add curry powder or a combination of coriander, cayenne, cardamom, cinnamon, and turmeric for even stronger South Asian flavor.

Makes 4 servings (285g each), 1½ cups each

⊛ Vegetarian   ⊓ Good for leftovers

¾ cup (144g) dried brown lentils, rinsed

4 teaspoons (18g) vegetable oil

1 (3g) garlic clove, peeled and finely chopped

2 tablespoons (12g) finely chopped peeled fresh ginger

1 tablespoon (7g) ground cumin

1 large (245g) leek, white and light green parts only, finely chopped (see note)

1 medium (100g) carrot, peeled and diced

2 tablespoons (30g) red wine vinegar

½ teaspoon (3g) Dijon mustard

Salt and freshly ground black pepper to taste (optional)

One 6-ounce (170g) bag baby spinach (about 8 cups)

1. Place the lentils and 1½ cups of water in a medium saucepan. Bring to a boil, then reduce the heat, cover, and simmer until just tender, about 30 minutes. Drain.

2. Meanwhile, heat 2 teaspoons of the oil in a large nonstick skillet over medium-low heat. Add the garlic, ginger, and cumin and cook for 2 minutes. Add the leek, carrot, and 2 tablespoons water and cook until the vegetables are soft and lightly browned, about 8 minutes; drizzle with a couple of tablespoons of water if they get too dry and start to stick. Transfer from the skillet to a medium bowl and add the cooked lentils.

3. Whisk together the vinegar, the remaining oil, and the mustard in a small bowl. Drizzle over the lentil mixture and season with salt and pepper if desired. Stir gently to mix well.

4. Heat the skillet over medium heat and add the spinach. Cook until the spinach barely softens, 2 to 4 minutes. Place on a small platter and top with the lentils.

NOTE: Clean the leek by slicing it in half lengthwise and rinsing all layers in a colander under cold running water.

Nutritional Information per Serving
Calories 235 • CD 0.82 • Carbohydrate 36g • Fat 6g • Protein 12g • Fiber 14g

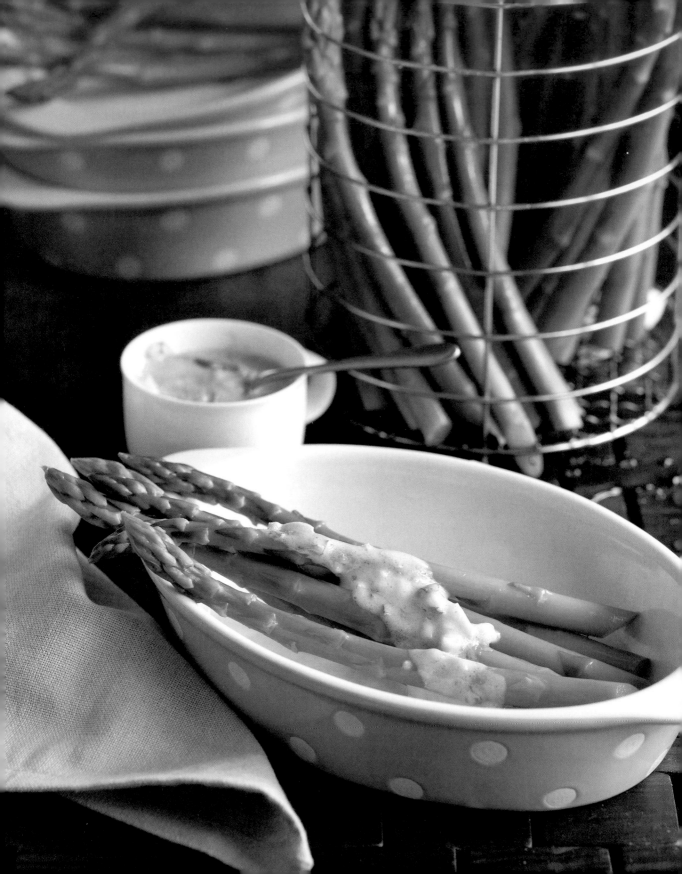

Asparagus with Tarragon-Mustard Vinaigrette

This chilled asparagus dish can be served as a first course or a side salad. Each time I take it to a potluck, friends demand the recipe. Substituting lemon juice for the vinegar and garnishing with grated lemon peel adds to the springtime flavors of this light dish.

Makes 4 servings (105g each), about ¼ pound asparagus and 1½ tablespoons dressing each

 Vegetarian

Table salt

1½ pounds (670g) asparagus spears, washed and trimmed to remove tough base

1 tablespoon (14g) olive oil

3 tablespoons (45g) tarragon or white balsamic vinegar, or lemon juice

1 small (10g) shallot, peeled and finely chopped

2 teaspoons (10g) Dijon mustard

2 teaspoons (2g) chopped fresh tarragon

Grated lemon peel (optional)

Freshly ground black pepper to taste

1. Place about 2 cups water and 1 tablespoon salt in a medium pot. Stand or lean the asparagus spears in the pot, cover, and cook on medium-high heat until the base of the spears can be pierced easily with a sharp knife, about 5 minutes, depending on the thickness of the spears. You may need to cook them in batches.

2. Transfer the spears from the boiling water to a colander and run under cold water to stop the cooking process. Set aside.

3. Meanwhile, to make the vinaigrette, in a small bowl whisk together the oil, vinegar, shallot, mustard, tarragon, lemon peel if using, and salt and pepper, or shake together in a small jar.

4. Arrange the chilled asparagus spears on a platter and drizzle with the vinaigrette.

Nutritional Information per Serving

Calories 55 • CD 0.52 • Carbohydrate 5g • Fat 4g • Protein 2g • Fiber 2g

Main Course Salads

Rainbow Chef's Salad

The specific combination of lettuce, vegetables, lean meats, and reduced-fat cheese is up to you, as long as your salad is full of color and variety. I add chopped fresh herbs to brighten the flavor.

Makes 4 servings (385g each), about 3½ cups each

6 cups (440g) torn or shredded romaine lettuce (see note)

1 medium (100g) carrot, peeled and grated

1 medium (180g) tomato, chopped

1 cup (96g) sliced mushrooms

1 medium (200g) cucumber, sliced

1 cup (90g) broccoli florets

4 (60g) green onions (scallions), white and light green parts, sliced

Chopped fresh herbs such as basil, cilantro, or dill (optional)

8 ounces (227g) lean deli meat of your choice, such as turkey breast, ham, and roast beef, cut into slivers

2 ounces (56g) reduced-fat cheese, cut into slivers or shredded

6 tablespoons (90g) red wine vinegar

2 tablespoons (28g) olive oil

¼ teaspoon (1g) table salt

Freshly ground black pepper to taste

1. Toss the lettuce, carrot, tomato, mushrooms, cucumber, broccoli, green onions, and herbs, if using, in a large bowl. Top with the meat and cheese.
2. Whisk together the vinegar, oil, salt, and pepper and serve on the side.

   NOTE: To shred leaves, stack them on a cutting board and thinly slice crosswise.

   VARIATION: To make this vegetarian, replace the meat with chickpeas or other beans.

Nutritional Information per Serving
Calories 230 • CD 0.60 • Carbohydrate 15g • Fat 12g • Protein 19g • Fiber 5g

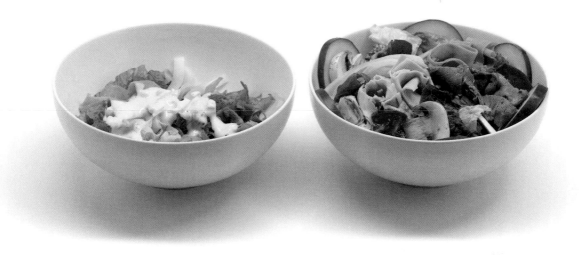

Traditional	How we lowered the CD	Volumetrics
Chef's salad	• Added more vegetables • Switched to lean meats and reduced-fat cheese • Made a lower-fat dressing	Rainbow Chef's Salad

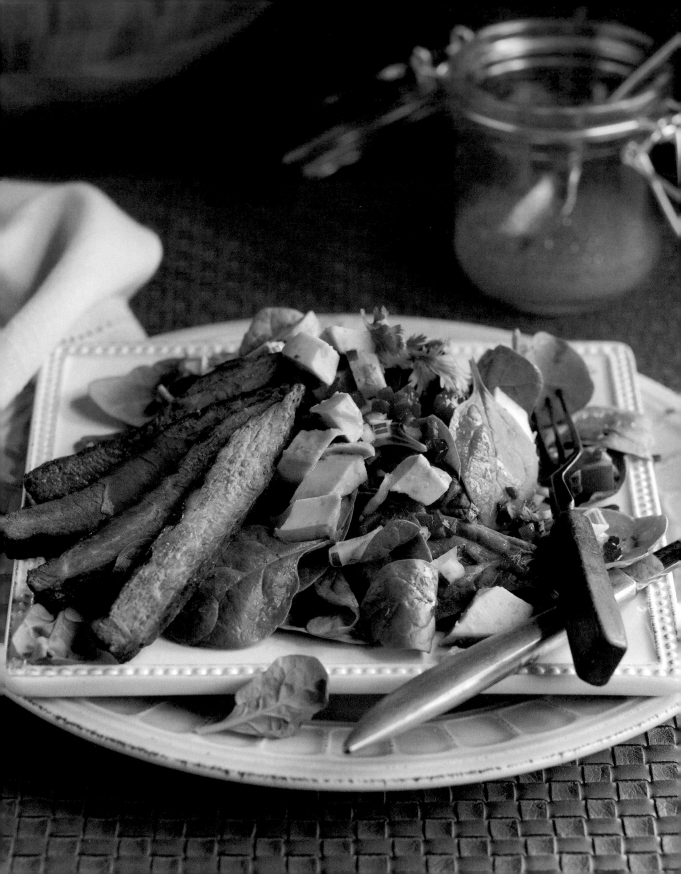

Chili-Rubbed Steak on a Deconstructed Guacamole Salad

For this salad, I got my inspiration from the individual components of guacamole—avocado, tomato, cilantro, onion, and lime juice—and put them on top of the salad individually instead of mixing them together.

Makes 4 servings (210g each), 3 cups salad plus 1½ ounces steak each

1 tablespoon (8g) chili powder

¼ teaspoon (1g) table salt

8 ounces (227g) strip steak, about 1½ inches thick

One 6-ounce (170g) bag baby spinach (about 8 cups)

1 medium (200g) avocado, split, pitted, peeled, and cubed

1 medium (119g) or 4 baby red bell peppers, seeded and finely chopped

1 medium (180g) tomato, chopped

½ cup (8g) chopped fresh cilantro

1 small (115g) red onion, peeled and chopped

3 tablespoons (46g) lime juice (from 1 to 2 limes)

1 tablespoon (14g) olive oil

¼ teaspoon (1g) hot sauce

Salt and freshly ground black pepper to taste

1. Heat a stovetop grill pan over medium heat or set the oven broiler on high.

2. Combine the chili powder and salt in a small bowl. Rub on both sides of the meat. Cook in the grill pan or under the broiler, turning over once, until the surfaces are browned and the interior temperature reaches 145° to 150°F on an instant-read thermometer, about 8 minutes per side. Remove from the heat, put on a cutting board, and cover lightly with foil.

3. Place the spinach on a large platter or bowl. Top with the avocado, red pepper, tomato, cilantro, and onion.

4. Whisk together the lime juice, oil, and hot sauce in a small bowl. Add salt and pepper to taste. Drizzle over the salad.

5. Slice the steak into thin slices and place on top of the salad.

Nutritional Information per Serving

Calories 270 • CD 1.3 • Carbohydrate 15g • Fat 18g • Protein 15g • Fiber 7g

Salade Niçoise

This salad brings back memories of lunch on a warm summer day in France. Tossing salad greens and vegetables first with oil provides a light coating that allows the lemon juice to flavor them more evenly. Other types of oil such as walnut, pecan, or flavored olive oil will impart a subtly different flavor.

Makes 4 servings (290g each), about 2½ cups each

8 (227g) small white or red potatoes (about 8 ounces), scrubbed

2 cups (250g) fresh green beans cut into 2-inch pieces

4 cups (80g) baby arugula (3 ounces)

Two 5-ounce (280g) cans water-packed solid white tuna, drained well and broken into chunks

1 medium (130g) tomato, cut into wedges

2 (100g) hard-cooked eggs, peeled and sliced

½ cup (67g) pitted niçoise or Kalamata olives

1 tablespoon (9g) capers, rinsed and drained (optional)

2 tablespoons (28g) olive oil

Juice of 1 lemon (47g)

½ teaspoon (3g) Dijon mustard

Salt and freshly ground black pepper to taste

1. Place the potatoes in a medium pot with enough water to cover. Bring to a boil, reduce the heat to medium-low, and simmer for 15 minutes or until almost tender.

2. Add the green beans and simmer for 5 minutes. Drain well in a colander and rinse with cold water to cool.

3. Place the arugula on a large platter. Arrange the tuna, tomato, eggs, potatoes, and beans on the arugula. Garnish with the olives and capers, if desired.

4. Whisk together the olive oil, lemon juice, mustard, and salt and pepper in a small bowl. Drizzle over the salad.

Nutritional Information per Serving
Calories 270 • CD 0.93 • Carbohydrate 21g • Fat 12g • Protein 21g • Fiber 4g

MAIN COURSE
Salad Sandwiches

Tuna-Apple Salad Sandwich

Make this sandwich with either light tuna, which has a stronger flavor and is very low in fat, or white albacore, with its milder flavor and small amount of healthy fat. I add curry powder and apple to give this lunch classic a flavor boost.

Makes 4 servings (235g each), 1 sandwich each

Two 5-ounce (280g) cans water-packed light or white tuna, drained well

1/3 cup (79g) light mayonnaise

1/2 medium (75g) apple, finely chopped

1 (40g) celery stalk, finely chopped

2 tablespoons (30g) pickle relish

1 tablespoon (7g) mild curry powder (optional)

Salt and freshly ground black pepper to taste

8 slices (304g) 100% whole-wheat bread, toasted if desired

4 (40g) lettuce leaves

4 slices (123g) tomato

12 thin slices apple, for garnish (optional)

1. Combine the tuna, mayonnaise, apple, celery, relish, and curry powder, if using, in a medium bowl. Season with salt and pepper.
2. Divide the salad evenly among 4 slices of bread. Top each with a lettuce leaf, tomato slice, and a second slice of bread. Garnish with apple slices, if desired.

Nutritional Information per Serving
Calories 350 • CD 1.5 • Carbohydrate 44g • Fat 9g • Protein 28g • Fiber 6g

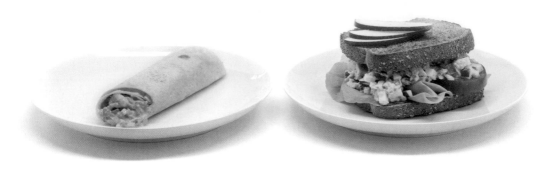

Traditional	How we lowered the CD	Volumetrics
Tuna salad wrap	• Added vegetables and fruit • Switched to light mayonnaise • Switched from a wrap to whole-grain bread	Tuna-Apple Salad Sandwich

Egg and Veggie Salad Sandwich

Most of the calories in eggs come from the yolk, so I eliminated half the yolks in order to bring down the CD. The onion complements the flavor of the eggs but you may prefer tomato slices instead. Vegans can substitute crumbled firm tofu for the eggs and soy mayo for regular mayo.

Makes 4 servings (205g each), 2 pita halves each

 Vegetarian

4 (200g) chilled hard-cooked eggs, peeled and chopped

4 (132g) chilled hard-cooked egg whites, chopped

⅓ cup (79g) light mayonnaise

4 (60g) green onions (scallions), white and light green parts, chopped

½ cup (55g) shredded carrots

Salt and freshly ground black pepper to taste

Four (228g) 6-inch whole-wheat pita breads

8 (80g) lettuce leaves

8 (30g) thin slices red onion

1. Combine the eggs, egg whites, mayonnaise, green onions, and carrots in a medium bowl. Season with salt and pepper.

2. Cut each pita in half to make two pockets. Divide the egg mixture evenly into the eight halves, about ⅓ cup egg mixture per pita half. Tuck a lettuce leaf and onion slice in each half.

Nutritional Information per Serving
Calories 305 • CD 1.5 • Carbohydrate 34g • Fat 13g • Protein 18g • Fiber 6g

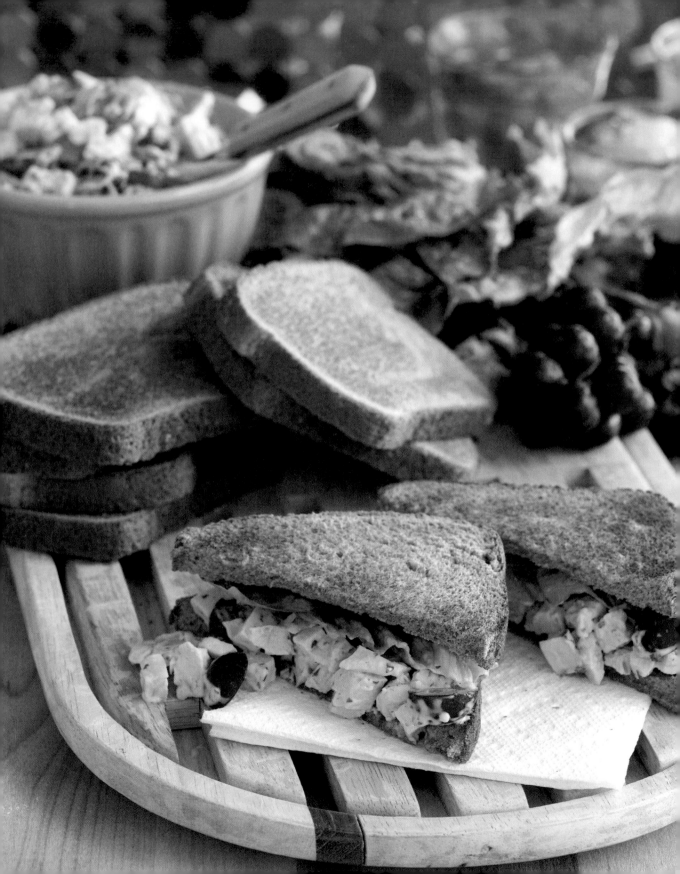

Chicken Salad Sandwich

I prefer making my sandwich with chicken breast for its lower CD, but you can also use thigh meat. The water chestnuts, cilantro, and sriracha sauce add Asian flavor notes. Sriracha sauce is an all-purpose spicy Asian-style condiment that can be found in the international aisle of most markets.

Makes 4 servings (235g each), 1 sandwich each

2 cups (280g) diced cooked skinless chicken

⅓ cup (79g) light mayonnaise

½ cup (76g) seedless red grapes, cut in half

½ cup (88g) canned, drained, sliced or diced water chestnuts

1 tablespoon (15g) Dijon mustard

¼ cup (6g) finely chopped fresh cilantro, parsley, or dill

2 teaspoons (12g) sriracha or chili-garlic sauce (optional)

Salt and freshly ground black pepper to taste

8 slices (304g) 100% whole-wheat bread, toasted if desired

4 (40g) lettuce leaves

1. Combine the chicken, mayonnaise, grapes, water chestnuts, mustard, cilantro, and sriracha sauce, if using, in a medium bowl. Season with salt and pepper.
2. Divide the salad evenly among 4 slices of bread. Top each with a lettuce leaf and a second slice of bread.

Nutritional Information per Serving
Calories 400 • CD 1.7 • Carbohydrate 45g • Fat 11g • Protein 30g • Fiber 6g

Sandwiches

Chicken Caesar Panini

I like to prepare panini sandwiches at home in a nonstick pan or cast-iron skillet. To make your own signature panini, choose your favorite bread, vegetable, meat, and cheese combination.

Makes 4 servings (250g each), ½ sandwich each

4 (12g) unpeeled garlic cloves

2 teaspoons (8g) olive oil

4 teaspoons (20g) Dijon mustard

4 (212g) whole-grain flatbreads (about 100 calories each)

8 ounces (227g) cooked skinless, boneless chicken breast, sliced thin, about 1 large or 2 small fillets

2 cups (112g) shredded romaine lettuce or baby spinach leaves (see note)

8 (246g) medium tomato slices

8 (30g) thin red onion slices

4 (56g) thin slices Muenster or Jack cheese (about 2 ounces total)

1. Microwave the garlic cloves until soft, 10 to 15 seconds. Peel. Press through a garlic press into a small bowl or mash with a fork. Add the oil and mustard and mash into a paste.

2. Heat a large nonstick frying pan on the stove over medium-low heat. Spread half the garlic paste onto each of 2 flatbreads. Layer each with half the chicken, lettuce, tomato, onion, and cheese. Top with the other two flatbreads.

3. Cook each sandwich in the pan until lightly browned on the bottom, about 4 minutes. Turn over and cook the other side until lightly browned. Press the top of the sandwich with a spatula while it cooks.

4. Cut each sandwich in half before serving.

NOTE: To shred leaves, stack them on a cutting board and thinly slice crosswise.

Nutritional Information per Serving
Calories 290 • CD 1.2 • Carbohydrate 21g • Fat 11g • Protein 33g • Fiber 9g

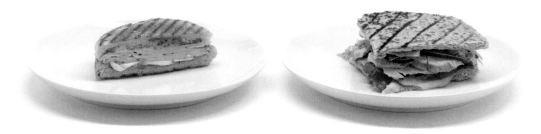

Traditional	How we lowered the CD	Volumetrics
Chicken-cheese panini	• Added more vegetables • Used less cheese • Used only a small amount of oil for the spread; no oil brushed on the outside	Chicken Caesar Panini

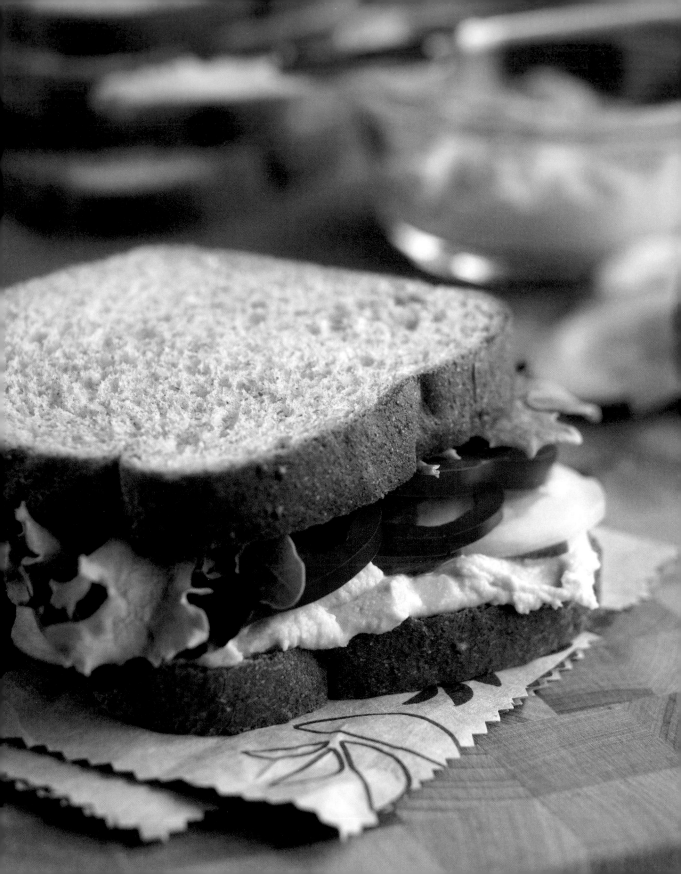

Hummus and Veggies: My Go-to Sandwich

It can be hard, when I am in a rush in the morning, to stop and pack a healthy lunch to take to work. My favorite super quick go-to sandwich is based on hummus and whatever salad veggies and bread I have on hand. This recipe is just one example. Hummus is easy to make yourself, but there are lots of ready-prepared choices. Pick whatever flavor you like, but check the CD as it can vary between brands.

Makes 1 serving, 1 sandwich (225g)

 Vegetarian

2 (64g) slices whole-grain bread

¼ cup (62g) hummus

4 (40g) round ¼-inch-thick cucumber slices

½ small (39g) red bell pepper, seeded and sliced

¼ cup (18g) baby salad greens

Spread 1 slice of bread with the hummus. Top with the vegetables, then the second slice of bread.

NOTE: If you're taking this to work, put the vegetables in a separate bag or container and add them to the sandwich right before eating. This prevents the bread from getting soggy.

Nutritional Information per Serving
Calories 290 • CD 1.3 • Carbohydrate 40g • Fat 9g • Protein 14g • Fiber 10g

Zesty Roast Beef and Veggie Pocket

I like the combination of vegetables in this sandwich and fit as much as I can into the pita. Add a zesty condiment—wing sauce is particularly good, but so are flavored mustards or chili-garlic sauce—for a flavor punch. Pictured on page 63.

Makes 4 servings (205g each), 2 pita halves each

½ cup (50g) thinly sliced red onion

2 tablespoons (30g) balsamic vinegar

2 tablespoons (30g) light mayonnaise

4 teaspoons (19g) Buffalo wings hot sauce

Four (228g) 6-inch whole-wheat pita breads

1 cup (30g) baby spinach

½ medium (90g) tomato, sliced

½ cup (100g) roasted red pepper in brine, rinsed, drained, and diced

12 ounces (340g) thinly sliced, lean deli roast beef, 9 to 12 slices

1. Combine the onions and vinegar in a small bowl and set aside.
2. Stir together the mayonnaise and hot sauce in another small bowl. Slice each pita in half and spread the insides with the mayonnaise-hot sauce mixture.
3. Divide the spinach, tomato, and red pepper among the pita halves. Top with the roast beef and then the onions.

Nutritional Information per Serving
Calories 290 • CD 1.4 • Carbohydrate 36g • Fat 6g • Protein 22g • Fiber 6g

Pizzas

Very Veggie Pizza

This is one of my favorite vegetable combinations for pizza. I like to use a lower-calorie flatbread in place of a traditional crust. It gives me a bigger portion of pizza and veggies for the calories.

Makes 4 servings (275g each), 1 flatbread each

 Vegetarian

Four (212g) whole-grain flatbreads (about 100 calories each)

1 cup (248g) jarred tomato-based pasta sauce

2 cups (272g) crumbled reduced-fat feta cheese (about 8 ounces)

2 cups (192g) sliced fresh mushrooms

One 14-ounce (392g) can artichoke hearts in brine or water, drained and cut into quarters

1 cup (134g) sliced black olives

1⅓ cups (43g) shredded or whole fresh baby spinach leaves (see note)

1. Preheat the oven to 450°F. Spray two baking sheets with cooking spray.
2. Place 2 flatbreads on each of the prepared sheets. Top each with ¼ cup sauce, ½ cup cheese, ½ cup mushrooms, 8 artichoke quarters, and ¼ cup olives. Sprinkle the remaining cheese on top of the pizzas.
3. Bake for 13 minutes, or until the cheese is melted.
4. Remove from the oven and top each pizza with ⅓ cup spinach. The spinach will wilt from the heat of the pizza.

NOTE: To shred leaves, stack them on a cutting board and thinly slice crosswise.

Nutritional Information per Serving

Calories 360 • CD 1.3 • Carbohydrate 41g • Fat 14g • Protein 22g • Fiber 13g

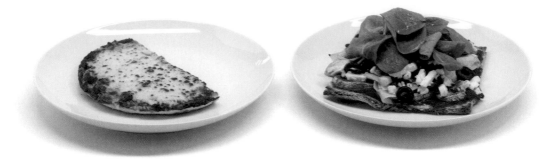

Traditional	How we lowered the CD	Volumetrics
Frozen pizza	• Added more vegetables and skipped the meat • Used less cheese • Switched to a whole-grain flatbread crust	Very Veggie Pizza

Hawaiian Pizza

This pizza shop favorite is very easy to re-create in a lower-CD way. The recipe works equally well made with refrigerated pizza dough.

Makes 8 servings (120g each), 1 slice each

✤ Vegetarian—Leave out ham

½ cup (124g) fat-free ricotta cheese

1 ounce (28g) grated Parmesan or Romano cheese (see note)

1 (3g) garlic clove, peeled and finely chopped

One baked 10-ounce (283g) whole-wheat pizza crust

One 12-ounce (340g) jar roasted red peppers in brine, rinsed, drained, patted dry, and finely chopped

One 8-ounce (227g) can crushed pineapple in juice, drained well

3 ounces (85g) lean deli ham, diced or slivered

Red pepper flakes or finely chopped jalapeño peppers to taste (optional)

1. Preheat the oven to 450°F.
2. Combine the ricotta and Parmesan cheeses with the garlic in a small bowl. Spread onto the crust. Top with the red peppers, followed by the pineapple and then the ham. Season with the pepper flakes or jalapeño peppers if desired.
3. Bake the pizza for 15 minutes, or until the cheese is bubbling.

NOTE: 1 ounce Parmesan equals about ½ cup freshly grated cheese or ¼ cup packaged grated cheese.

VARIATION: To make this vegetarian, omit the ham.

Nutritional Information per Serving
Calories 165 • CD 1.4 • Carbohydrate 23g • Fat 5g • Protein 9g • Fiber 3g

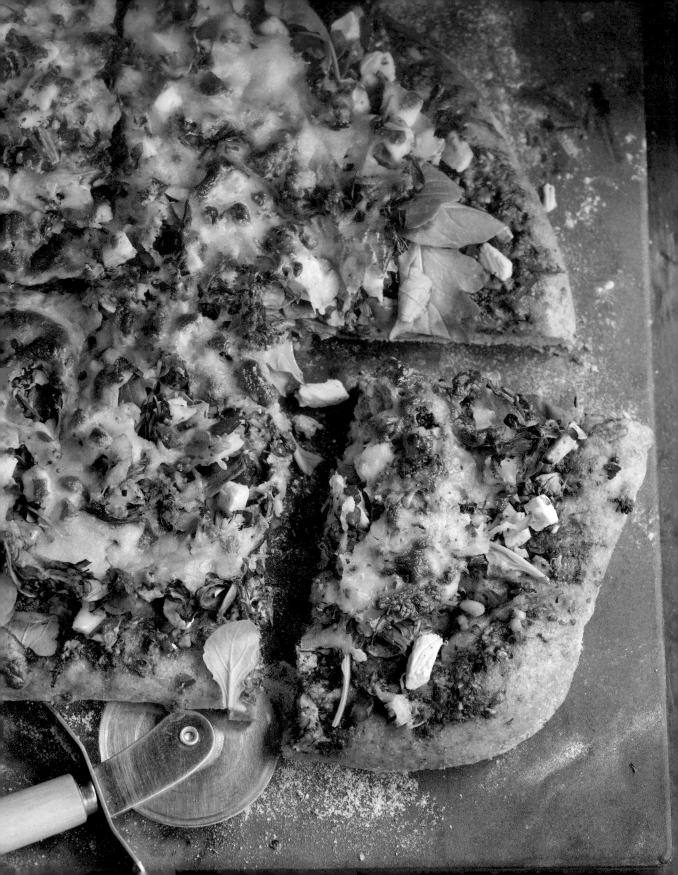

Pesto Pizza with Chicken and Vegetables

You can buy easy-to-use refrigerated pizza dough, including the whole-wheat variety, at most supermarkets. I enjoy putting together combinations of favorite vegetables. Here I used broccoli and arugula, with a touch of roasted red pepper for color.

Makes 6 servings (160g each), 1 slice each

🍅 Vegetarian—Make without chicken

One 15-ounce (428g) package refrigerated whole-wheat pizza dough

2 cups (142g) chopped fresh broccoli florets and stems

One 5-ounce (159g) container baby arugula

½ cup (130g) roasted red peppers in brine, rinsed, drained, and chopped

¼ cup (60g) pesto sauce

1 cup (140g) diced cooked chicken breast

¾ cup (84g) shredded part-skim mozzarella cheese (about 3 ounces)

1. Preheat the oven to 425°F. Pat out the pizza dough into a 12-inch round or square on a baking sheet.
2. Place the broccoli in a large microwaveable bowl with 2 tablespoons water. Cover and microwave until soft, about 2 minutes. Fold in the arugula, red peppers, pesto sauce, and chicken.
3. Top the crust with the vegetable-chicken mixture. Sprinkle with the cheese.
4. Bake for 10 minutes. Lightly cover with a piece of foil to keep the topping moist. Continue baking for about 5 minutes, until the crust is crisp and lightly browned. Cut into 6 wedges.

VARIATION: To make this vegetarian, omit the chicken.

Nutritional Information per Serving
Calories 300 • CD 1.9 • Carbohydrate 34g • Fat 11g • Protein 19g • Fiber 7g

Pastas

Volumetrics Spaghetti Bolognese

Spaghetti Bolognese was a favorite when I was studying in England—everyone there calls it "Spag Bol." This recipe calls for very lean meat, eliminating the need to drain off fat during cooking. You can substitute ground turkey, ground chicken, or meatless crumbles with equally good results.

Makes 6 servings (340g each), 1¼ cups sauce plus ½ cup pasta

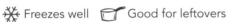 Freezes well 　　 Good for leftovers

SAUCE

1 tablespoon (14g) olive oil

3 (9g) garlic cloves, peeled and chopped

1 medium (119g) onion, peeled and chopped

1 (41g) celery stalk, chopped

1 small (43g) carrot, peeled and chopped

1 medium (119g) green bell pepper, seeded and chopped

12 ounces (340g) lean ground beef (at least 90% lean)

One 28-ounce (794g) can or two 14.5-ounce cans diced tomatoes with basil, garlic, and oregano

One 6-ounce (170g) can tomato paste

½ cup (120g) dry red wine or water

1 teaspoon (1g) dried basil

1 teaspoon (1g) dried oregano

Salt and freshly ground black pepper to taste (optional)

PASTA

6 ounces (170g) whole-wheat spaghetti

1 ounce (28g) grated Parmesan cheese (see note)

1. Heat the olive oil in a medium saucepan over medium heat. Add the garlic, onion, celery, carrot, and green pepper and cook, stirring occasionally, for 10 minutes,

until soft. Add the beef, break up with a spoon, and cook, stirring often, until the beef no longer is pink, about 5 minutes.

2. Stir in the tomatoes, tomato paste, wine, basil, and oregano. Bring to a boil, then reduce heat to medium-low, cover, and simmer for at least 30 minutes, stirring occasionally. Add salt and pepper, if desired.

3. Meanwhile, cook the spaghetti according to package directions. Drain.

4. Serve the sauce over the spaghetti, topped with Parmesan cheese.

NOTE: 1 ounce Parmesan equals about ½ cup freshly grated cheese or ¼ cup packaged grated cheese.

Nutritional Information per Serving
Calories 335 • CD 0.98 • Carbohydrate 40g • Fat 10g • Protein 20g • Fiber 7g

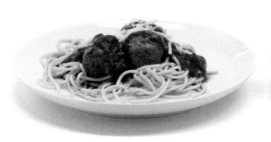 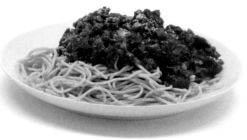

Traditional	How we lowered the CD	Volumetrics
Spaghetti Bolognese	• Added more vegetables • Increased the volume of sauce • Used leaner ground beef • Switched to whole-wheat pasta	Volumetrics Spaghetti Bolognese

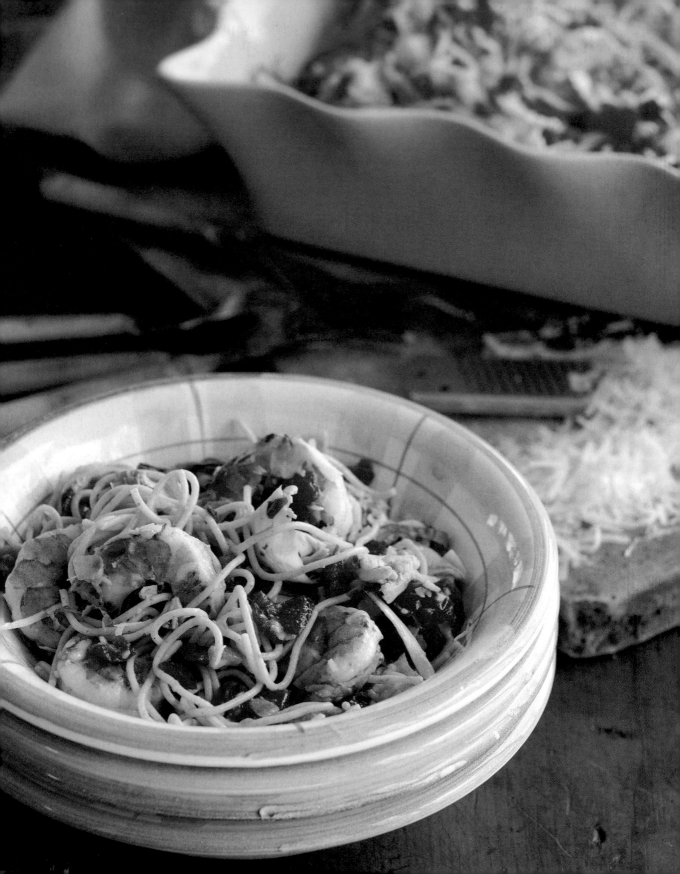

Diane's Basil Shrimp and Pasta

My friend Diane was given the recipe for this special occasion dish by a food editor whom she met in France. It's okay to switch to canned diced tomatoes—drain them well before adding—if tasty fresh tomatoes are not available or are expensive. I substituted the more flavorful Asiago cheese for the feta in her original recipe, but it is delicious either way.

Makes 4 servings (500g each), 2 cups shrimp and vegetables plus ¾ cup cooked pasta

6 ounces (170g) whole-wheat linguine or spaghetti

1 teaspoon (4g) olive oil

1 medium (119g) onion, peeled and chopped

5 (15g) garlic cloves, peeled and finely chopped

1 pound (454g) large shrimp, peeled and deveined (fresh or frozen, raw or precooked, see notes)

4 cups (720g) diced plum tomatoes (about 1¾ pounds)

½ cup (120g) dry white wine

Juice of half a lemon (25g)

One 12-ounce (340g) package frozen artichoke hearts (see notes)

¼ cup (10g) chopped fresh basil (see notes)

¼ teaspoon (1g) red pepper flakes

2 ounces (56g) shredded Asiago cheese (about ½ cup)

1. Cook the pasta according to the package directions. Drain and set aside.

2. Meanwhile, heat the oil in a large skillet over medium heat. (The skillet should be large enough to hold all ingredients.) Add the onions and cook, stirring occasionally, until soft, about 5 minutes. Add the garlic and raw shrimp and cook until the shrimp turn pink, about 3 minutes. Transfer the shrimp to a small bowl or plate and set aside.

3. Add the tomatoes, wine, and lemon juice to the vegetables in the skillet. Cook until the tomatoes are soft, about 5 minutes. Add the artichoke hearts, basil, and pepper flakes and cook until the artichokes have thawed and the mixture is simmering, about 5 minutes.

4. Fold in the pasta and shrimp and simmer gently for about 2 minutes. Top each serving with 2 tablespoons Asiago cheese.

NOTES: If using frozen shrimp, thaw the shrimp completely before using.

If using precooked shrimp, add at step 4.

If frozen artichoke hearts are not available, substitute one 14-ounce can of artichoke hearts in brine, rinsed and drained, and add in step 3.

Do not substitute dried basil for fresh because the flavor is different.

Nutritional Information per Serving
Calories 440 • CD 0.88 • Carbohydrate 52g • Fat 9g • Protein 42g • Fiber 6g

Creamy Pork Tenderloin with Mushrooms over Egg Noodles

This dish is so creamy and flavorful that you'd never guess I used light cream cheese, lean pork, and double the mushrooms to bring down the CD from my original 1970s recipe. Skinless, boneless chicken breast can be substituted for the pork.

Makes 4 servings (345g each), 1¼ cups meat and vegetables plus ½ cup noodles

 Good for leftovers

- 1 tablespoon (14g) vegetable oil
- 2 medium (268g) yellow onions, peeled and chopped
- 1 (3g) garlic clove, peeled and finely chopped
- 12 ounces (340g) mushrooms, sliced
- 1 cup (240g) dry white wine
- 4 ounces (113g) light cream cheese, cut into ½-inch cubes
- 1 pound (454g) pork tenderloin, trimmed of visible fat, cut into ½-inch-thick slices
- Salt and freshly ground black pepper to taste
- 6½ ounces (185g) egg noodles
- ¼ cup (12g) finely chopped chives

1. Heat the oil in a large skillet over medium-high heat until the oil begins to shimmer. Add the onion and garlic and cook for 2 minutes to soften.
2. Add the mushrooms and cook until the mushrooms release their juices, about 5 minutes.
3. Add the wine and bring to a boil. Reduce the heat to low and simmer for 5 minutes.
4. Gently stir in the cream cheese until the sauce is smooth. Add the pork, stir to combine, cover, and gently simmer for 10 minutes. (Keep the heat low after adding the pork to prevent it from overcooking and becoming tough.) Remove the cover and simmer 5 minutes more or until the pork is cooked through and the sauce thickens somewhat.
5. Meanwhile, cook the noodles according to the package directions. Drain.
6. Divide the egg noodles among the four plates and top with the pork and sauce. Garnish with the chives.

Nutritional Information per Serving
Calories 450 • CD 1.3 • Carbohydrate 31g • Fat 16g • Protein 35g • Fiber 3g

Meatless Pastas

Pasta Tricolore

Here, the three colors come from the combination of veggies. You can mix any three colors you like.

Makes 4 servings (255g each), 2 cups each

 Vegetarian 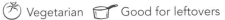 Good for leftovers

1 medium (253g) zucchini

1 medium (191g) yellow squash

8 ounces (227g) whole-wheat fusilli or penne pasta

1 large (189g) red bell pepper, seeded and cut into thin strips

Juice and grated zest from 1 lemon (50g)

1 tablespoon (14g) olive oil

½ cup (67g) pitted Kalamata or other Italian or Greek black olives, sliced

½ cup (25g) chopped fresh basil

1 ounce (28g) grated Parmesan cheese (see note)

Salt and freshly ground black pepper to taste (optional)

4 sprigs fresh basil

1. Cut the zucchini and squash in half lengthwise. Use a teaspoon to scrape the seeds out of each half. Cut crosswise into ½-inch-thick crescents.
2. Cook the pasta according to the package directions, adding the red pepper when 5 minutes remain to cook the pasta and adding the zucchini and squash with 2 minutes remaining. Drain the pasta and vegetables and place in a large bowl.
3. Meanwhile, whisk the lemon juice and zest with the olive oil.
4. Add the lemon juice–oil mixture, olives, basil, and cheese and toss to combine. Season with salt and pepper if desired. Garnish each serving with a sprig of basil.

NOTE: 1 ounce Parmesan equals about ½ cup freshly grated cheese or ¼ cup packaged grated cheese.

Nutritional Information per Serving
Calories 310 • CD 1.2 • Carbohydrate 51g • Fat 8g • Protein 13g • Fiber 7g

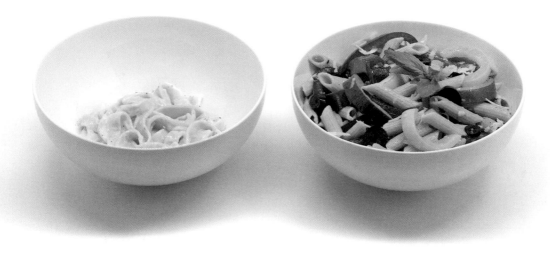

Traditional	How we lowered the CD	Volumetrics
Fettuccine Alfredo	• Switched from a cream sauce to a small amount of olive oil plus vegetables • Used whole-wheat pasta in place of white and decreased the portion size	Pasta Tricolore

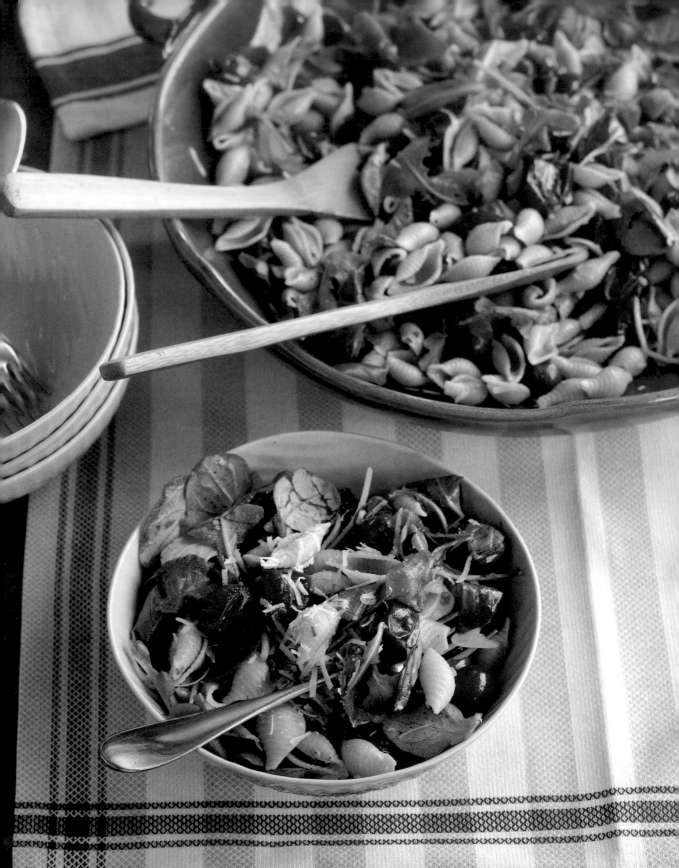

Pasta with Exploding Tomatoes and Arugula

Cherry and grape tomatoes are available year-round, but the members of my lab staff especially love to make "exploding tomatoes" in the summer when farm-fresh tomatoes hit the local market. For a slightly different flavor, try this recipe with baby spinach or mixed spicy baby greens and change to Parmesan or part-skim mozzarella cheese. The arugula and tomato mixture, without the pasta, also makes a delicious topping for a prepared pizza crust.

Makes 4 servings (280g each), about 2 cups each

 Vegetarian

8 ounces (227g) whole-wheat pasta shells

2 pints (560g) cherry or grape tomatoes

3 (9g) garlic cloves, peeled and thinly sliced

2 teaspoons (8g) olive oil

2½ ounces (70g) baby arugula (about 4 cups)

½ cup (28g) shredded Romano cheese (1 ounce)

¼ teaspoon (1g) red pepper flakes

Salt and freshly ground black pepper to taste

1. Preheat the oven to 400°F. Spray a large baking sheet with cooking spray.
2. Cook the pasta according to the package directions. Drain and keep warm.
3. Meanwhile, place the tomatoes and garlic on the baking sheet and drizzle the oil over them. Bake for 15 minutes, until the tomatoes are lightly browned and break open.
4. Toss the tomatoes and accumulated juices, warm pasta, and arugula in a large bowl. Sprinkle with the cheese and pepper flakes, and season with salt and pepper.

Nutritional Information per Serving

Calories 275 • CD 0.98 • Carbohydrate 50g • Fat 5g • Protein 12g • Fiber 7g

Melissa's Leek Lasagna

My daughter Melissa makes this dish for the vegetarians at our family celebrations. She bumped up the vegetables and cut back the cheese while keeping the delicious flavor and texture of traditional lasagna. Melissa tried several different vegetables in the filling before settling on leeks for the best flavor. She recommends fresh lasagna noodles if you can find them; here, I suggest no-boil noodles.

Makes 6 servings (425g), one 4½-inch square each

 Vegetarian Freezes well 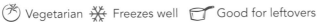 Good for leftovers

SAUCE

1 tablespoon (14g) olive oil

1 large (184g) onion, peeled and chopped

6 (18g) garlic cloves, peeled and finely chopped

2 large (225g) portobello mushroom caps, chopped

1 large (160g) red bell pepper, seeded and chopped

One 28-ounce (794g) can crushed tomatoes

1 tablespoon (1g) finely chopped fresh oregano leaves or 1 teaspoon dried oregano

1 tablespoon (14g) sugar

Salt and freshly ground black pepper to taste (optional)

FILLING

3 medium (314g) leeks, white parts only

Two 10-ounce (567g) boxes frozen chopped spinach

One 15-ounce (430g) container part-skim ricotta

2 tablespoons (17g) grated Parmesan cheese

One 8-ounce (230g) box no-boil lasagna noodles

½ cup (57g) shredded part-skim mozzarella cheese

1. To make the sauce, heat the olive oil in a medium saucepan on medium heat. Add the onion and cook, stirring occasionally, until soft, about 5 minutes. Add the garlic, mushrooms, and red pepper and cook for 5 to 10 minutes, stirring occasionally, until the mushrooms give up their liquid and are soft. Add the tomatoes, oregano, and sugar and simmer for 15 minutes, uncovered. Season with salt and pepper, if desired.

2. Meanwhile, to make the filling, clean the leeks by slicing them in half lengthwise and rinsing all layers in a colander under cold running water. Slice the leeks into ½-inch pieces and put in a medium microwaveable bowl with 2 tablespoons water. Cover and microwave 4 minutes, until soft.

3. Put the spinach in a separate medium microwaveable bowl. Cover and microwave in 2-minute intervals until thawed, about 10 minutes. Drain as much liquid as possible. Add to the leeks along with the ricotta and Parmesan and mix well.

4. Preheat the oven to 400°F. Spray a 9 by 13-inch glass baking dish with cooking spray.

5. To assemble the lasagna, spread 1 cup of the sauce in the bottom of the dish. Add a layer of noodles. Spread half of the ricotta filling in an even layer on top of the noodles. Add another layer of noodles. Spread half of the remaining sauce on top. Add another layer of noodles. Spread the rest of the ricotta filling on top. Add a layer of noodles. Cover with the remaining sauce and sprinkle with the mozzarella cheese.

6. Cover with foil and bake for 15 minutes. Uncover and bake for 20 minutes more, or until the lasagna is bubbling and the cheese topping is lightly browned. Allow to cool for 5 minutes before cutting and serving.

Nutritional Information per Serving
Calories 425 • CD 1.0 • Carbohydrate 60g • Fat 12g • Protein 24g • Fiber 9g

Stir-Fry Entrées

Chicken-Broccoli Stir-Fry with Water Chestnuts and Carrots

I enjoy making stir-fry dishes because they cook up so quickly and can be made with whatever combination of vegetables I have in my refrigerator. Don't be afraid to get the wok or skillet nice and hot.

Makes 4 servings (390g each), 1½ cups chicken and vegetables plus ½ cup rice each

🍲 Good for leftovers

⅔ cup (125g) brown rice

2 large (950g) heads broccoli, cut into florets (about 6 cups)

2 medium (201g) carrots, peeled and cut into thin rounds

¾ cup (180g) low-sodium chicken broth

2 teaspoons (8g) canola oil

1 tablespoon (10g) finely chopped peeled fresh ginger

3 (9g) garlic cloves, peeled and finely chopped

12 ounces (340g) skinless, boneless chicken breast, cut into 1-inch pieces

2 tablespoons (31g) reduced-sodium soy sauce

1 tablespoon (20g) hoisin sauce

1 tablespoon (8g) cornstarch

One 8-ounce (227g) can sliced water chestnuts, drained

½ teaspoon (3g) sesame oil

3 (45g) green onions (scallions), white and light green parts, thinly sliced

1. Cook the rice according to the package directions. Keep warm.

2. Meanwhile, microwave the broccoli, carrots, and ¼ cup of the chicken broth in a large bowl, covered, for 3 minutes. Set aside.

3. Spray a wok or large skillet with cooking spray. Heat the canola oil in the wok over medium-high heat. Stir-fry the ginger and garlic for 30 seconds to soften. Add the broccoli, carrots, and liquid from the bowl and stir-fry for 5 minutes, until just tender.

4. Add the chicken, the remaining broth, the soy sauce, and hoisin sauce. Cook for 4 minutes, stirring often.

5. Combine the cornstarch with 2 tablespoons water in a small bowl. Add to the wok along with the water chestnuts. Simmer for 2 minutes. Drizzle with the sesame oil and garnish with the green onions. Serve with the rice.

Nutritional Information per Serving
Calories 330 • CD 0.85 • Carbohydrate 43g • Fat 7g • Protein 26g • Fiber 8g

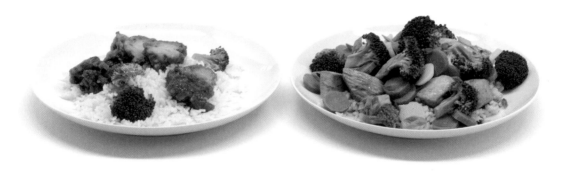

Traditional	How we lowered the CD	Volumetrics
General Tsao's chicken	• Added more vegetables • Reduced fat and sugar in the sauce • Switched from fried, skin-on chicken pieces to chicken breast fillet • Decreased the portion of rice and switched to brown rice	Chicken-Broccoli Stir-Fry with Water Chestnuts and Carrots

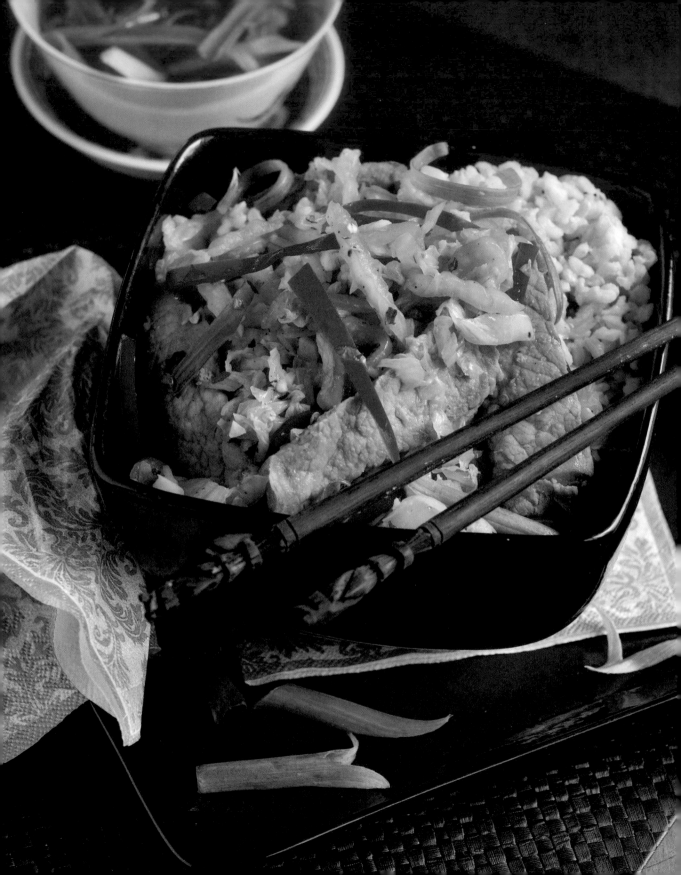

Pork Stir-Fry with Asian Cabbage and Red Pepper

I like to use napa cabbage for its mild flavor and soft texture when cooked. The red pepper adds color and helps lower the CD. This recipe is extremely adaptable, so try chicken in place of the pork, switch to a pepper of a different color, and use other Asian greens.

Makes 4 servings (385g each), 1½ cups meat and vegetables plus ½ cup rice

Good for leftovers

⅔ cup (125g) brown rice

12 ounces (340g) boneless pork loin, trimmed of visible fat and cut into ½-inch-thick strips

3 tablespoons (45g) reduced-sodium soy sauce

1 teaspoon (4g) sesame oil

2 teaspoons (8g) canola oil

1 tablespoon (10g) finely chopped peeled fresh ginger

3 (9g) garlic cloves, peeled and finely chopped

1 large (164g) red bell pepper, seeded and cut into thin strips

1 small (651g) head napa cabbage, about 1½ pounds, cut crosswise into thin strips

2 tablespoons (30g) dry sherry or white wine

1 tablespoon (15g) rice vinegar

1 teaspoon (6g) light brown sugar

1 tablespoon (8g) cornstarch

½ teaspoon (1g) red pepper flakes

1. Cook the rice according to the package directions. Keep warm.

2. Meanwhile, marinate the pork for 10 minutes in a medium bowl with 1 tablespoon of the soy sauce and ½ teaspoon of the sesame oil.

3. Spray a regular or nonstick wok with cooking spray, add 1 teaspoon of the canola oil, and heat over medium-high heat. Add the pork and marinade and stir-fry until lightly browned but still slightly pink in the middle, about 5 minutes. Transfer from the wok to a plate or bowl and set aside. Do not clean the wok.

4. Return the wok to the stove over medium-high heat and add the remaining canola oil. Add the ginger, garlic, and red pepper and stir-fry for 2 minutes. Add half the cabbage and stir-fry until the cabbage begins to wilt, about 2 minutes. Add the remaining cabbage, cover, reduce the heat to medium, and cook until the cabbage is tender, about 6 minutes.

5. Stir together the remaining 2 tablespoons of soy sauce, sherry, vinegar, brown sugar, and cornstarch in a small bowl. Add to the wok along with the pork and any accumulated juices and simmer for 2 minutes, until the sauce thickens.

6. Drizzle with the remaining sesame oil and sprinkle with the pepper flakes. Serve with the rice.

Nutritional Information per Serving
Calories 345 • CD 0.90 • Carbohydrate 35g • Fat 12g • Protein 24g • Fiber 5g

Spicy Tofu with Peppers and Snow Peas

Tofu, a soybean product, is sold in varying degrees of firmness. Firm and extra firm tofus are my favorites for stir-frying because they hold their shape well. Tofu absorbs the spicy flavor of the sauce.

Makes 4 servings (285g each), 1¾ cups plus ½ cup pasta

 Vegetarian   Good for leftovers

4 ounces (114g) whole-wheat spaghetti

2 teaspoons (8g) canola oil

1 tablespoon (10g) finely chopped peeled fresh ginger

3 (9g) garlic cloves, peeled and finely chopped

One 15-ounce (425g) carton firm or extra firm tofu, drained, patted dry with a paper towel, and cut into ½-inch cubes

2 medium (278g) green peppers, seeded and cut into thin strips

12 ounces (340g) fresh or frozen sugar snap peas or snow peas

½ cup (120g) vegetable broth

1 tablespoon (8g) cornstarch

¼ cup (72g) bottled Szechuan sauce

Chili-garlic or sriracha sauce to taste (optional)

1 tablespoon (9g) sesame seeds

1. Cook the spaghetti according to package directions. Drain and keep warm.
2. Meanwhile, heat the oil in a wok over medium-high heat until it begins to shimmer. Add the ginger and garlic and stir-fry for 1 minute. Add the tofu and stir-fry for about 5 minutes, until the tofu begins to develop a light crust. Add the peppers and peas and stir-fry for 5 to 8 minutes, until just tender.
3. Whisk together the broth, cornstarch, Szechuan sauce, and chili-garlic sauce, if using, in a medium bowl. Add to the wok, stir to combine, and simmer until the liquid thickens, about 1 minute. Sprinkle with sesame seeds before serving with the pasta.

Nutritional Information per Serving
Calories 275 • CD 0.96 • Carbohydrate 36g • Fat 9g • Protein 16g • Fiber 8g

Stews

French Beef Stew

The combination of tomatoes, red wine, olives, and thyme gives this dish a hearty and decidedly French flavor. The dried mushrooms add an earthiness that complements the meat.

Makes 6 servings (410g each), 1½ cups each

 Freezes well 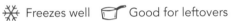 Good for leftovers

1 tablespoon (14g) olive oil

1 medium (119g) onion, peeled and chopped

2 (6g) garlic cloves, peeled and finely chopped

2 tablespoons (16g) all-purpose flour

¼ teaspoon (1g) table salt

¼ teaspoon (1g) freshly ground black pepper

1 pound (454g) chuck shoulder pot roast, trimmed of fat and cut into 1-inch cubes

½ cup (120g) dry red wine

Two 14.5-ounce (822g) cans reduced-sodium beef broth

One 14.5-ounce (411g) can diced tomatoes with basil, garlic, and oregano

½ ounce (15g) dried porcini mushrooms (½ cup)

½ teaspoon (1g) dried thyme

2 medium (259g) Yukon gold potatoes, scrubbed and cut into eighths

3 medium (234g) carrots, peeled and cut into 1-inch lengths

3 (120g) celery stalks, cut into 1-inch lengths

½ cup (67g) pitted niçoise or Kalamata olives

¼ cup (10g) chopped fresh basil

1. Heat 1 teaspoon of the oil in a large pot over medium heat. Add the onion and garlic to the pot and cook for 5 minutes, stirring often, until soft. Transfer to a small bowl. Do not clean the pot.

2. Meanwhile, combine the flour, salt, and pepper in a resealable plastic bag. Add the

beef. Seal the bag and shake to coat the beef with the flour and seasonings. Remove the beef from the bag, shaking off the excess flour mixture back into the bag. Set aside the bag.

3. Add the remaining oil to the pot. Add the beef and cook on medium-low heat, stirring frequently, until lightly browned on all sides, about 5 minutes.

4. Add back the cooked onion and garlic. Stir in the wine, broth, tomatoes, mushrooms, thyme, and reserved flour mixture. Bring to a boil, reduce the heat to simmer, cover, and cook for 20 minutes.

5. Add the potatoes, carrots, and celery, cover, and cook for 20 to 30 minutes more, until the vegetables are fully cooked. Stir in the olives and cook for 5 minutes. Garnish with the basil.

Nutritional Information per Serving
Calories 300 • CD 0.73 • Carbohydrate 28g • Fat 9g • Protein 22g • Fiber 6g

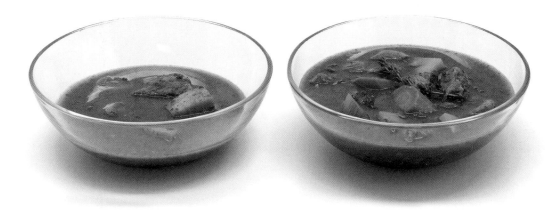

Traditional	How we lowered the CD	Volumetrics
Beef stew	• Cooked the onions and garlic in less oil • Chose a leaner cut of beef • Browned the beef in less oil • Added more vegetables • Added more liquid	French Beef Stew

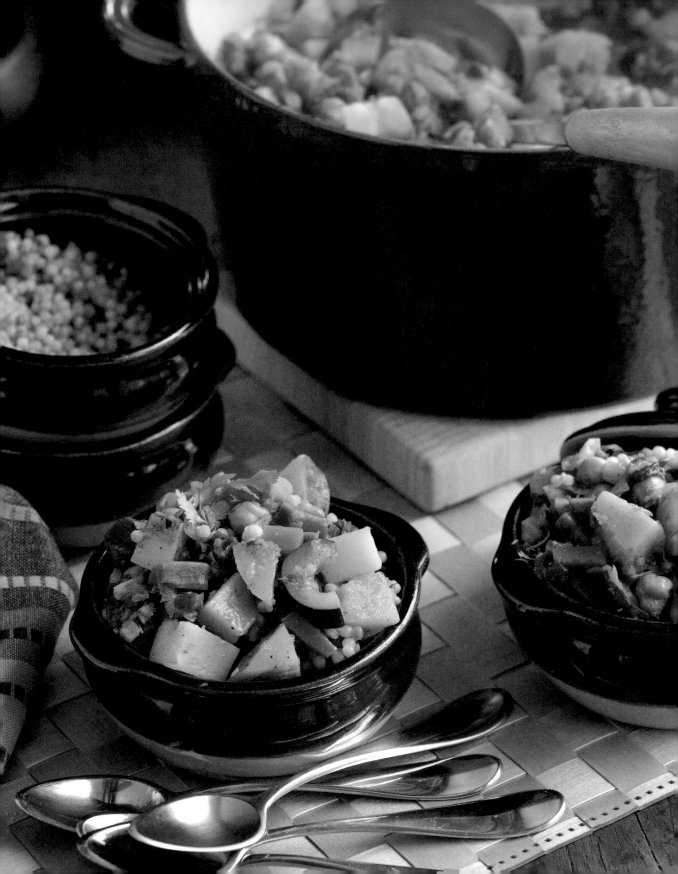

Couscous with Middle Eastern Vegetable Stew

Couscous, a form of pasta, is popular in North Africa, where it is topped with a fragrant vegetable stew made with or without meat. I enjoy this stew best over large Israeli or Moroccan couscous but regular, whole-wheat, or seasoned couscous can be used instead.

Makes 4 servings (600g each), 2 cups vegetables with ¾ cup couscous each

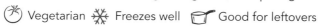 Vegetarian ❄ Freezes well ☕ Good for leftovers

1 medium (119g) onion, peeled and cut into small pieces

3 (9g) garlic cloves, peeled and finely chopped

2 small (122g) carrots, peeled and cut into ½-inch pieces

One 14.5-ounce (411g) can plain or seasoned diced tomatoes

2 teaspoons (4g) ground cinnamon

2 teaspoons (4g) ground ginger

1 teaspoon (2g) ground turmeric

One 14.5-ounce (411g) can vegetable or reduced-sodium chicken broth

1 cup (112g) Israeli or Moroccan couscous

1 large (213g) Yukon gold potato, scrubbed and cut into ½-inch cubes

1 large (700g) (about 1½ pounds) butternut squash, peeled, seeded, and cut into ½-inch cubes

1 small (136g) zucchini, cut in half lengthwise, then into ¼-inch slices

One 15.5-ounce (439g) can chickpeas, rinsed and drained

½ cup (8g) finely chopped fresh cilantro

Salt, freshly ground black pepper, and cayenne pepper to taste

1. Combine the onion, garlic, carrots, tomatoes, cinnamon, ginger, turmeric, and broth in a medium pot over medium-high heat. Bring to a boil, reduce the heat to low, cover, and simmer for 25 minutes.

2. Meanwhile, cook the couscous according to package directions. Keep warm.

3. Add the potato, squash, zucchini, and chickpeas and simmer uncovered for 15 minutes, adding water if necessary to keep the vegetables just covered with liquid.

4. Stir in the cilantro and season with salt, pepper, and cayenne before serving over the couscous.

Nutritional Information per Serving
Calories 355 • CD 0.59 • Carbohydrate 77g • Fat 2g • Protein 13g • Fiber 11g

Irish Lamb Stew

The beer gives this stew a deep, rich flavor that pairs well with the lamb. I call for potatoes to keep this stew traditional but also add other root vegetables, such as carrots.

Makes 6 servings (320g each), 1½ cups each

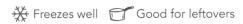 ❄ Freezes well   ☐ Good for leftovers

2 tablespoons (16g) all-purpose flour

¼ teaspoon (1g) table salt

¼ teaspoon (1g) black pepper

1 pound (454g) boneless, trimmed lamb shoulder, cut into 1-inch cubes

2 teaspoons (8g) vegetable oil

1 large (170g) onion, peeled and chopped

3 (9g) garlic cloves, peeled and finely chopped

One 12-ounce (355g) bottle dark beer or stout, or 1½ cups water

One 14.5-ounce (411g) can reduced-sodium beef broth

3 large (460g) carrots (about 1 pound), peeled and cut into 1-inch pieces

3 medium (438g) Yukon gold or red potatoes (about 1 pound), scrubbed and cut into 8 to 12 pieces each

1 teaspoon (0.5g) dried thyme

2 bay leaves

1. Combine the flour, salt, and pepper in a resealable plastic bag. Add the lamb. Seal and shake to coat the lamb with the flour mixture. Remove the lamb pieces from the bag, shaking off the excess flour back into the bag. Set aside the bag.

2. Heat 1 teaspoon of oil in a medium pot over medium heat. Add the lamb and cook, stirring, for about 6 minutes or until the pieces are lightly browned. Transfer the lamb to a plate and set aside. Do not clean the pot.

3. Heat the remaining oil in the pot over medium heat. Add the onion and garlic and cook for about 3 minutes, until soft. Add the beer and simmer for 2 minutes while scraping up the browned bits from the bottom of the pot.

4. Return the lamb and accumulated juices to the pot. Stir in the reserved flour, the broth, carrots, potatoes, thyme, and bay leaves. Bring to a boil, then reduce the heat, cover, and simmer until the vegetables are soft, at least 30 minutes. Uncover for the last 10 minutes to thicken the stew. Remove the bay leaves before serving.

Nutritional Information per Serving
Calories 280 • CD 0.88 • Carbohydrate 28g • Fat 8g • Protein 19g • Fiber 4g

Comfort Foods

Volumetrics Gumbo

The name gumbo comes from the African word for okra, the primary vegetable in this soup-like stew. Its combination of onions, celery, and green bell peppers is classic Cajun. Traditional gumbo is thickened with a large amount of roux, a high-calorie flour and fat mixture that can be used in smaller amounts for an equally tasty dish.

Makes 8 servings (450g), 1½ cups gumbo plus ½ cup rice each

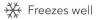 Freezes well 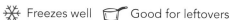 Good for leftovers

1⅓ cups (247g) brown rice

4 teaspoons (16g) vegetable oil

2 medium (232g) yellow onions, peeled and chopped

4 (12g) garlic cloves, peeled and chopped

3 (152g) celery stalks, chopped

2 large (328g) green bell peppers, seeded and chopped

3 tablespoons (24g) all-purpose flour

One 16-ounce (454g) bag frozen cut okra

One 14-ounce (397g) package turkey kielbasa, cut into ½-inch pieces

One 32-ounce (946g) carton or can reduced-sodium chicken broth

One 14.5-ounce (411g) can no-salt-added diced tomatoes

1 tablespoon (8g) paprika

1 bay leaf

1 pound (454g) shrimp, peeled, deveined, and tails removed (fresh or frozen, raw or precooked)

Salt, freshly ground black pepper, and cayenne pepper to taste

1. Cook the rice according to the package directions. Keep warm.
2. Meanwhile, heat 2 teaspoons of the oil in a large pot or Dutch oven over medium-high heat. Cook the onions, garlic, celery, and green peppers, stirring occasionally, until soft, about 10 minutes. Transfer to a bowl and set aside. Do not clean the pot.

3. Heat the remaining oil in the pot over medium heat. Add the flour and cook, stirring, until the flour turns light brown, about 30 seconds. Stir in the onion mixture, okra, kielbasa, chicken broth, tomatoes, paprika, and bay leaf. Bring to a boil, then reduce heat, cover, and simmer for 30 minutes, stirring occasionally.

4. Add the shrimp and cook for 5 to 10 minutes, until the shrimp are fully cooked. Season to taste with salt, pepper, and cayenne. Remove the bay leaf before serving. Serve over the rice.

NOTES: If using frozen shrimp, thaw the shrimp completely before adding in step 4.

If using precooked shrimp, cook only until they are heated through, about 2 minutes.

Nutritional Information per Serving
Calories 320 • CD 0.71 • Carbohydrate 38g • Fat 8g • Protein 23g • Fiber 5g

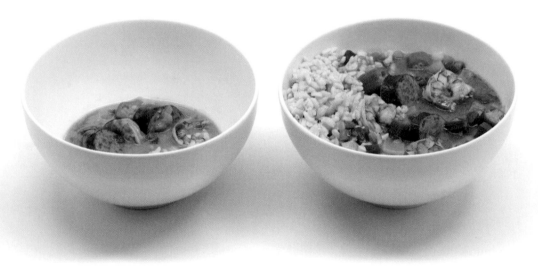

Traditional	How we lowered the CD	Volumetrics
Louisiana gumbo	• Cut down on the amount of roux • Added more vegetables • Increased liquid • Substituted turkey kielbasa for sausage	Volumetrics Gumbo

Enchilada Casserole

This casserole is particularly well-suited for leftovers. I like to vary the spiciness with mild, medium, or hot salsa and plain or spicy refried beans.

Makes 8 servings (365g each), 3 by 4 inches each

 Vegetarian ✳ Freezes well 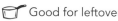 Good for leftovers

One 16-ounce (454g) jar salsa

One 14.5-ounce (411g) can crushed tomatoes

12 (288g) corn tortillas, cut in half

One 16-ounce (454g) can fat-free refried beans

One 15.5-ounce (439g) can pinto beans, rinsed and drained

2 small (170g) or 1 large onion, peeled and finely chopped

2 small (240g) zucchini, diced

1 large (213g) red bell pepper, seeded and diced

1 cup (165g) frozen corn kernels

1 cup (112g) shredded reduced-fat Mexican blend cheese (4 ounces)

½ cup (120g) fat-free sour cream, for garnish

1. Preheat the oven to 400°F. Spray a 9 by 13-inch baking pan with cooking spray.
2. Combine the salsa and tomatoes with ¾ cup water in a medium bowl.
3. Cover the bottom of the pan with 8 tortilla halves; the tortillas may overlap. Top the tortillas with the refried beans, onions, and 1½ cups of the salsa mixture.
4. Cover with another 8 tortilla halves. Top with the zucchini, red pepper, corn, and 1 cup of the salsa mixture.
5. Cover with the remaining 8 tortilla halves. Top with the remaining salsa mixture.
6. Loosely cover with foil and bake for 45 minutes, until bubbling. Uncover, top with the cheese, and bake until the cheese melts, about 5 minutes. Let cool for a few minutes, then cut into portions. Serve with the sour cream.

Nutritional Information per Serving
Calories 265 • CD 0.73 • Carbohydrate 48g • Fat 3g • Protein 14g • Fiber 10g

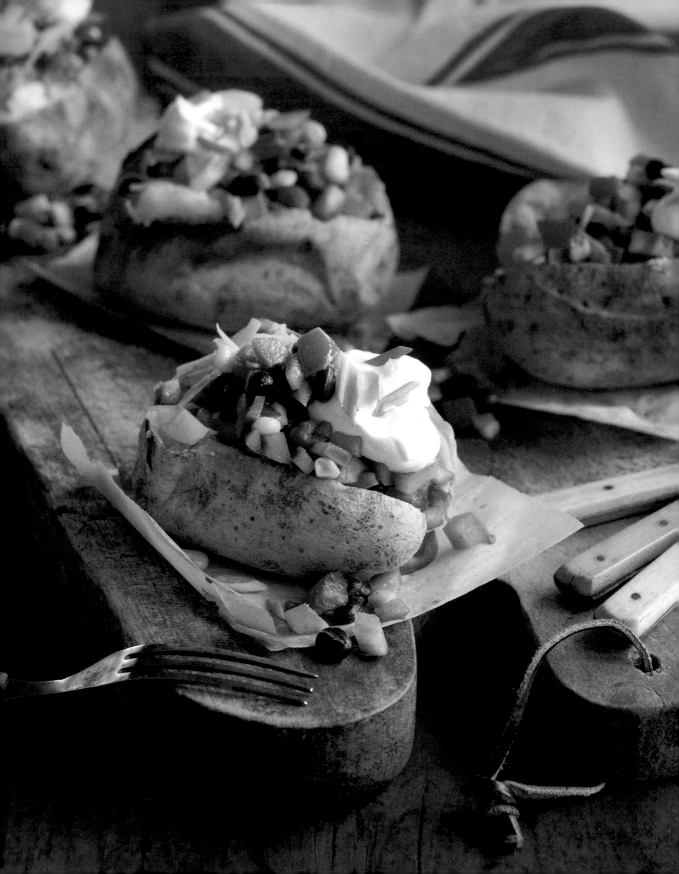

Baked Potato with Black Bean and Pepper Salsa

This is a perfect comfort food for me—easy and delicious. You don't have to bake all six potatoes—just save the extra salsa to put over salad or pasta or use as a dip for vegetables.

Makes 6 servings (360g each), 1 baked potato topped with ¾ cup salsa each

 Vegetarian

One 15.5-ounce (439g) can black beans, rinsed and drained

⅔ cup (112g) frozen white or yellow corn kernels

¾ cup (135g) diced fresh tomato

1 (15g) green onion (scallion), thinly sliced

1 medium (119g) green bell pepper, seeded and diced

1 medium (130g) yellow or orange bell pepper, seeded and diced

2 tablespoons (28g) olive oil

¼ cup (60g) red wine vinegar

1½ teaspoons (8g) Worcestershire sauce

1½ teaspoons (7g) Tabasco sauce

1 teaspoon (3g) ground cumin

Salt and ground white pepper to taste

6 medium (1,038g) baking potatoes (about 6 ounces each)

6 tablespoons (42g) shredded reduced-fat cheddar cheese

6 tablespoons (90g) reduced-fat sour cream

1. To make the salsa, combine the black beans, corn, tomato, green onion, peppers, olive oil, vinegar, Worcestershire sauce, Tabasco sauce, cumin, salt, and white pepper in a large bowl. Mix well. Cover and refrigerate for 2 hours.

2. An hour before you are ready to eat, preheat the oven to 400°F. Scrub the potatoes well with a potato brush and water. Pierce each potato with a fork three or four times. Place the potatoes on a baking sheet and bake for 45 to 60 minutes, until potatoes are tender when pierced with a fork.

3. Cut each potato in half lengthwise. Use a fork to gently break up the flesh. Top each potato with ¾ cup of the salsa, 1 tablespoon cheese, and 1 tablespoon sour cream.

Nutritional Information per Serving
Calories 325 • CD 0.90 • Carbohydrate 53g • Fat 8g • Protein 11g • Fiber 8g

Poultry Entrées

Volumetrics Chicken Cacciatore

My version of chicken cacciatore—hunter's chicken in English—has plenty of vegetables and a splash of red wine to round out the flavor. I use almost the same recipe to make chicken Provençal, switching the red wine to white and adding a few olives.

Makes 4 servings (395g each), 1½ cups chicken and vegetables plus ½ cup pasta each

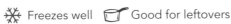 Freezes well 　 Good for leftovers

4 ounces (114g) whole-wheat penne

3 tablespoons (28g) all-purpose flour

½ teaspoon (2g) table salt

¼ teaspoon (1g) freshly ground black pepper

1 pound (454g) skinless, boneless chicken breast fillets, cut into 1-inch cubes

1 tablespoon (14g) olive oil

1 medium (137g) onion, peeled and chopped

1 medium (140g) green bell pepper, seeded and chopped

3 (9g) garlic cloves, peeled and finely chopped

10 ounces (284g) button mushrooms, sliced

One 14.5-ounce (411g) can crushed tomatoes with basil

½ cup (120g) dry red wine

2 teaspoons (3g) dried oregano

1. Cook the pasta according to the package directions. Drain and keep warm.
2. Meanwhile, combine the flour, salt, and pepper in a resealable plastic bag. Add the chicken and seal the bag. Shake to coat the chicken with the flour mixture. Remove the chicken pieces from the bag and shake off the excess flour back into the bag. Discard any remaining flour.
3. Spray the bottom of a large saucepan with cooking spray. Heat the oil in the

saucepan over medium heat. Add the chicken and cook, stirring, for about 5 minutes or until the sides of the chicken pieces are lightly browned. Transfer the chicken to a plate or bowl and set aside. Do not clean the pot.

4. Add the onion, bell pepper, and garlic to the saucepan and cook, stirring occasionally, until almost soft, about 5 minutes. Add the mushrooms and cook for 7 minutes, until the mushrooms have released their liquid and are soft. Add the tomatoes, wine, and oregano and cook over medium heat, stirring occasionally, for 5 minutes.

5. Add back the chicken and accumulated juices and cook for 5 to 7 minutes, stirring, until the chicken is fully cooked. Serve with the pasta.

Nutritional Information per Serving
Calories 360 • CD 0.91 • Carbohydrate 38g • Fat 7g • Protein 33g • Fiber 6g

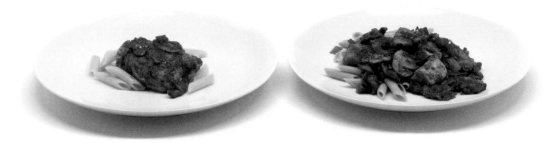

Traditional	How we lowered the CD	Volumetrics
Classic chicken cacciatore	• Switched to chicken breast fillets from skin-on chicken parts • Decreased oil for sautéing • Added more vegetables	Volumetrics Chicken Cacciatore

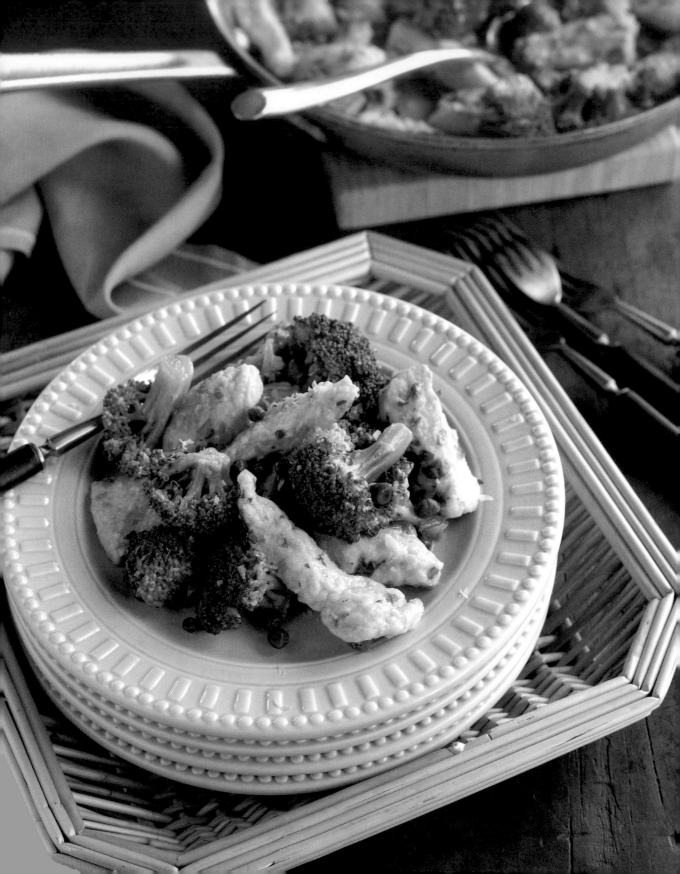

Turkey Piccata with Broccoli

Turkey breast cutlets are available year-round—no need to limit turkey to Thanksgiving. I keep a jar of capers in the refrigerator to brighten the flavor of dishes like this.

Makes 4 servings (210g each), 1½ cups each

Good for leftovers

3 tablespoons (28g) all-purpose flour

¼ teaspoon (1g) table salt

¼ teaspoon (1g) freshly ground black pepper

1 pound (454g) turkey cutlets, cut into 1-inch strips

1 tablespoon (14g) olive oil

1 (3g) garlic clove, peeled and finely chopped

½ cup (120g) dry white wine or reduced-sodium chicken broth

Juice of 1 lemon (50g)

2 tablespoons capers (18g), rinsed and drained

½ teaspoon (2g) sugar

4 cups (284g) broccoli florets

¼ cup (15g) chopped fresh parsley

1. Combine the flour, salt, and pepper in a resealable plastic bag. Add the turkey. Seal and shake to coat the turkey with the flour mixture. Remove the turkey pieces and shake off the excess flour back into the bag.

2. Spray the bottom of a large nonstick skillet with cooking spray. Heat 2 teaspoons of the oil in the skillet over medium heat. Add the turkey and cook, stirring, for about 5 minutes, until all sides of the turkey pieces are lightly browned. Transfer the turkey to a plate or bowl and set it aside. Do not clean the skillet.

3. Heat the remaining oil in the skillet over medium-low heat. Add the garlic and cook for about 1 minute. Add the wine, lemon juice, capers, and sugar and bring to a simmer. Add the turkey and any accumulated juices and cook until it is cooked through and no longer pink and the sauce begins to thicken, about 5 minutes.

4. Meanwhile, steam the broccoli on the stove or in the microwave until just soft and still bright green, about 5 minutes.

5. Combine the turkey and broccoli in a serving bowl. Sprinkle with the parsley.

Nutritional Information per Serving
Calories 230 • CD 1.1 • Carbohydrate 11g • Fat 4g • Protein 31g • Fiber 3g

Jennifer's Orange Chicken

This quick and easy child-friendly chicken dish was developed by my lab manager, Jennifer. Serve with your choice of vegetables—the Asian Green Beans are a favorite of Jennifer's kids.

Makes 4 servings (170g each), about 1 cup each

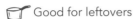 Good for leftovers

¼ cup (30g) all-purpose flour

¼ cup (27g) plain dry bread crumbs

¼ teaspoon (1g) table salt

¼ teaspoon (1g) freshly ground black pepper

1 pound (454g) skinless, boneless chicken breast, cut into ½-inch slices

1½ tablespoons (20g) vegetable oil

1½ cups (372g) orange juice

3 tablespoons (60g) apricot, peach, or orange preserves

1. Combine the flour, bread crumbs, salt and pepper in a medium bowl. Coat each piece of chicken in the flour mixture and set aside on a large plate in one layer.

2. Heat the oil in a large, nonstick skillet over medium-high heat. Cook the chicken pieces, turning them over occasionally, until they are browned, about 5 minutes. Add the orange juice and preserves. Stir gently to prevent the chicken from sticking to the skillet. Reduce the heat to medium-low, cover, and simmer gently for 15 minutes.

3. Uncover and simmer for an additional 3 to 4 minutes to thicken the sauce.

Nutritional Information per Serving
Calories 290 • CD 1.7 • Carbohydrate 28g • Fat 7g • Protein 28g • Fiber 1g

Protein Packet Entrées

Steak and Onions in a Packet

I suggest flank steak for this recipe but you can choose whichever type of lean steak you like best. Cooking in parchment gives this dish an elegant look.

Makes 4 servings (210g each), 1 packet each

3 medium (390g) red onions, peeled and sliced thin

1 pound (454g) flank steak, cut into 4 equal pieces

2 tablespoons (30g) Dijon mustard

1 tablespoon (18g) maple syrup

½ teaspoon (2g) paprika, preferably smoked

½ teaspoon (2g) freshly ground black pepper

¼ teaspoon (1g) table salt

1. Preheat the oven to 400°F. Cut parchment paper or heavy-duty foil into four 12- to 15-inch squares.
2. Microwave the onion slices in a covered bowl for 3 minutes to soften.
3. Place one-quarter of the onions on each parchment sheet. Top each with a piece of flank steak. Whisk together the mustard, syrup, paprika, pepper, and salt in a small bowl. Spoon about 2 teaspoons of the sauce on top of each steak.
4. Bring together the two sides of parchment that parallel the edges of the steak and fold over several times to seal. Fold in the parchment at each open end several times to seal.
5. Place the packets on a baking sheet, leaving at least 1 inch between packets. Bake about 25 minutes, until the internal temperature of the steak reaches 145° to 150° on an instant-read thermometer.
6. Cut a slit in the top of each packet to release the steam. Remove the steak and onions from the packets before serving. Drizzle with the accumulated juices.

Nutritional Information per Serving

Calories 230 • CD 1.1 • Carbohydrate 13g • Fat 8g • Protein 25g • Fiber 2g

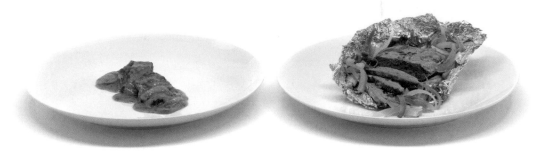

Traditional	How we lowered the CD	Volumetrics
Steak and onions with gravy	• Used a leaner cut of beef • Increased vegetables • Created a flavorful low-CD sauce by cooking in a packet	Steak and Onions in a Packet

Chicken and Seasonal Tomatoes in a Packet

I love making this dish in the summer, when my local farmers' market is filled with tomatoes of different colors. Be sure to fold over and crimp the parchment or foil tightly to avoid leaks. Pictured on page xvii.

Makes 4 servings (295g each), 1 packet each

4 cups (680g) diced red, orange, yellow, and/or heirloom tomatoes (1½ pounds)

½ cup (21g) chopped fresh basil

2 teaspoons (10g) balsamic vinegar

2 teaspoons (8g) olive oil

½ teaspoon (3g) table salt

Four 4-ounce (454g) skinless, boneless chicken breast fillets

1. Preheat the oven to 450°F. Cut parchment paper or heavy-duty foil into four 12- to 15-inch squares.
2. Combine the tomatoes, basil, vinegar, oil, and salt in a medium bowl.
3. Place each fillet on a piece of parchment. Top with about 1 cup of the tomato mixture; use all the mixture.
4. Bring together the two sides of parchment that parallel the edges of the fillet and fold over several times to seal. Fold in the parchment at each open end several times to seal. Place the packets on a baking sheet. Bake 15 minutes for thin fillets or 18 minutes for thicker fillets.
5. Cut a slit in the top of each packet to release the steam. Remove the chicken and tomatoes from the packets before serving. Drizzle with the accumulated juices.

Nutritional Information per Serving
Calories 185 • CD 0.63 • Carbohydrate 7g • Fat 6g • Protein 26g • Fiber 2g

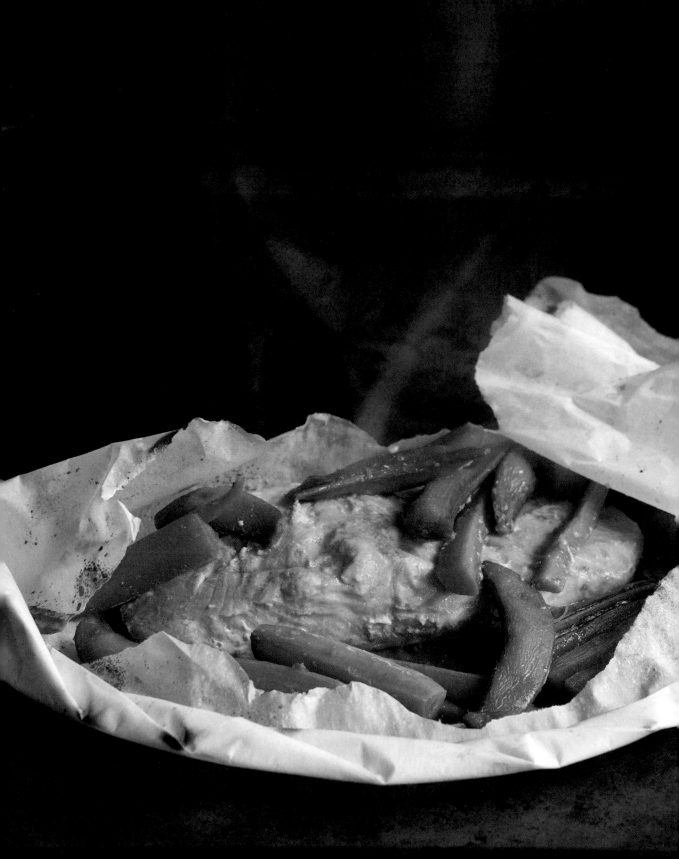

Asian Salmon in a Packet

Salmon is one of my favorite types of fish to pair with Asian flavors. I like the color contrast of the bright green pea pods and the bright orange carrots against the salmon. Tilapia and snapper also work well in this recipe.

Makes 4 servings (255g each), 1 packet each

2 cups (299g) baby carrots, cut lengthwise in quarters

Half of a 1-pound (240g) bag frozen sugar snap peas or snow peas, thawed

Four 4-ounce (454g) skinless salmon fillets

2 tablespoons (30g) reduced-sodium soy sauce

2 tablespoons (30g) rice vinegar

2 teaspoons (7g) grated peeled fresh ginger

2 teaspoons (12g) light brown sugar

1 teaspoon (4g) sesame oil

1 teaspoon (3g) cornstarch

1. Preheat the oven to 400°F. Cut parchment paper or heavy-duty foil into four 12- to 15-inch squares.
2. Microwave the carrots in a covered bowl for 5 minutes to soften.
3. Put one-quarter each of the peas and carrots on each parchment sheet. Top with a salmon fillet. Whisk together the soy sauce, vinegar, ginger, sugar, sesame oil, and cornstarch in a small bowl. Spoon about 1½ tablespoons of the sauce on top of each fillet.
4. Bring together the two sides of parchment that parallel the edges of the fillet and fold over several times to seal. Fold in the parchment at each open end several times to seal.
5. Place the packets on a baking sheet, leaving at least 1 inch between packets. Bake until the salmon is just cooked through, about 25 minutes, until the internal temperature of the salmon reaches 145° on an instant-read thermometer.
6. Cut a slit in the top of each packet to release the steam. Remove the salmon and vegetables from the packets before serving. Drizzle with the accumulated juices.

Nutritional Information per Serving
Calories 315 • CD 1.2 • Carbohydrate 14g • Fat 16g • Protein 25g • Fiber 4g

Seafood Entrées

Crab-Asparagus Quiche

I like to serve baked brunch and lunch dishes like this since I can do most of the work ahead of time. To lower the CD, I used a flavorful filling and skipped the typical quiche crust. Serve with a big tossed salad and crusty whole-grain rolls.

Makes 6 servings (190g each), 1 wedge each

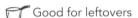 Good for leftovers

2 teaspoons (8g) olive oil

1 medium (120g) onion, peeled and chopped

1 large (150g) red bell pepper, seeded and chopped

1 pound (454g) asparagus, washed, trimmed to remove the tough base, and cut on the diagonal into 1-inch pieces

3 large (150g) eggs

1½ cups (339g) 1% fat cottage cheese

½ cup (123g) nonfat plain yogurt

½ cup (60g) all-purpose flour

½ ounce (14g) grated Parmesan cheese (see note)

¼ teaspoon (0.5g) cayenne pepper

¼ teaspoon (1g) table salt

¼ teaspoon (1g) ground black pepper

¼ cup (15g) chopped scallions

½ cup (56g) shredded reduced-fat cheddar cheese (2 ounces)

8 ounces (227g) cooked lump crab meat, drained and picked over to remove any shell

1. Preheat the oven to 350°F. Spray a 10-inch pie plate or quiche dish with cooking spray.

2. Heat the oil in a large nonstick skillet over medium-high heat. Add the onion, red pepper, and asparagus and cook, stirring occasionally, until soft, about 5 minutes.

3. In a blender or food processor, blend the eggs, cottage cheese, yogurt, flour, Parmesan, cayenne, salt, and black pepper until smooth.

4. Transfer egg mixture to a large bowl. Stir in the cooked vegetables.

5. With a rubber spatula, fold in the scallions, cheddar, and crab. Pour into the prepared dish.

6. Bake for 50 minutes or until a knife inserted into the center comes out clean.

7. Remove from the oven and allow the quiche to sit for 5 minutes before cutting into 6 wedges.

NOTE: ½ ounce Parmesan equals about ¼ cup freshly grated cheese or 2 tablespoons packaged grated cheese.

Nutritional Information per Serving
Calories 225 • CD 1.2 • Carbohydrate 13g • Fat 8g • Protein 24g • Fiber 2g

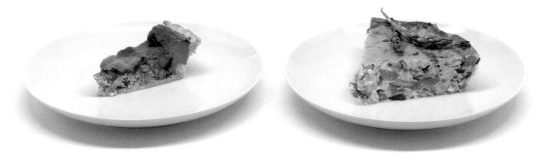

Traditional	How we lowered the CD	Volumetrics
Seafood quiche	• Created a flavorful filling that doesn't need a crust • Added more vegetables • Used low-fat cheese and nonfat yogurt in place of cream • Decreased the amount of cheese	Crab-Asparagus Quiche

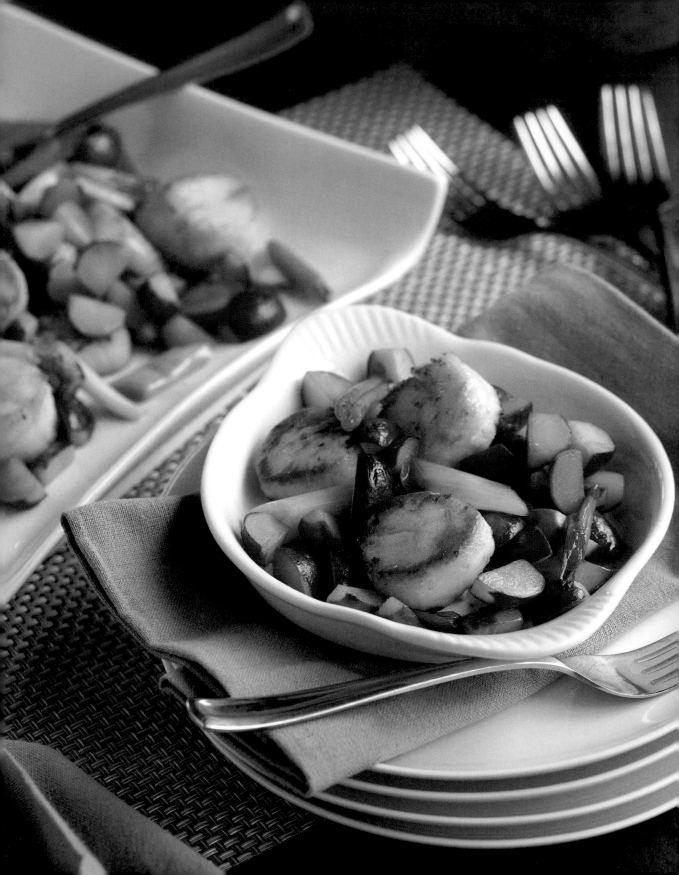

Anne's Sea Scallops with Radishes and Spring Onions

My colleague Anne is a chef who teaches culinary skills to both undergraduates and teens. The rice vinegar reduction forms a flavorful glaze on the lightly cooked, brightly colored vegetables.

Makes 4 servings (265g each), 1½ cups each

1 pound (454g) fresh sea scallops, tough muscle tabs removed

2 tablespoons (16g) all-purpose flour

¼ teaspoon (1g) table salt

½ teaspoon (0.5g) ground coriander

1 tablespoon (14g) vegetable oil

One 1-pound (454g) bag red radishes, cut in quarters

2 bunches (110g) green onions (scallions), white and light green parts, cut into 1-inch lengths

2 tablespoons (30g) rice vinegar

Salt and freshly ground black pepper to taste (optional)

1. Rinse the scallops and pat dry. Place the flour, salt, and coriander in a resealable plastic bag. Add the scallops, seal, and shake to coat completely.

2. Heat 2 teaspoons of the oil in a large nonstick skillet over medium heat. Add the scallops and cook until the bottoms are light brown, about 3 minutes. Turn over the scallops and cook 3 minutes until the other side is light brown. Remove from the pan and set aside on a plate. Do not clean the skillet.

3. Add the remaining oil to the skillet. Add the radishes and green onions and sauté for 30 seconds. Add the vinegar and ¼ cup water and stir to scrape up the browned bits on the bottom of the skillet. Cook the radishes and onions for 2 minutes more. Add the scallops and any accumulated juices, stir gently to combine, and season with salt and pepper if desired.

Nutritional Information per Serving
Calories 180 • CD 0.68 • Carbohydrate 13g • Fat 5g • Protein 21g • Fiber 4g

Greek Tilapia Fillets with Olives and Oregano

Tilapia holds its shape well and has a mild flavor that pairs well with different seasoning combinations. This recipe reminds me of the delicious fish that is served in outdoor cafés throughout Greece.

Makes 4 servings (150g each), 1 fillet each

Four 4-ounce (454g) tilapia fillets

½ cup (67g) sliced pitted Kalamata olives

1 tablespoon (9g) capers, rinsed and drained (optional)

1 medium (17g) shallot, peeled and finely chopped

Juice of ½ lemon (28g)

¼ cup (60g) white wine

1 tablespoon (1g) finely chopped fresh oregano

2 teaspoons (8g) melted butter

Salt and freshly ground black pepper to taste (optional)

4 oregano sprigs, for garnish

1. Preheat the oven to 400°F. Spray a baking dish with cooking spray; make sure the dish is large enough to hold the fish in a single layer.
2. Place the fish in the baking dish. Sprinkle with the olives and the capers, if using. Whisk together the shallot, lemon juice, wine, chopped oregano, and butter in a small bowl and pour over the fish. Season with salt and pepper, if desired.
3. Bake for 15 to 20 minutes, until the fish flakes easily with a fork. Garnish each fillet with an oregano sprig.

Nutritional Information per Serving
Calories 165 • CD 1.1 • Carbohydrate 3g • Fat 6g • Protein 23g • Fiber 1g

Grilled Dishes

Korean-Style Steak Fajitas

Mexican-Korean fusion food is popular in Los Angeles and other cities where chefs have taken the best of each cuisine and created new combination dishes. I followed suit—the filling of this dish is entirely Mexican while the Volumetrics-friendly lettuce wrap is common in Korean grilled dishes.

Makes 4 servings (275g each), 3 or 4 fajita wraps each

🥘 Good for leftovers

12 ounces (340g) lean flank steak, trimmed of visible fat, cut into ½-inch-wide strips

2 medium (238g) red bell peppers, seeded and sliced into rings

2 small (220g) onions, peeled and sliced into rings

1 cup (264g) red or green salsa

1 head (238g) red or green leaf lettuce, separated into leaves, washed, and dried

½ cup (8g) chopped fresh cilantro

8 (36g) red radishes, finely chopped

4 (60g) green onions (scallions), white and light green parts only, sliced into thin rounds

1. Combine the steak, red peppers, onions, and ¼ cup of the salsa in a medium bowl. Stir to combine. Refrigerate for 15 minutes.

2. Heat a grill pan or nonstick skillet over medium-high heat. Remove the steak and vegetables from the salsa, shaking off and discarding the extra salsa, and cook, stirring occasionally, until the steak is fully cooked and the vegetables are soft, about 7 minutes. Remove the steak from the pan if it is done before the vegetables.

3. Serve the steak and vegetables on a platter, with a plate of lettuce leaves and bowls of the remaining salsa, cilantro, radishes, and green onions as condiments to be added by each diner at the table.

Nutritional Information per Serving

Calories 205 • CD 0.75 • Carbohydrate 15g • Fat 7g • Protein 21g • Fiber 4g

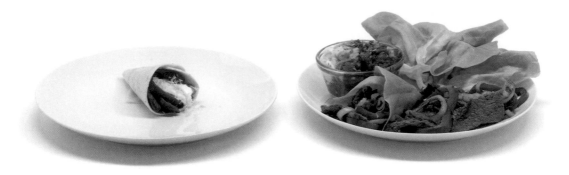

Traditional	How we lowered the CD	Volumetrics
Steak fajitas	• Used lettuce instead of tortillas • Chose a lean cut of beef	Korean-Style Steak Fajitas

Chicken and Zucchini Skewers with Peanut Dipping Sauce

This quick and easy dish is so versatile that you can make it with chicken breast or thigh meat, beef, or turkey, and use any vegetable that you can thread onto a skewer, including mushrooms, peppers, and pearl onions. I serve it as a main course or an appetizer. Pictured on page 143.

Makes 4 main course servings (175g each), 2 skewers each

SKEWERS

1 pound (454g) skinless, boneless chicken breast, cut into 1-inch cubes

1 medium (225g) zucchini, cut in half lengthwise, then crosswise into ½-inch slices

¼ cup (60g) orange juice

1 tablespoon (15g) reduced-sodium soy sauce

1 (3g) garlic clove, peeled and finely chopped

8 wooden skewers

SAUCE

¼ cup (64g) peanut butter

¼ cup (61g) nonfat plain yogurt

Juice of ½ lime (22g)

1 small (10g) shallot, peeled and finely chopped

½ teaspoon (3g) reduced-sodium soy sauce

Pinch of cayenne pepper

1. Combine the chicken, zucchini, orange juice, soy sauce, and garlic in a medium bowl. Mix to coat, cover, and refrigerate for at least 1 hour. Soak the skewers in water for at least 1 hour.

2. Preheat the oven to 400°F. Spray a 9 by 13-inch baking pan with cooking spray.

3. Remove the chicken and zucchini from the marinade and thread alternately onto the skewers. (Discard leftover marinade.) Place the skewers in the pan in a single layer. Bake for 20 minutes, turning over once, until the chicken is lightly browned and sizzling.

4. Meanwhile, stir together the peanut butter, yogurt, lime juice, shallot, soy sauce, and cayenne in a small bowl.

5. Serve the skewers hot, with the dipping sauce.

Nutritional Information per Serving
Calories 245 • CD 1.4 • Carbohydrate 7g • Fat 11g • Protein 30g • Fiber 1g

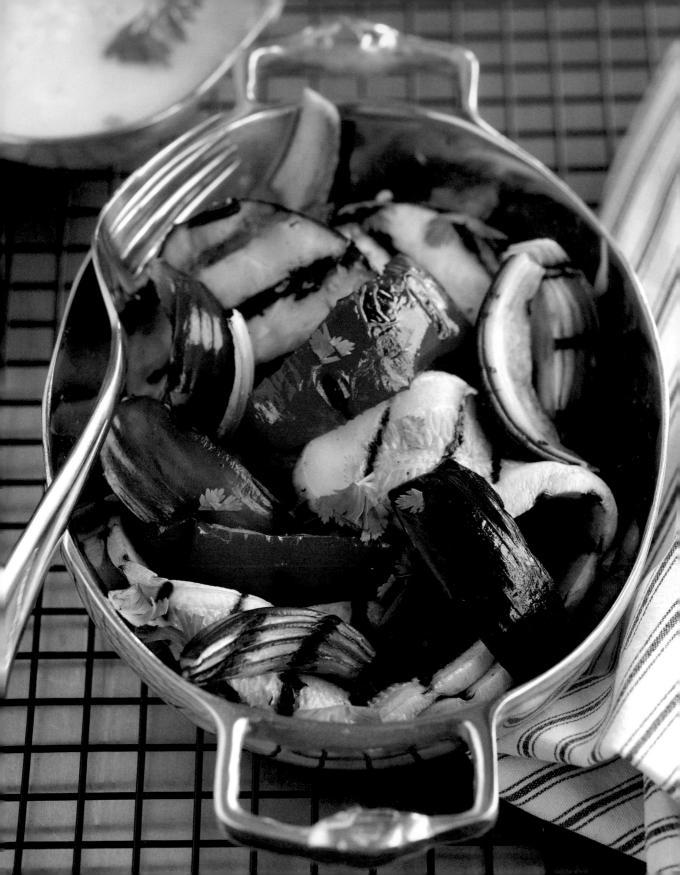

Persian-Style Grilled Vegetables

I enjoy preparing a combination of vegetables of different colors, with classic yogurt and Persian herb condiments, to give this dish a festive feel. The vegetables can be broiled or grilled in a grill pan when an outdoor grill is not available. Use any leftover vegetables as a tasty Volumetrics sandwich filling.

Makes 6 servings (175g each), about 7 pieces each

 Vegetarian 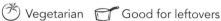 Good for leftovers

1 medium (548g) eggplant, sliced into ½-inch rounds

1 medium (196g) summer squash, sliced lengthwise into ½-inch strips

2 medium (238g) bell peppers, any color, seeded and sliced lengthwise into 8 strips each

1 large (150g) red onion, peeled and cut into 8 wedges

Juice of 2 lemons (96g)

Zest of 1 lemon

1½ tablespoons (20g) olive oil

1 tablespoon (15g) Dijon mustard

3 (9g) garlic cloves, peeled and finely chopped

¾ cup (184g) nonfat plain yogurt

1 cup (46g) finely chopped fresh mint, cilantro, or basil

1. Place the eggplant, squash, peppers, and onion in a large bowl. Whisk together the lemon juice, lemon zest, olive oil, mustard, and garlic in a small bowl. Add salt to taste. Stir 2 tablespoons into the yogurt and refrigerate. Pour the remainder over the vegetables. Stir to coat and marinate for 30 minutes.

2. Meanwhile, preheat a gas or charcoal grill on one side only.

3. Grill the vegetables over indirect heat for about 10 minutes, or until the cooked surface softens and grill marks develop, brushing once with the leftover marinade. Turn over and grill for 5 to 10 minutes more, brushing with the leftover marinade, until the vegetables are soft. Remove each vegetable when done and place on a platter. They may cook at different rates.

4. Serve the vegetables with the yogurt dip and chopped mint on the side.

Nutritional Information per Serving
Calories 110 • CD 0.63 • Carbohydrate 16g • Fat 4g • Protein 4g • Fiber 5g

Chilis

Volumetrics Chili con Carne

I added cocoa powder and cinnamon to give depth to the flavor of this hearty chili. If my market doesn't have chili-seasoned beans, I switch to regular canned beans.

Makes 6 servings (445g each), about 1½ cups chili plus ½ cup rice each

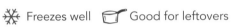 ❄ Freezes well   ⌇ Good for leftovers

2 teaspoons (8g) olive oil

12 ounces (340g) lean ground beef (at least 90% lean)

1 medium (119g) onion, peeled and chopped

2 (6g) garlic cloves, peeled and finely chopped

2 medium (238g) red bell peppers, seeded and chopped

One 1.25-ounce (34g) packet chili seasoning

2 teaspoons (4g) unsweetened cocoa powder

½ teaspoon (1g) ground cinnamon

One 15-ounce (425g) can chili-seasoned pinto beans

Two 14.5-ounce (822g) cans tomatoes with green chiles

1 cup (165g) frozen corn kernels

Salt and freshly ground pepper to taste

1 cup (185g) brown rice

6 tablespoons (42g) shredded reduced-fat cheddar cheese

3 (45g) green onions (scallions), white and light green parts, sliced into thin rounds

2 tablespoons (31g) reduced-fat sour cream

1. Heat the oil in a large saucepan over medium heat. Add the beef and cook, stirring to break up large clumps, until lightly browned, about 5 minutes. Remove from the pan and keep warm.

2. Add the onion, garlic, red peppers, and chili seasoning to the oil and cook for 3 minutes, until the vegetables begin to soften.

3. Add the beef back and any accumulated juices. Stir in the cocoa, cinnamon, beans, tomatoes, and corn. Bring to a boil, then reduce the heat to a simmer, partially cover, and cook for 20 to 30 minutes, stirring occasionally, until the chili is at the desired thickness. Season with salt and pepper.

4. Meanwhile, cook the rice according to package directions.

5. Serve the chili in bowls over the rice, garnished with the cheese, green onions, and sour cream.

Nutritional Information per Serving
Calories 425 • CD 0.96 • Carbohydrate 59g • Fat 12g • Protein 23g • Fiber 10g

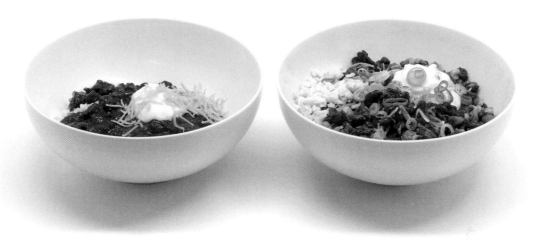

Traditional	How we lowered the CD	Volumetrics
Chili con carne	• Chose lean ground beef instead of higher-fat beef chunks • Cooked the onions and garlic in liquid from the beef • Added more vegetables and canned tomatoes • Included beans • Used reduced-fat cheese and sour cream	Volumetrics Chili con Carne

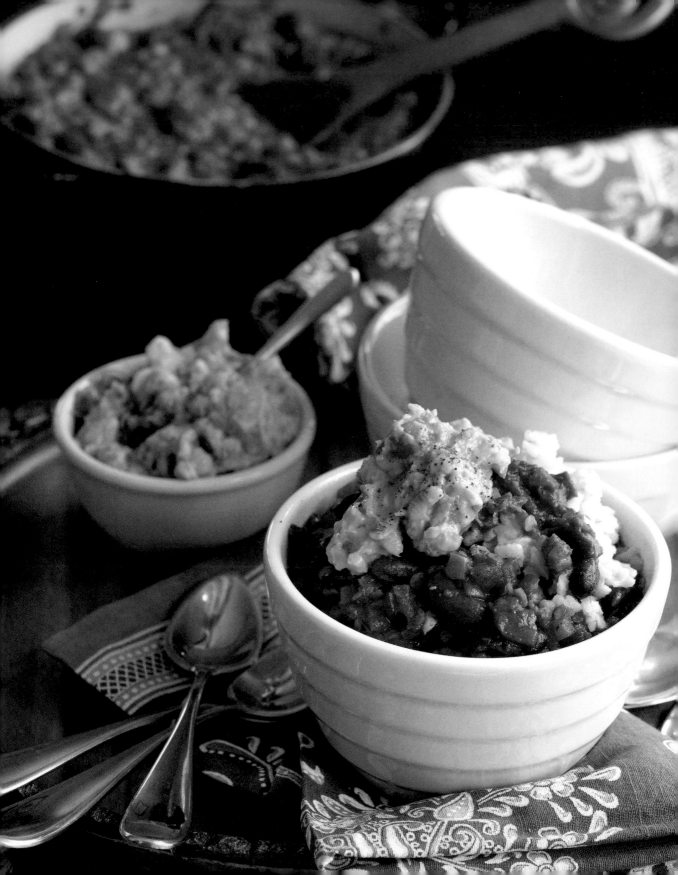

Juliet's Vegetarian Chili

My daughter Juliet and I created this recipe with a surprise ingredient: red lentils. They add thickness and protein while completely breaking down so that you don't notice they are there. Add whatever vegetables are in your refrigerator, such as zucchini, butternut squash, mushrooms, or green beans. To turn up the heat, replace the bell pepper with a hot fresh pepper, canned green chiles, or canned chipotles.

Makes 6 servings (465g each), about 1½ cups chili plus ½ cup rice each

⊙ Vegetarian ❄ Freezes well ▭ Good for leftovers

2 teaspoons (8g) olive oil

1 medium (119g) onion, peeled and finely chopped

2 (6g) garlic cloves, peeled and finely chopped

2 tablespoons (16g) chili powder

1 teaspoon (2g) ground cumin

3 (120g) celery stalks, diced

1 large (144g) carrot, peeled and diced

1 medium (119g) red bell pepper, seeded and diced

One 28-ounce (794g) can crushed tomatoes

Two 15.5-ounce (878g) cans red kidney beans, rinsed and drained

½ cup (96g) red lentils

1 tablespoon (15g) light brown sugar

Salt and freshly ground black pepper to taste (optional)

1 cup (195g) brown rice

6 tablespoons (87g) guacamole

½ teaspoon (1g) cayenne pepper

1. Heat the oil in a large saucepan over medium heat. Add the onions, garlic, chili powder, and cumin and cook, stirring occasionally, for 3 minutes, until the onions begin to soften. Add the celery, carrot, and red pepper and cook for 5 minutes.

2. Add the tomatoes, 1 cup water, the kidney beans, lentils, and brown sugar. Bring to a boil, then reduce the heat to a simmer, partially cover, and cook for 20 to 30 minutes, stirring occasionally and adding extra water as needed, until the vegetables are tender. Season with salt and pepper if desired.

3. Meanwhile, cook the rice according to package directions.

4. Serve the chili in bowls over the rice, topped with 1 tablespoon guacamole and dusted with cayenne pepper.

Nutritional Information per Serving

Calories 375 • CD 0.81 • Carbohydrate 68g • Fat 6g • Protein 16g • Fiber 14g

White Turkey Chili

This dish gets its name from the light-colored turkey and beans and the absence of tomato sauce. The split peas round out the flavor and thicken the chili.

Makes 4 servings (520g each), about 1¼ cups chili plus ½ cup bulgur wheat each

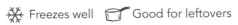 ❄ Freezes well   🍲 Good for leftovers

2 teaspoons (8g) olive oil

1 medium (119g) onion, peeled and finely chopped

2 (6g) garlic cloves, peeled and finely chopped

1 medium (119g) green bell pepper, seeded and finely chopped

1 tablespoon (8g) chili powder

1 teaspoon (2g) ground cumin

12 ounces (340g) skinless raw turkey breast, diced

One 15.5-ounce (439g) can white kidney or cannellini beans, rinsed and drained

One 14.5-ounce (411g) can reduced-sodium chicken broth

½ cup (98g) dried yellow or green split peas

1 teaspoon (2g) dried oregano

Salt and freshly ground black pepper and cayenne pepper to taste (optional)

1 cup (140g) bulgur wheat

½ cup (132g) green or tomatillo salsa

1. Heat the oil in a large saucepan over medium heat. Add the onions, garlic, green pepper, chili powder, and cumin and cook for 7 minutes, stirring often, until the vegetables begin to soften.
2. Add the turkey, beans, broth, ½ cup water, the split peas, and oregano. Bring to a boil, then reduce the heat to a simmer, partially cover, and cook for 20 to 30 minutes, stirring occasionally, until the peas soften. Season with salt, pepper, and cayenne if desired.
3. Meanwhile, prepare the bulgur wheat according to package directions.
4. Serve in bowls over the bulgur wheat and topped with salsa.

Nutritional Information per Serving
Calories 440 • CD 0.85 • Carbohydrate 62g • Fat 4g • Protein 40g • Fiber 18g

SIDE DISHES
Grain Salads

Quinoa Tabbouleh Salad

This colorful dish, developed by Jackie, a postdoctoral fellow in my department, is a favorite for picnics and parties. I use whichever vinegar I have on hand—cider, white or red wine, white balsamic, or champagne.

Makes 8 servings (210g each), 1½ cups each

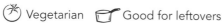 Vegetarian   Good for leftovers

1 cup (170g) quinoa

Juice of 1 lemon (48g)

2 tablespoons (30g) cider vinegar

1 (3g) garlic clove, peeled and finely chopped

1 teaspoon (2g) dried oregano

1 tablespoon (14g) olive oil

1 bunch (36g) radishes (about 8), trimmed and thinly sliced

1 small (74g) green bell pepper, seeded and finely chopped

Half of a 10-ounce (142g) bag matchstick carrots (about 2 cups)

1 bunch (120g) green onions (scallions), white and light green parts, sliced

1 pint (280g) cherry tomatoes, cut in half

1 medium (201g) cucumber, seeded if desired, finely chopped

1 cup (60g) chopped fresh parsley

1. Prepare the quinoa according to the package directions. Place in a large bowl and allow to cool for 30 minutes.

2. Meanwhile, whisk together the lemon juice, vinegar, garlic, and oregano in a small bowl.

3. Drizzle the quinoa with the olive oil and stir gently to combine. Fold in the radishes, green pepper, carrots, green onions, tomatoes, cucumber, and parsley. Add the lemon juice mixture and fold to combine. Serve at room temperature or chilled.

Nutritional Information per Serving

Calories 125 • CD 0.60 • Carbohydrate 20g • Fat 3g • Protein 4g • Fiber 4g

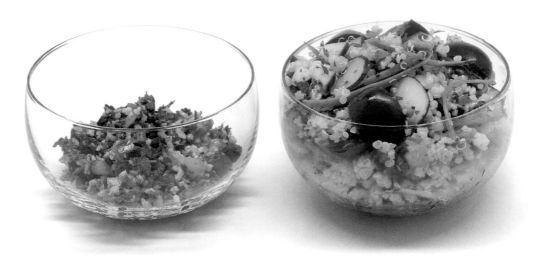

Traditional	How we lowered the CD	Volumetrics
Tabbouleh	• Increased the amount and variety of vegetables • Used much less oil	Quinoa Tabbouleh Salad

Kim's Black Bean and Barley Salad

Kim, my administrative assistant, says that she brings this salad to picnics and potlucks because everyone loves it and asks for the recipe. I love its versatility—any combination of beans and vegetables makes an equally delicious salad. The barley is a must for texture.

Makes 4 servings (255g each), 1 cup each

🍅 Vegetarian   🍲 Good for leftovers

⅓ cup (66g) pearled barley

Juice of 1 orange (80g) or ¼ cup orange juice

2 tablespoons (30g) white balsamic vinegar

2 tablespoons (28g) olive oil

1½ teaspoons (3g) ground cumin

1 teaspoon (2g) dried oregano

1 (3g) garlic clove, peeled and finely chopped

Salt and freshly ground black pepper to taste (optional)

One 15.5 ounce (439g) can black beans, rinsed and drained

1 cup (145g) fresh or frozen corn kernels

2 (30g) green onions (scallions), white and light green parts only, finely chopped

1 small (74g) red bell pepper, seeded and finely chopped

1 small (100g) avocado, split, pitted, peeled, and diced

½ cup (8g) chopped fresh cilantro

1 small lime, cut into 8 wedges

1. Combine the barley and 1 cup water in a small saucepan. Bring to a boil, then reduce heat, cover, and simmer until the barley is just tender, about 40 minutes. Drain off any remaining water.

2. Meanwhile, make the dressing by whisking together the orange juice, vinegar, olive oil, cumin, oregano, garlic, and salt and pepper if using.

3. Gently combine the beans, corn, green onions, red pepper, avocado, cilantro, and cooked barley in a medium bowl. Add the dressing and toss to combine. Serve warm or chilled, garnishing each serving with 2 lime wedges.

Nutritional Information per Serving
Calories 280 • CD 1.1 • Carbohydrate 39g • Fat 12g • Protein 8g • Fiber 9g

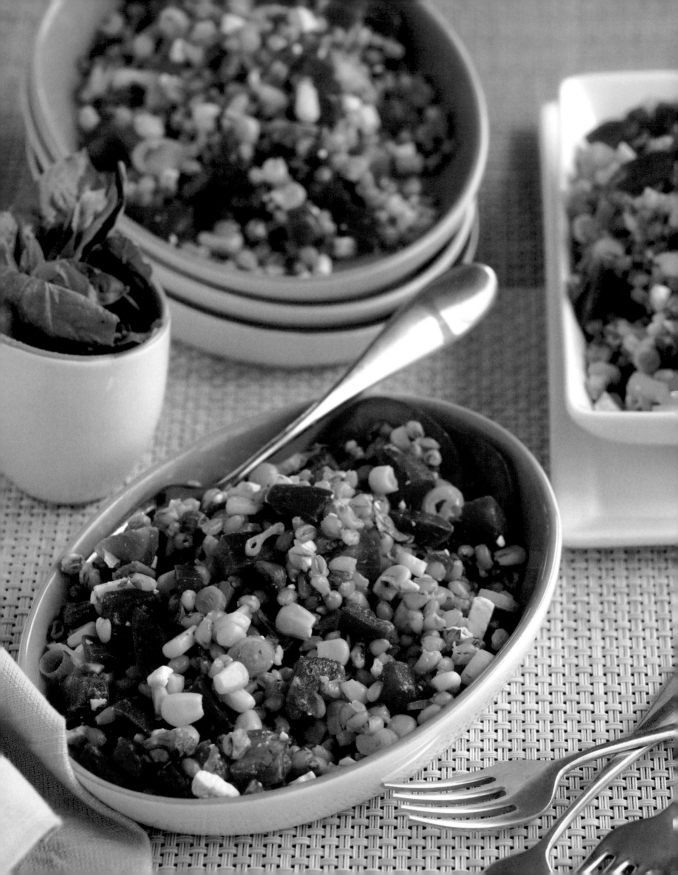

Wheatberry Salad

Wheatberries have a delicious nutty flavor that gives you a delicious way to get whole grains. I love them combined with the zestiness of the balsamic vinegar and feta cheese. Both my daughter Melissa and I bring this to buffets and potlucks, where it is a favorite.

Makes 6 servings (160g each), about 1 cup each

 Vegetarian 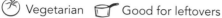 Good for leftovers

1 cup (184g) wheatberries

½ cup (82g) fresh or thawed frozen corn kernels (see note)

3 tablespoons (45g) balsamic vinegar

1 tablespoon (14g) olive oil

3 medium (369g) tomatoes, chopped

2 (30g) green onions (scallions), white and light green parts only, sliced into thin rounds

¼ cup (34g) crumbled fat-free Mediterranean herb feta cheese

2 tablespoons (30g) capers, drained (optional)

¼ cup (10g) finely chopped fresh basil

Salt and freshly ground black pepper to taste

1. Cook the wheatberries according to package instructions. Drain, place in a large bowl, and while the wheatberries still are hot, stir in the corn, vinegar, and olive oil. Allow to cool to room temperature.

2. Add the tomatoes, green onions, cheese, capers if using, and basil and toss gently. Season with salt and pepper. Serve at room temperature or chill before serving.

NOTE: Adding the corn to the hot wheatberries will cook the corn.

Nutritional Information per Serving
Calories 155 • CD 0.97 • Carbohydrate 28g • Fat 3g • Protein 8g • Fiber 5g

Vegetables

Asian Green Beans

Jennifer, my lab manager, says that this recipe turns most kids into vegetable lovers. It's so popular that you may need to double the quantities!

Makes 4 servings (130g each), 1 cup each

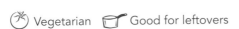 Vegetarian　　 Good for leftovers

1 pound (454g) green beans, ends trimmed, snapped in half

1 tablespoon (16g) hoisin sauce

2 tablespoons (30g) reduced-sodium soy sauce

1 teaspoon (4g) sesame oil

One 8-ounce (227g) can sliced water chestnuts, drained

1 tablespoon (15g) rice vinegar

1 tablespoon (10g) finely diced red bell pepper, for garnish (optional)

1. Place the green beans in a microwaveable bowl with ½ inch water. Cover and microwave on high for 4 minutes or until beans are just tender. Drain.
2. Meanwhile, combine the hoisin sauce, soy sauce, and sesame oil in a small bowl.
3. Spray a medium skillet or wok with cooking spray. Place over medium-high heat and add the green beans, sauce mixture, and water chestnuts. Cook for 3 minutes, stirring, until the green beans and water chestnuts are hot and coated with sauce. Add the vinegar and stir until coated. Garnish with the red pepper, if desired.

Nutritional Information per Serving
Calories 65 • CD 0.50 • Carbohydrate 14g • Fat 1g • Protein 3g • Fiber 4g

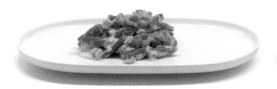 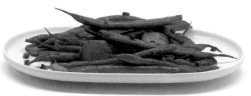

Traditional	How we lowered the CD	Volumetrics
Green bean casserole	• Eliminated the creamy mushroom sauce • Steamed the green beans rather than cooking with fat • Used sesame oil for flavor	Asian Green Beans

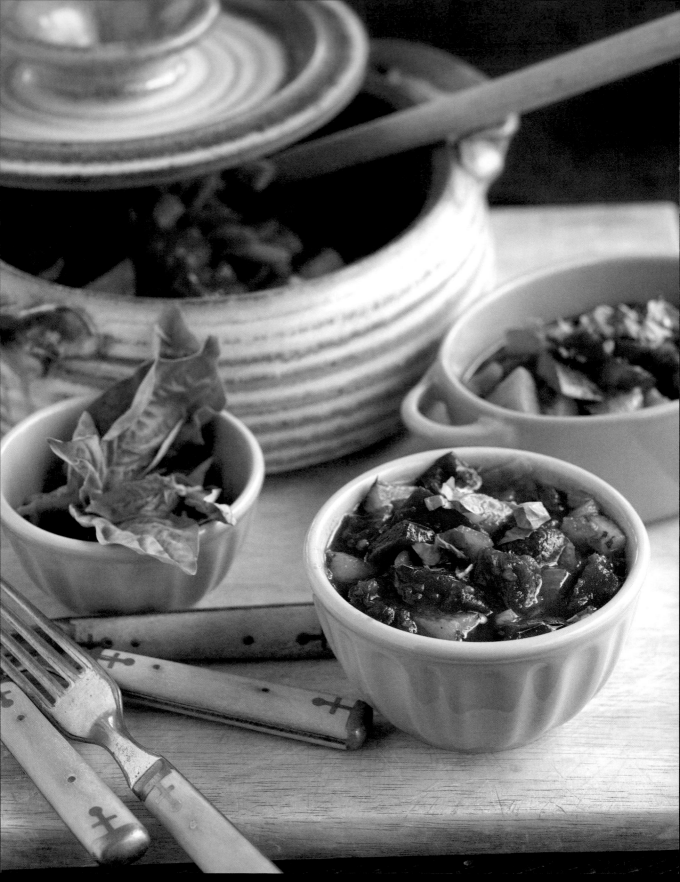

South-of-France Ratatouille

I love the versatility of ratatouille. A classic side dish, ratatouille also enhances sandwiches and is a flavorful topping for fish, chicken, baked potato, or pasta. This recipe differs from the traditional in that it does not include eggplant; feel free to add it in place of or in addition to some of the other vegetables.

Makes 4 servings (225g each), 1 cup each

🍅 Vegetarian   🍲 Good for leftovers

1 tablespoon (14g) olive oil

1 (3g) garlic clove, peeled and finely chopped

1 medium (119g) yellow onion, peeled and chopped

1 medium (119g) red bell pepper, seeded and cut into ¾-inch pieces

1 medium (119g) orange, yellow, or green bell pepper, seeded and cut into ¾-inch pieces

1 medium (196g) zucchini or yellow summer squash, cut into ¾-inch cubes

One 14.5-ounce (411g) can plain or seasoned diced tomatoes, or 1 pound fresh tomatoes, diced

½ cup (120g) vegetable broth or water

2 tablespoons (33g) tomato paste

1 tablespoon (3g) chopped fresh thyme or basil or 1 teaspoon dried thyme or basil

Salt and freshly ground black pepper to taste

Red pepper flakes (optional)

1. Heat the olive oil in a large skillet over medium heat. Cook the garlic and onion for 5 minutes, stirring occasionally, until the onions are soft and translucent. Add the peppers and cook for 10 minutes, stirring occasionally. Add the zucchini and cook for 5 minutes. Drain the canned tomatoes, if using, and reserve the juice. Add the tomatoes, broth, tomato paste, and thyme and stir to combine.

2. Reduce the heat to low, cover, and simmer for 20 minutes. Simmer longer if you prefer a thicker consistency or add some of the reserved tomato juice for a moister ratatouille. Season with salt and pepper, and pepper flakes, if desired.

Nutritional Information per Serving
Calories 110 • CD 0.49 • Carbohydrate 16g • Fat 4g • Protein 3g • Fiber 3g

Grilled Portobello Mushroom Caps

With two daughters who are vegetarians, I am always making dishes that they can eat at a cookout or barbecue. I either leave the mushrooms whole for vegetarians to use in place of a burger patty or slice them after cooking to serve as a flavorful side dish.

Makes 4 servings (85g each), 1 cap each

 Vegetarian

4 teaspoons (20g) olive oil

¼ cup (60g) red wine vinegar

4 (12g) garlic cloves, peeled and finely chopped

1 tablespoon (4g) dried basil

Salt and freshly ground black pepper to taste

4 (454g) portobello mushroom caps (about 1 pound total)

1. Whisk together the oil, vinegar, garlic, basil, and salt and pepper in a medium bowl. Place the mushroom caps next to each other, gill side up, in a glass baking dish. Pour the oil and vinegar mixture evenly into the caps. Allow the mushrooms to marinate at room temperature for at least 10 minutes.

2. Meanwhile heat an outdoor grill to medium or heat a grill pan on the stove over medium heat.

3. Grill the mushrooms gill side up for 15 to 20 minutes, until the oil and vinegar mixture is bubbling and the tops of mushroom caps have grill marks. Turn the mushrooms over and grill for 10 minutes more.

4. Serve whole or sliced, hot or at room temperature.

Nutritional Information per Serving
Calories 75 • CD 0.86 • Carbohydrate 6g • Fat 5g • Protein 3g • Fiber 2g

Sweet Potato Casserole

I prefer this lightened-up holiday classic to overly sweet casseroles. I use fresh sweet potatoes and a crispy sweet topping with just enough crunch and nutty flavor to contrast the flavor and texture of the sweet potatoes.

Makes 10 servings (100g each), about ½ cup each

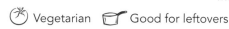 Vegetarian 🍲 Good for leftovers

SWEET POTATOES

4 cups (800g) mashed sweet potatoes (about 3 pounds raw; see note)

½ cup (122g) low-fat milk

1 tablespoon (14g) butter

½ teaspoon (3g) table salt

½ teaspoon (1g) ground cinnamon

½ teaspoon (0.5g) ground nutmeg

TOPPING

¼ cup (10g) bran flake cereal, crushed

¼ cup (55g) packed light brown sugar

¼ cup (27g) pecans, finely chopped

1 tablespoon (14g) butter, melted

1. Preheat the oven to 350°F. Spray a 2- or 3-quart glass dish or an 8-inch square baking pan with cooking spray.

2. Combine the potatoes, milk, butter, salt, cinnamon, and nutmeg in a medium bowl. Spoon the mixture into the prepared pan.

3. To make the topping, combine the cereal, sugar, pecans, and melted butter. Sprinkle evenly over the potato mixture.

4. Bake for 30 minutes or until the casserole begins to bubble at the edges.

NOTE: Either bake the sweet potatoes in the oven and peel them when cool enough to handle or boil with the skin on for about 20 minutes or until soft and then remove the skin. If you prefer a chunky consistency, mash the potatoes with a hand masher; for a smoother consistency, use a hand mixer.

Nutritional Information per Serving
Calories 140 • CD 1.4 • Carbohydrate 24g • Fat 5g • Protein 2g • Fiber 3g

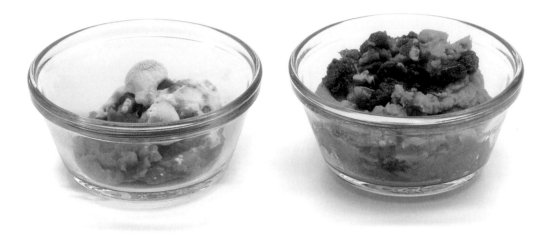

Traditional	How we lowered the CD	Volumetrics
Candied sweet potatoes	• Used fresh sweet potatoes in place of canned sweet potatoes in syrup • Mashed the sweet potatoes with milk and a small amount of butter instead of cream	Sweet Potato Casserole

Balsamic-Glazed Carrots

Balsamic vinegar takes on a sweet-and-sour flavor when it is reduced down to the thickness of syrup. Regular and white balsamic vinegars work equally well. I use this recipe for other root vegetables, including parsnips, turnips, and onions.

Makes 4 servings (130g each), 1 cup each

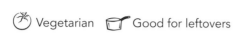 Vegetarian   Good for leftovers

1 pound (454g) carrots, peeled and cut into 1-inch pieces

½ small (33g) onion, peeled and finely chopped

2 (6g) garlic cloves, peeled and finely chopped

¼ cup (60g) balsamic vinegar

2 teaspoons (8g) olive oil

½ teaspoon (2g) sugar

Salt and freshly ground black pepper to taste

1. Place the carrots, onion, garlic, vinegar, olive oil, sugar, and ½ cup water in a small saucepan over medium heat. Bring to a boil, then reduce the heat, cover, and simmer for 20 to 30 minutes, until the carrots are almost tender.

2. Uncover the saucepan and simmer the carrots until the liquid in the pan is reduced to a light glaze, about 15 minutes. Season with salt and pepper.

Nutritional Information per Serving

Calories 85 • CD 0.65 • Carbohydrate 14g • Fat 3g • Protein 1g • Fiber 3g

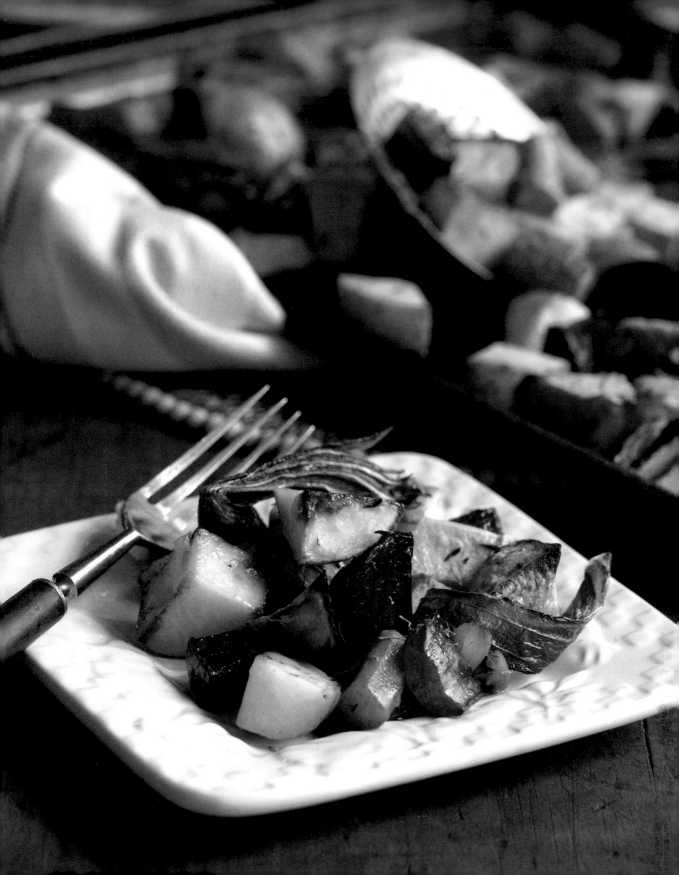

Roasted Diced Fall Vegetables

I choose root vegetables of as many different colors as possible to enhance the appeal of this festive fall dish. The vegetables steam for the first half of the cooking period to make them soft. Baking uncovered then allows them to roast and caramelize.

Makes 6 servings (180g each), about 1 cup each

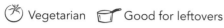 Vegetarian   Good for leftovers

2 cups (244g) 1-inch-thick pieces carrot

2 cups (290g) peeled 1-inch cubes white and/or sweet potato

2 cups (280g) peeled 1-inch cubes butternut or other squash

1 medium (119g) yellow and/or red onion, cut into 8 wedges

1 cup (210g) peeled 1-inch cubes parsnip, turnip, beet, and/or celery root

8 (24g) garlic cloves, peeled

¼ cup (60g) vegetable, chicken, or beef broth, preferably low-sodium

2 tablespoons (28g) olive oil

1 teaspoon (2g) dried herbes de Provence or dried thyme

½ teaspoon (3g) table salt

Freshly ground black pepper to taste

1. Preheat the oven to 425°F. Spray a 9- by 13-inch baking pan with cooking spray.
2. Combine the carrots, potatoes, squash, onion, parsnips, garlic, broth, oil, herbs, salt, and pepper in a large bowl. Transter to the prepared pan and cover with heavy-duty aluminum foil. Bake for 30 minutes.
3. Uncover the pan and bake for 30 minutes more or until the vegetables are soft and the liquid in the pan has evaporated.
4. Turn the oven heat to broil. Place the pan on the top oven rack and broil the vegetables for 2 to 3 minutes until slightly browned.

Nutritional Information per Serving
Calories 180 • CD 1.0 • Carbohydrate 32g • Fat 5g • Protein 4g • Fiber 4g

Mixed Vegetable Salads

Lemony New Potato Salad

The light freshness of this salad is a welcome change from heavy mayonnaise-laden potato salad. Double, triple, or even quadruple this recipe to serve a crowd, and use small red, white, and blue potatoes to make it more festive.

Makes 4 servings (135g each), 1 cup each

🍅 Vegetarian   🥘 Good for leftovers

1 pound (454g) small red potatoes, scrubbed well

1 large (45g) shallot, peeled and finely chopped

Juice of 1 lemon (50g)

1 tablespoon (14g) vegetable oil

1 teaspoon (4g) sugar

1 teaspoon (5g) Dijon mustard

Salt and freshly ground black pepper to taste (optional)

¼ cup (12g) finely chopped chives

1. Place the potatoes in a small saucepan and cover with water. Bring to a boil over medium-high heat, reduce heat to simmer, cover, and cook for 20 minutes or until potatoes feel cooked but firm when tested with a fork. Drain the water, slice the potatoes in half, and place in a medium bowl.

2. Whisk together the shallot, lemon juice, oil, sugar, and mustard. Pour over the warm potatoes and toss gently to combine. Season with salt and pepper if desired. Chill. Sprinkle with the chives before serving.

Nutritional Information per Serving
Calories 125 • CD 0. 93 • Carbohydrate 22g • Fat 4g • Protein 3g • Fiber 2g

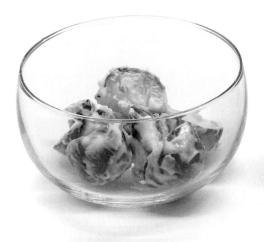 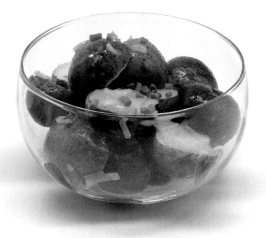

Traditional	How we lowered the CD	Volumetrics
Potato salad	• Cut out mayonnaise • Dressed the potatoes with a lemon juice dressing containing only a small amount of oil	Lemony New Potato Salad

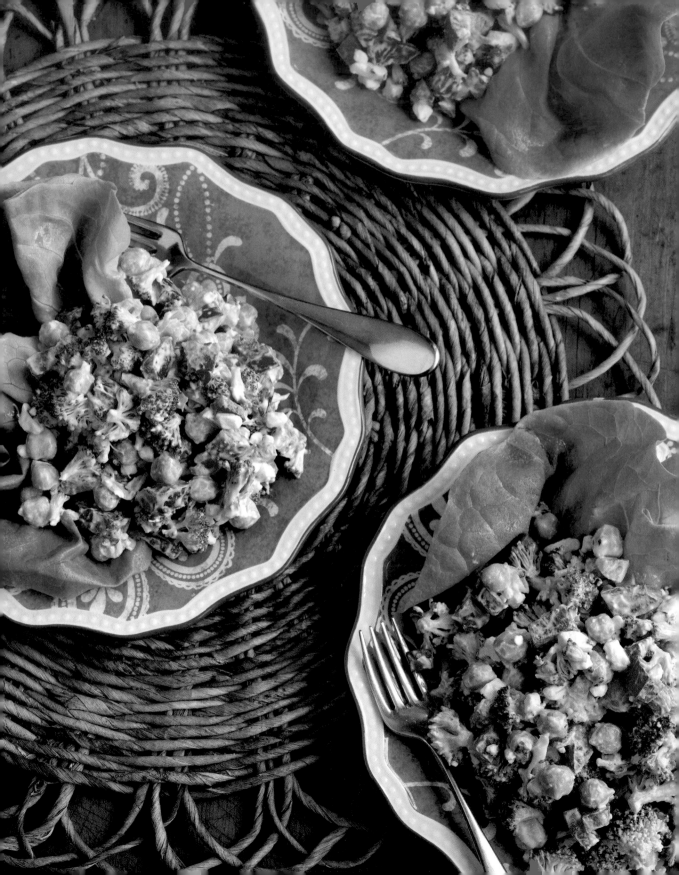

Creamy Broccoli-Feta Salad

This is one of my favorites to take to a picnic—it is colorful and holds up well without wilting. Double the recipe so that you don't run out!

Makes 6 servings (160g each), 1 cup each

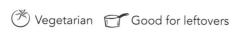 Vegetarian　　Good for leftovers

¾ cup (184g) nonfat plain yogurt

½ cup (68g) crumbled plain or flavored reduced-fat feta cheese

2 tablespoons (30g) lemon juice

1 tablespoon (1g) finely chopped fresh dill or basil

1 (3g) garlic clove, peeled and finely chopped

8 ounces (227g) broccoli florets (from 2 bunches), chopped into small pieces

One 15.5-ounce (439g) can chickpeas, rinsed and drained

1 medium (119g) red bell pepper, seeded and chopped

Salt and freshly ground black pepper to taste (optional)

1. Combine the yogurt, feta, lemon juice, dill, and garlic in a medium bowl.
2. Toss the broccoli, chickpeas, and red pepper with the yogurt dressing in a serving bowl. Season with salt and pepper if desired.

Nutritional Information per Serving
Calories 125 • CD 0.78 • Carbohydrate 19g • Fat 2g • Protein 8g • Fiber 4g

Succotash Salad

Succotash, a combination of corn and lima beans, is a favorite side dish of mine that is not as common as it was when I was a child. I added lima beans but you may prefer using shelled edamame (soybeans). For great flavor, substitute the kernels cut from 8 ears of fresh corn in season for the frozen corn.

Makes 12 servings (105g each), ⅔ cup each

 Vegetarian   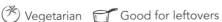 Good for leftovers

⅓ cup (80g) cider vinegar

¼ cup (56g) canola oil

1 tablespoon (15g) lemon juice

⅓ cup (20g) finely chopped fresh parsley

2 tablespoons (5g) chopped fresh basil

1 teaspoon (4g) sugar

½ teaspoon (3g) table salt

⅛ teaspoon (1g) cayenne pepper

1 medium (119g) green bell pepper, seeded and chopped

1 medium (119g) red bell pepper, seeded and chopped

4 cups (656g) frozen corn, thawed

1 cup (164g) frozen lima beans, thawed

1 small (70g) red onion, peeled and chopped

Whisk together the vinegar, oil, lemon juice, parsley, basil, sugar, salt, and cayenne in a large bowl. Add the green and red peppers, corn, lima beans, and onion and mix well. Cover and chill for several hours or overnight.

Nutritional Information per Serving
Calories 125 • CD 1.2 • Carbohydrate 19g • Fat 5g • Protein 3g • Fiber 3g

Rice

Squash Risotto

Traditional risotto requires standing in front of the stove for close to an hour, so when short on time, I prefer this faster, no-fuss recipe. The quick-cooking brown rice makes it less authentic but it is equally tasty. I like to make this with a variety of types of winter squash that grow locally, and all work well in this creamy dish. When *really* short on time, I have even used frozen winter squash.

Makes 6 servings (190g each), 1 cup each

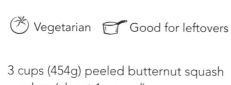 Vegetarian   Good for leftovers

3 cups (454g) peeled butternut squash cubes (about 1 pound)

One 14.5-ounce (411g) can vegetable broth

2 teaspoons (8g) olive oil

2 medium (238g) onions, peeled and chopped

3 (9g) garlic cloves, peeled and finely chopped

1 cup (86g) instant brown rice

½ cup (120g) dry white wine

¼ teaspoon (0.5g) ground nutmeg

1 ounce (28g) grated Parmesan cheese (see note)

3 tablespoons (6g) chopped fresh sage, cilantro, or other herb

Salt and freshly ground pepper to taste

1. Combine 2 cups of the squash with 1 cup of the vegetable broth in a microwaveable bowl, cover, and microwave until the squash is very soft, about 10 minutes. Allow to cool for 10 minutes, then mash or blend until smooth.

2. Meanwhile, finely chop the remaining cup of squash into very small pieces. Heat the olive oil in a medium pot over medium heat. Cook the chopped squash, onion, and garlic until soft, stirring often, about 6 minutes. Stir in the rice, ½ cup of the

vegetable broth, and the wine. Bring to a boil, then reduce the heat and simmer uncovered until almost all the liquid has been absorbed, about 5 minutes.

3. Add the remaining broth and simmer uncovered until almost all the liquid has been absorbed, about 5 minutes.

4. Add the mashed squash and simmer until all the liquid evaporates and the rice is fully cooked, about 8 minutes. Stir in the nutmeg and cheese. Season with salt and pepper to taste. Top each serving with a sprinkle of sage or other herb.

NOTE: 1 ounce Parmesan equals about ½ cup freshly grated cheese or ¼ cup packaged grated cheese.

Nutritional Information per Serving
Calories 160 • CD 0.84 • Carbohydrate 25g • Fat 4g • Protein 5g • Fiber 3g

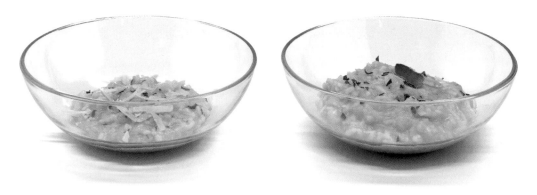

Traditional	How we lowered the CD	Volumetrics
Risotto	• Switched to brown rice • Added squash in place of some of the rice • Decreased the amount of cheese	Squash Risotto

Cauliflower Rice

My daughter Melissa serves this Volumetrics rice with Indian dishes and stews. This is a good recipe for sneaking vegetables into a side dish. Leave out the coconut and cardamom if you're serving this with chili or other stews.

Makes 8 servings (165g each), 1 cup each

Vegetarian   Good for leftovers

1 cup (185g) white basmati rice

¼ cup (20g) shredded unsweetened coconut

5 cardamom pods (optional)

¼ teaspoon (1g) table salt

1 small (454g) head cauliflower (about 1 pound), chopped into small pieces

Half of a 16-ounce (227g) bag frozen peas

1. Place the rice, 2 cups water, the coconut, cardamom if using, and salt in a large pot over medium-high heat. Bring to a boil, place the cauliflower on top of the rice, reduce the heat, cover, and simmer for 10 minutes.

2. Layer the peas on top of the cauliflower, cover, and simmer for 5 to 10 minutes, until all the water is absorbed. Turn off the heat and let pot sit covered for 10 more minutes.

3. Mix to combine. Remove the cardamom pods before serving.

Nutritional Information per Serving
Calories 135 • CD 0.82 • Carbohydrate 26g • Fat 2g • Protein 4g • Fiber 3g

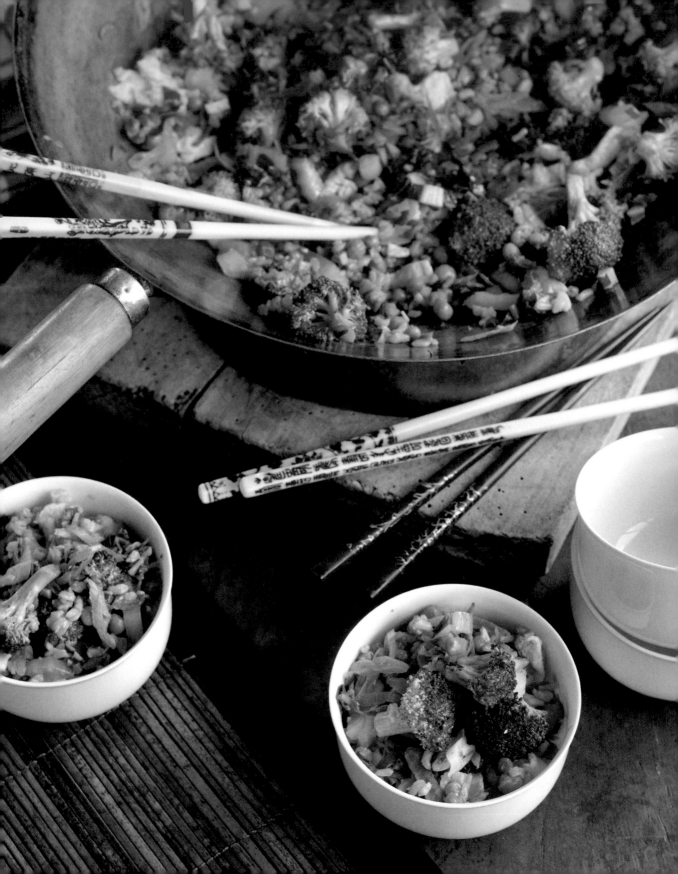

Volumetrics Vegetable Fried Rice

Here's what I love about vegetable fried rice—there are no set rules. I grab vegetables from my fridge, chop them into very small pieces, and cook them in a very hot wok.

Makes 4 servings (230g each), 1 cup each

Vegetarian   Good for leftovers

2 teaspoons (8g) canola oil

1 large (50g) egg

1 tablespoon (10g) finely chopped peeled fresh ginger

2 (6g) garlic cloves, peeled and finely chopped

1 small (61g) carrot, peeled and grated

2 cups (140g) finely chopped Chinese cabbage, such as napa or bok choy

2 cups (142g) small fresh or frozen broccoli florets

1 cup (145g) frozen peas

2 cups (390g) cooked brown rice (see note)

2 tablespoons (30g) reduced-sodium soy sauce

½ teaspoon (2g) sesame oil

2 (30g) green onions (scallions), white and light green parts, sliced into thin rounds

1. Heat 1 teaspoon of the canola oil in a wok or large nonstick skillet over medium-high heat. Break the egg into a small bowl, whisk with a fork, and cook in the wok for 30 seconds. Add the ginger and garlic and cook for 30 seconds to soften.

2. Add the remaining canola oil. Add the carrots and cabbage and stir-fry until the cabbage wilts, about 3 minutes. Add the broccoli and stir-fry until the color turns to bright green, about 2 minutes. Add the peas and rice and gently stir-fry until the rice becomes crisp, about 4 minutes.

3. Whisk together the soy sauce, sesame oil, and 2 tablespoons water. Pour over the rice mixture and toss to combine. Garnish with the green onion.

NOTE: This dish can be made with hot rice—cook ⅔ cup brown rice with 1⅓ cups water—before you cook the egg and vegetables, but cold rice is preferable. Plan ahead by refrigerating leftover rice a day or two before so that it's ready for this recipe.

Nutritional Information per Serving
Calories 210 • CD 0.91 • Carbohydrate 34g • Fat 5g • Protein 8g • Fiber 6g

PARTY DISHES

Jennifer's Buffalo Party Dip

This is a new twist on traditional Buffalo chicken wings. The idea came to my lab manager, Jennifer, one day when she was trying to think of a way to sneak in vegetables at her next party. She substituted cooked chopped cauliflower for the chicken and none of the guests noticed. It was eaten so quickly that she doubled the recipe the next time!

Makes 6 servings (185g each), ½ cup dip plus 6 celery pieces each

 Vegetarian

One 8-ounce (227g) package light cream cheese

½ cup (128g) reduced-fat blue cheese dressing

½ cup (113g) Buffalo wing sauce or hot pepper sauce

¾ cup (185g) shredded reduced-fat cheddar cheese

1 cup (124g) finely chopped cooked cauliflower

12 (480g) celery stalks, for dipping (about 1 bunch)

1. Preheat the oven to 350°F. Spray a medium ovenproof dish with cooking spray.
2. Combine the cream cheese and dressing in a medium skillet over medium heat. Stir frequently until the cream cheese melts. Add the hot sauce and ½ cup of the cheddar. Stir until the cheese is melted. Stir in the cauliflower and remove from the heat.
3. Pour the mixture into the prepared dish. Sprinkle with the remaining cheese.
4. Bake for 25 to 30 minutes, or until bubbly.
5. Meanwhile, wash and trim the celery. Cut each stalk into 3 pieces for serving.

Nutritional Information per Serving
Calories 165 • CD 0.89 • Carbohydrate 10g • Fat 10g • Protein 9g • Fiber 2g

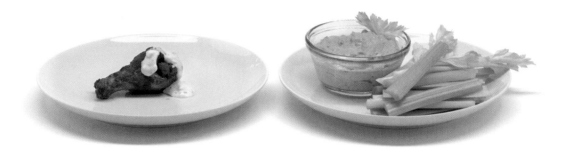

Traditional	How we lowered the CD	Volumetrics
Buffalo chicken wings with blue cheese dressing	• Substituted vegetables for the wings • Used reduced-fat cheeses to make a lower-CD dip • Sneaked in cauliflower	Jennifer's Buffalo Party Dip

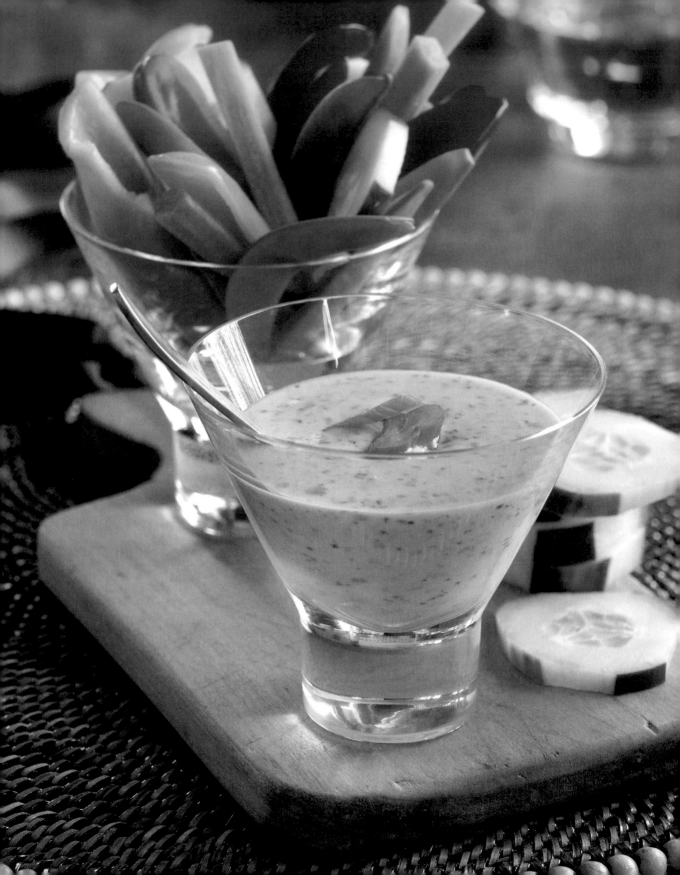

Crudités with Cilantro-Lime Ranch Dip

This dip was created by Kitti, a dietitian in my lab, and quickly became a lab favorite. It is versatile and works as a dip for vegetables, a topping for tacos or fajitas, or even a salad dressing. Tomatillo, a distant member of the tomato family, is a staple in Mexican cooking and adds tanginess to the dressing. Pictured on page 143.

Makes 15 servings (155g each), ¼ cup dip plus ½ cup vegetables each

Vegetarian

4 (136g) tomatillos

1 cup (244g) fat-free milk

Juice of 1 lime (30g)

1 cup (240g) reduced-fat sour cream

1 cup (240g) fat-free mayonnaise

1 small packet (28g) buttermilk ranch dressing mix

¼ teaspoon garlic powder

Small pinch cayenne powder

1 cup (16g) chopped cilantro, or more if you like a strong cilantro taste

FOR DIPPING

2 large (298g) red, yellow, or orange peppers, cut into 8 strips each

2 cups (244g) baby carrots

1 medium (208g) cucumber, cut into slices

2 cups (227g) snow peas or sugar snap peas (about 8 ounces)

1. Remove the paper-like skin from the tomatillos. Broil the tomatillos in a small ovenproof dish until browned on all sides, turning them every couple of minutes. Tomatillos will be soft and flattened.

2. Place the milk in the blender. Add the lime juice; the milk will begin to curdle. Add the tomatillos and any accumulated juices, the sour cream, mayonnaise, dressing mix, garlic, cayenne, and cilantro. Blend until smooth.

3. Refrigerate at least 1 hour. The dressing will thicken upon standing.

4. Arrange the vegetables on platter and serve with dressing in a bowl on the side.

Nutritional Information per Serving
Calories 75 • CD 0.48 • Carbohydrate 10g • Fat 3g • Protein 3g • Fiber 2g

Nutritional Information per Serving, dip alone
Calories 50 • CD 0.83 • Carbohydrate 5g • Fat 3g • Protein 2g • Fiber 0g

Chicken Breast Strips with Smoky Orange Dipping Sauce

The smoky flavor in this dish comes from the chipotle chiles in the orange sauce. The sauce also can stand alone as a grilling sauce for beef, salmon, or tofu.

Makes 8 servings (75g each), 2 strips plus 2 tablespoons sauce each

½ cup (28g) panko bread crumbs

2 teaspoons (4g) paprika

¼ teaspoon (1g) table salt

1 large (50g) egg

SAUCE

½ cup (124g) orange juice

2 tablespoons (30g) cider vinegar

1 tablespoon (16g) light brown sugar

1 tablespoon (16g) chopped canned chipotle chiles, or to taste

1 teaspoon (5g) Dijon mustard

1 pound (454g) skinless, boneless chicken breast, cut into ½-inch-thick strips

1 (3g) garlic clove, peeled and finely chopped

1 tablespoon (8g) cornstarch dissolved in 2 tablespoons (30g) water

1. Preheat the oven to 400°F. Spray a baking sheet with cooking spray or use a nonstick baking sheet.
2. Mix together the bread crumbs, paprika, and salt in a resealable plastic bag. Whisk together the egg and mustard in a medium bowl.
3. Place the chicken strips in the bowl with the egg-mustard mixture and stir until the chicken strips are evenly coated. Transfer the chicken strips to the plastic bag with the bread crumb mixture and shake to coat on all sides. Place on the baking sheet in a single layer.
4. Bake for 25 minutes, turning the strips over after 15 minutes, until the chicken is sizzling and lightly browned.
5. Meanwhile, combine the orange juice, vinegar, sugar, chiles, garlic, and cornstarch mixture in a small microwaveable bowl. Microwave at 30-second intervals, stirring between intervals, until the sauce thickens, about 2 minutes.

Nutritional Information per Serving

Calories 110 • CD 1.5 • Carbohydrate 8g • Fat 2g • Protein 13g • Fiber 0g

POTLUCK DISHES

Melissa's Peanut-Udon Salad

This is great to take to parties—it is the dish I am most frequently requested to make. Definitely double the recipe or you may be sent home to make more! Try asking the guests what makes the noodles so creamy. I bet no one will come up with the secret ingredient: tofu! If you prefer, use broccoli slaw (or other crunchy vegetables) instead of bean sprouts.

Makes 6 servings (190g each), 1½ cups each

 Vegetarian

One 8.8-ounce (250g) package udon noodles (see note)

7 ounces (198g) soft or silken tofu (½ package)

¼ cup (60g) rice vinegar

3 tablespoons (42g) peanut butter

1½ tablespoons (15g) chopped peeled fresh ginger

1 tablespoon (15g) reduced-sodium soy sauce

1 tablespoon (13g) sugar

2 teaspoons (8g) sesame oil

1 teaspoon (5g) Dijon mustard

1 (3g) garlic clove, peeled

2 tablespoons (28g) canola oil

½ cup (8g) cilantro stems and leaves

One 8-ounce (227g) package bean sprouts (3 cups)

Salt to taste

1. Cook the udon noodles according to the package directions. Drain and rinse in a colander under cold water until cool. Set aside.

2. Meanwhile, to prepare the sauce, purée the tofu, vinegar, peanut butter, ginger, soy sauce, sugar, sesame oil, mustard, and garlic in a blender or food processor. Slowly add the canola oil while blending or processing.

3. Place the noodles, cilantro, and bean sprouts into a large bowl and add the sauce.

Mix using a large fork or spaghetti server to coat the noodles and vegetables evenly. Add salt and serve at room temperature.

NOTE: Udon noodles come in different thicknesses; I prefer the thickest. Cooking time will depend on the type you choose.

Nutritional Information per Serving
Calories 260 • CD 1.4 • Carbohydrate 31g • Fat 12g • Protein 8g • Fiber 1g

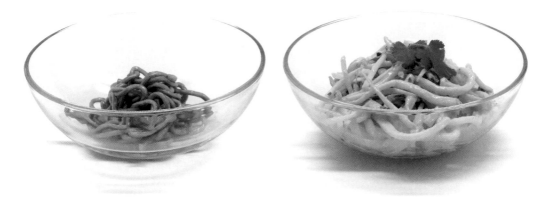

Traditional	How we lowered the CD	Volumetrics
Sesame noodles	• Added tofu for creaminess • Reduced the amounts of peanut butter and sesame oil • Added more vegetables	Melissa's Peanut-Udon Salad

Volumetrics Macaroni and Cheese

My lab staff has been innovative in creating recipes with hidden vegetables. The colors of the cauliflower and summer squash blend in with the macaroni and cheese. This creamy version of the popular comfort food is the type of dish our study participants love.

Makes 6 servings (240g each), 1¼ cups each

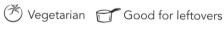 Vegetarian   Good for leftovers

8 ounces (227g) dry macaroni

1 tablespoon (14g) butter

2 tablespoons (16g) flour

½ teaspoon (3g) table salt

1 cup (244g) fat-free milk

8 ounces (227g) shredded reduced-fat sharp cheddar cheese (about 2 cups)

1¾ cups (225g) frozen cauliflower, cooked and puréed (see note)

1¾ cups (225g) frozen summer squash, cooked and puréed (see note)

1. Preheat the oven to 350°F. Spray a 2- or 3-quart casserole with cooking spray.

2. Cook the macaroni according to package directions. Drain in a colander and set aside.

3. Melt the butter in medium saucepan over medium-low heat. Stir in the flour and salt. Gradually stir in the milk. Cook, stirring constantly, until thickened. Add the cheese and stir until melted. Add the puréed vegetables and macaroni and stir until well combined.

4. Pour into the prepared pan and bake, covered, for 35 to 40 minutes, until bubbling.

NOTE: Puréed vegetables can be prepared from cooked frozen or fresh vegetables. Use about 1 cup of each of the puréed vegetables.

Nutritional Information per Serving
Calories 315 • CD 1.3 • Carbohydrate 36g • Fat 11g • Protein 17g • Fiber 2g

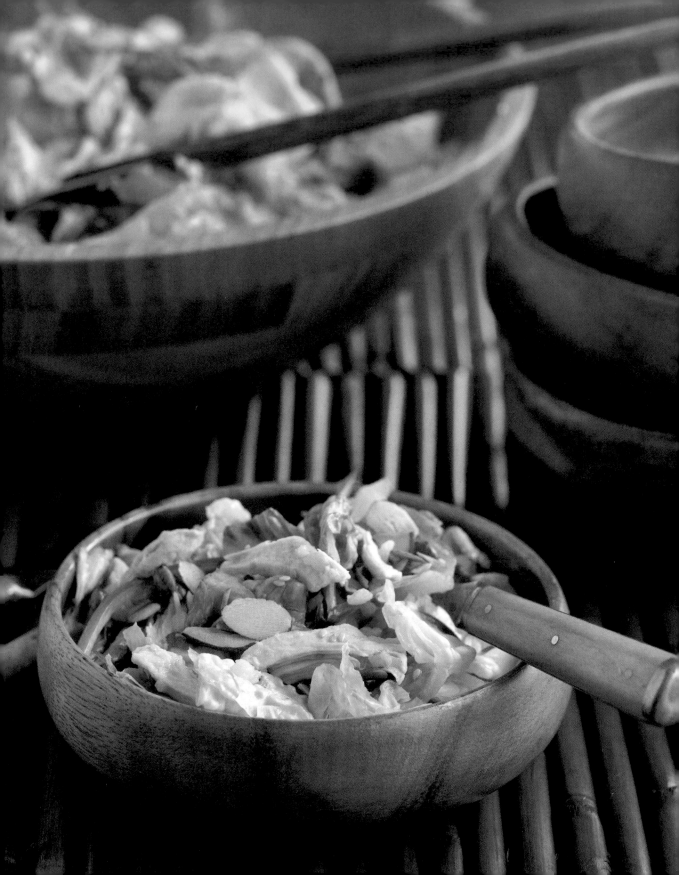

Asian Chicken Salad

This great big salad was a huge hit at the bridal shower for one of my staff members. The sweet and tangy dressing pairs well with the chicken and almonds.

Makes 8 servings (165g each), 1½ cups each

2 large (424g) heads romaine lettuce, rinsed, dried, and shredded

3 cups (420g) shredded cooked chicken breast

1 cup (195g) cooked brown long-grain rice

½ cup (46g) toasted sliced almonds

¼ cup (36g) toasted sesame seeds

2 (30g) green onions (scallions), sliced into thin rounds

½ cup (120g) rice vinegar

¼ cup (56g) canola oil

¼ cup (50g) sugar

1 teaspoon (5g) table salt

½ teaspoon (2g) freshly ground black pepper

1. Toss together the lettuce, chicken, rice, almonds, sesame seeds, and green onions in a large bowl until thoroughly mixed.

2. Whisk or shake together the vinegar, oil, sugar, salt, and pepper until well combined. Pour over the salad and toss.

Nutritional Information per Serving
Calories 275 • CD 1.7 • Carbohydrate 16g • Fat 15g • Protein 20g • Fiber 3g

SNACKS
Dips

Volumetrics Spinach-Artichoke Dip

Traditional spinach-artichoke dip is a party favorite of mine, but its CD is high. You can spice this dip up by adding seasonings such as Creole spices or cayenne pepper.

Makes 8 servings (240g each),

½ cup dip plus about 10 carrot sticks and ½ pita

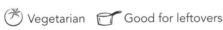 Vegetarian 　Good for leftovers

One 14-ounce (397g) can artichoke hearts in water or brine, drained and chopped

One 10-ounce (280g) box frozen chopped spinach, thawed and squeezed to remove liquid

1 cup (256g) fat-free sour cream

½ cup (120g) light mayonnaise

FOR DIPPING
2 pounds (908g) carrots, peeled, cut in half lengthwise, and then into 3-inch pieces

1 ounce (28g) grated Parmesan cheese (see note)

1 (3g) garlic clove, peeled and finely chopped

1 teaspoon (1g) dried basil, chili powder, or Italian seasoning (optional)

⅛ teaspoon (0.5g) table salt

1 tablespoon (10g) finely chopped carrot, for garnish (optional)

4 (228g) whole-wheat pita breads, cut into wedges

1. Preheat the oven to 350°F. Spray a small ovenproof baking dish with cooking spray.

2. Stir together the artichoke hearts, spinach, sour cream, mayonnaise, cheese, garlic, seasoning, if using, and salt in a medium bowl until well blended. Transfer to the

prepared dish and bake for 35 to 40 minutes, until the edges are bubbling. Garnish with the chopped carrot if desired.

3. Serve warm or at room temperature with the carrots and pita wedges for dipping.

NOTE: 1 ounce Parmesan equals about ½ cup freshly grated cheese or ¼ cup packaged grated cheese.

Nutritional Information per Serving of dip with carrots and pita bread
Calories 215 • CD 0.90 • Carbohydrate 33g • Fat 7g • Protein 8g • Fiber 7g

Nutritional Information per Serving of dip alone
Calories 110 • CD 1.1 • Carbohydrate 9g • Fat 6g • Protein 4g • Fiber 1g

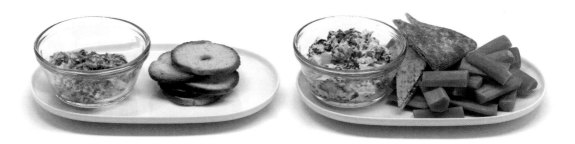

Traditional	How we lowered the CD	Volumetrics
Spinach-artichoke dip	• Switched to fat-free sour cream • Reduced the amount of mayonnaise and used light instead of regular	Volumetrics Spinach-Artichoke Dip

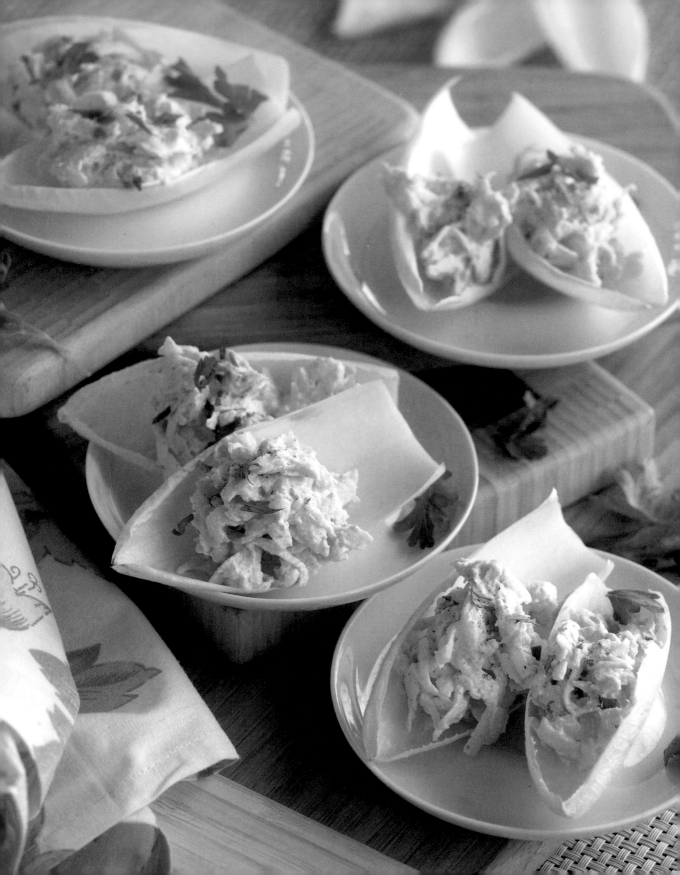

Apple–Goat Cheese Dip with Endive Leaves

I needed to make a quick but elegant appetizer for guests and decided to combine goat cheese, light cream cheese, and curry powder. To add texture, moisture, and flavor while lowering CD, I mixed in shredded apple. The Belgian endive leaves make this dish particularly festive.

Makes 4 servings (165g each), 2 stuffed leaves each

 Vegetarian

2 ounces (57g) soft goat cheese (about ¼ cup)

2 tablespoons (30g) light cream cheese

1 large (170g) Granny Smith or other tart apple, peeled, cored, and shredded

1 teaspoon (2g) curry powder

8 (424g) Belgian endive leaves

Parsley leaves to garnish

Mix together the goat cheese, cream cheese, apple, and curry powder in a small bowl. Spread 2 tablespoons of the dip onto each of the Belgian endive leaves. Garnish with parsley.

Nutritional Information per Serving
Calories 85 • CD 0.51 • Carbohydrate 10g • Fat 3g • Protein 6g • Fiber 4g

Kim's Cantina Night Bean Dip

This Mexican dip, contributed by Kim, my administrative assistant, always is a big hit at parties. Try it with different bean and vegetable combinations, your choice of salsa, and other types of cheese.

Makes 8 servings (205g each), 1 cup dip
plus 1 ounce chips each

 Vegetarian   Good for leftovers

One 16-ounce (454g) can fat-free refried beans

One 15.5-ounce (439g) can black beans, rinsed and drained

1 medium (180g) tomato, chopped

1 medium (119g) green or red bell pepper, seeded and chopped

½ large (80g) onion, peeled and chopped

½ cup (132g) mild, medium, or hot salsa

⅓ cup (44g) grated reduced-fat Mexican cheese blend

½ cup (122g) nonfat plain yogurt (optional)

8 ounces (227g) baked tortilla chips (about 8 cups)

1. Preheat the oven to 350°F.
2. Mix the refried and black beans, tomato, bell pepper, onion, and salsa in a medium bowl. Place in a 9-inch pie plate and sprinkle with the cheese. Bake for 25 to 30 minutes, until bubbly. Top with the yogurt, if desired, and serve with tortilla chips.

Nutritional Information per Serving
Calories 225 • CD 1.1 • Carbohydrate 43g • Fat 2g • Protein 11g • Fiber 7g

Finger Foods

Roasted Eggplant and Fennel Caponata

The beauty of this no-fuss recipe is that the vegetables can roast while I am busy getting ready for guests. Once they're cooked, it takes just minutes to mash them into a coarse dip or spread. Switch the fennel to a few celery stalks if you don't care for its licorice undertones.

Makes 6 servings (280g each), ½ cup caponata plus
5 slices red pepper and 3 slices breed

 Vegetarian 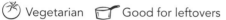 Good for leftovers

1 medium (490g) eggplant (about 1 pound), cut into 1-inch cubes

1 small (234g) fennel bulb (about 8 ounces), chopped

1 medium (160g) tomato, chopped

1 small (78g) red onion, peeled and chopped

4 (12g) garlic cloves, peeled

FOR DIPPING
4 red bell peppers, cut into strips

Small (8 ounce) (227g) whole-wheat baguette, cut into thin slices

¼ cup (60g) balsamic vinegar

2 teaspoons (8g) olive oil

1 teaspoon (4g) sugar

¼ teaspoon (1g) table salt

Freshly ground black pepper to taste

2 tablespoons (20g) golden raisins

6 sliced, pitted olives (optional)

1. Preheat the oven to 425°F. Spray a 9 by 13-inch baking pan with cooking spray.
2. Combine the eggplant, fennel, tomato, onion, garlic, vinegar, olive oil, sugar, salt, and pepper in a large bowl. Transfer to the prepared pan, cover with heavy-duty aluminum foil, and bake for 30 minutes.

3. Uncover the pan and bake for an additional 30 to 35 minutes, until the vegetables are soft and the liquid in the pan has evaporated.

4. Place the vegetables into a medium bowl and mash with a fork or potato masher or process in a food processor to the desired texture. Stir in the raisins. Garnish with olives if desired. Serve with red pepper and baguette slices.

Nutritional Information per Serving of dip with peppers and bread
Calories 195 • CD 0.70 • Carbohydrate 34g • Fat 3g • Protein 8g • Fiber 9g

Nutritional Information per Serving of dip alone
Calories 75 • CD 0.71 • Carbohydrate 14g • Fat 2g • Protein 2g • Fiber 4g

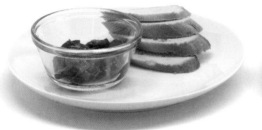 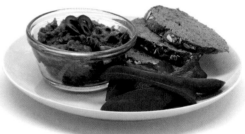

Traditional	How we lowered the CD	Volumetrics
Caponata	• Cut way back on oil • Roasted the eggplant instead of sautéing • Added vegetables	Roasted Eggplant and Fennel Caponata

Zesty Vegetable Pinwheels

This recipe is so popular at staff parties that the platter is empty within minutes. You can fit in a lot of veggies when you chop them finely. Roll the tortilla as tightly as you can to hold in the vegetables.

Makes 8 servings (125g each), 4 pieces each

 Vegetarian

One 8-ounce (227g) package light cream cheese, softened

½ cup (124g) reduced-fat sour cream

1 tablespoon (9g) taco seasoning

4 (232g) reduced-fat 10-inch whole-wheat tortillas, about 100 calories each

1 medium (119g) red or yellow pepper, seeded and chopped

1 cup (71g) finely chopped fresh broccoli florets

1 cup (110g) shredded peeled carrot

¼ cup (32g) finely chopped red onion

¼ cup (34g) sliced pitted Kalamata olives

1. Combine the cream cheese, sour cream, and taco seasoning.
2. Spread one-quarter of the mixture evenly on each of the tortillas, allowing a small border around the edge.
3. Top each tortilla with one-quarter of the vegetables. Starting at one edge, roll up each tortilla tightly. Wrap in plastic wrap and chill for at least 1 hour before slicing.
4. Before serving, cut ½ inch off each end and discard. Cut each tortilla into eight 1-inch-thick slices.

Nutritional Information per Serving
Calories 165 • CD 1.3 • Carbohydrate 20g • Fat 8g • Protein 7g • Fiber 5g

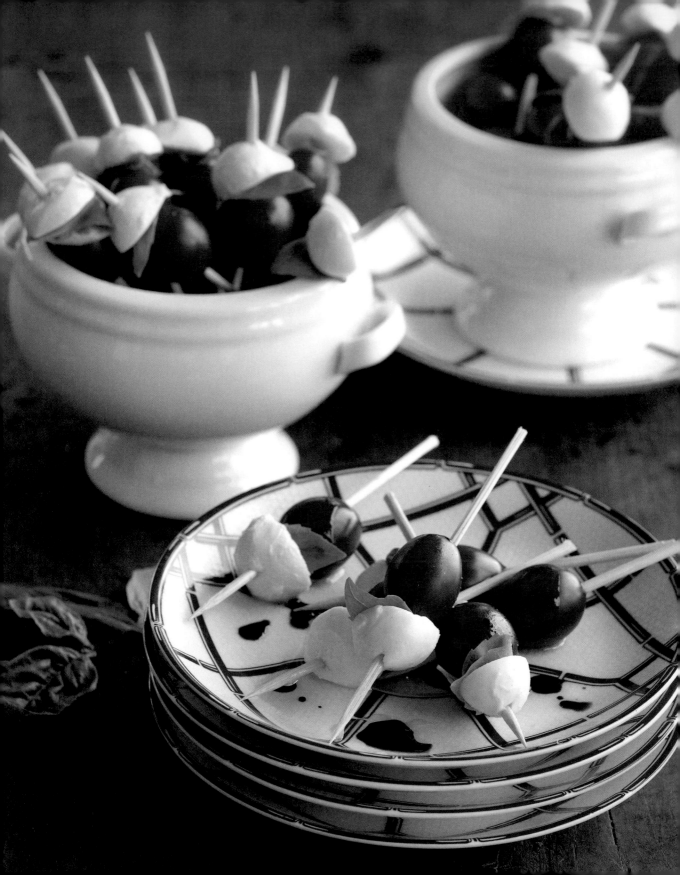

Tomato and Mozzarella Mini Sticks

This recipe is so simple that it's easy to put together for last-minute guests. I love making it with local tomatoes and basil from my garden in the summer. It is almost as good in the winter, with cherry tomatoes and basil now available year-round. Add pieces of canned artichoke hearts (not the marinated type) for variety.

Makes 8 servings (75g each), 6 toothpicks each

 Vegetarian

48 cocktail toothpicks

48 small (298g) cherry or grape tomatoes, 1 to 2 pints depending on size of the tomatoes

48 small (24g) basil leaves

One 8-ounce (227g) container fresh ciliegini or small bocconcini mozzarella balls (about ⅓ ounce each), cut in half (see note)

2 tablespoons (30g) regular or white balsamic vinegar

1 teaspoons (4g) olive oil

Thread each toothpick with tomato, a basil leaf, and half a cheese ball. Place the completed skewers on a platter. Drizzle with the vinegar and oil before serving.

NOTE: Some mozzarella balls are small enough to use whole.

Nutritional Information per Serving
Calories 95 • CD 1.3 • Carbohydrate 2g • Fat 7g • Protein 5g • Fiber 1g

Festive Fare

Spinach-Cheese Balls

Panko bread crumbs originated in Japan, where they are used in the crispy coating on tonkatsu dishes. Combined with Parmesan cheese and oregano, they give this party dish a tasty crunch. I serve these as is, or sometimes with my favorite tomato-based pasta sauce.

Makes 4 servings (115g each), 5 spinach-cheese balls each

 Vegetarian

One 10-ounce (280g) box frozen chopped spinach, thawed and squeezed to remove the liquid

½ cup (28g) freshly grated Parmesan cheese (1 ounce)

½ cup (124g) part-skim ricotta cheese

1 small (70g) onion, peeled and finely grated

1 (3g) garlic clove, peeled and finely chopped

1 slice (28g) whole-wheat bread, torn into small pieces

2 large (66g) egg whites

Salt and freshly ground black pepper to taste

Red pepper flakes to taste

½ cup (12g) panko bread crumbs

½ teaspoon (0.5g) dried oregano

1. Preheat the oven to 400°F. Spray a baking sheet with cooking spray.
2. Combine the spinach, ¼ cup of the Parmesan, the ricotta, onion, garlic, bread, egg whites, salt, and peppers in a large bowl. Combine the remaining Parmesan cheese with the panko crumbs, oregano, and salt and peppers in a small bowl.
3. Form the spinach mixture into small balls using two tablespoons or a 1-ounce scoop. Roll in the panko mixture to coat and place on the baking sheet.
4. Bake for 30 minutes or until crisp on the outside and lightly browned. Serve with toothpicks.

Nutritional Information per Serving

Calories 140 • CD 1.2 • Carbohydrate 12g • Fat 5g • Protein 12g • Fiber 3g

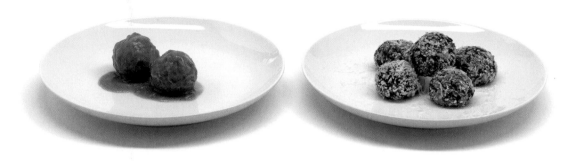

Traditional	How we lowered the CD	Volumetrics
Swedish meatballs	• Replaced the meat with a spinach-ricotta mixture • Eliminated the high-fat Swedish meatball sauce	Spinach-Cheese Balls

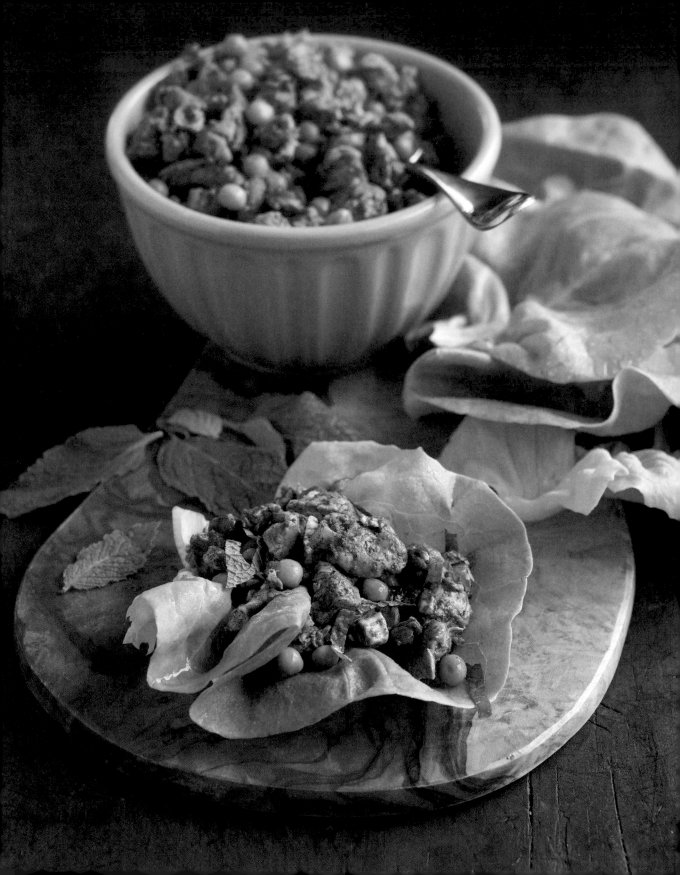

Curried Chicken Lettuce Cups

I double or even triple this recipe for a quick party dish. Make sure you use lettuce leaves that are large and soft so that they "cup" the chicken mixture without breaking. Choose a curry powder with the level of heat that you like.

Makes 8 servings (75g each), 1 lettuce cup with ½ cup filling each

2 teaspoons (8g) vegetable oil

1 tablespoon (8g) curry powder

1 medium (119g) onion, peeled and finely chopped

2 (6g) garlic cloves, peeled and finely chopped

12 ounces (340g) ground or chopped raw chicken breast

2 cups (290g) thawed frozen green peas

Salt and freshly ground black pepper to taste

8 large (120g) Boston lettuce leaves

¾ cup (45g) chopped mint, basil, cilantro, or watercress leaves

1. Spray a large skillet with cooking spray. Heat the oil in the skillet over medium heat. Add the curry powder and cook until fragrant, about 1 minute. Add the onion and garlic and cook, stirring occasionally, until soft, about 5 minutes. Add the chicken, cover, and simmer until fully cooked, 5 to 8 minutes. Fold in the peas.
2. Serve in a bowl with lettuce leaves and mint or other herb garnish on the side for guests to assemble their own.

VARIATION: To make this vegetarian, use crumbled tofu in place of the chicken.

Nutritional Information per Serving
Calories 105 • CD 1.4 • Carbohydrate 8g • Fat 3g • Protein 12g • Fiber 3g

Marinated Mushrooms

I like to vary the vinegar in this recipe, using white wine vinegar for a sharp, crisp flavor or white balsamic if I want the mushrooms to taste smoother and sweeter. Almost all of the marinade stays behind, so the CD of this dish is very low.

Makes 4 servings (75g each), ½ cup each

(🍅) Vegetarian

10 ounces (283g) baby bella or small button mushrooms, wiped clean, stems trimmed

¼ cup (60g) white wine vinegar or white balsamic vinegar

2 tablespoons (28g) olive oil

2 (6g) garlic cloves, peeled and finely chopped

1 tablespoon (1g) minced fresh tarragon

½ teaspoon (3g) Dijon mustard

¼ teaspoon (1g) table salt

¼ teaspoon (1g) freshly ground black pepper

1. Combine the mushrooms, vinegar, oil, garlic, tarragon, mustard, salt, and pepper in a resealable plastic container. Cover and gently shake the container to coat the mushrooms. Refrigerate at least 24 hours, gently shaking at least once to distribute the marinade.
2. Remove mushrooms from the marinade and serve with toothpicks.

Nutritional Information per Serving
Calories 25 • CD 0.33 • Carbohydrate 3g • Fat 1g • Protein 2g • Fiber 1g

DESSERTS
Cakes

Chocolate Chip–Zucchini Squares

My lab staff has mastered the art of adding lots of vegetables to baked goods. Most of our study subjects love our vegetable-rich versions because they are so moist. Even young children don't notice the veggies.

Makes 24 servings (85g each), one 2-inch square each

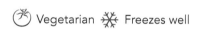 Vegetarian ❄ Freezes well

3 cups (360g) white whole-wheat flour

1 teaspoon (5g) table salt

1 teaspoon (2g) ground cinnamon

1 teaspoon (2g) ground nutmeg

1 teaspoon (5g) baking soda

½ teaspoon (1g) baking powder

¾ cup (183g) egg substitute

¾ cup (150g) granulated sugar

½ cup (110g) packed light brown sugar

½ cup (110g) vegetable oil

½ cup (122g) unsweetened applesauce

2 teaspoons (8g) pure vanilla extract

6 cups (678g) shredded zucchini, with skin (5 medium, about 1½ pounds)

1 cup (224g) semisweet chocolate mini morsels

1. Preheat the oven to 350°F. Spray a 9 by 13-inch glass baking pan with cooking spray.
2. Sift together the flour, salt, cinnamon, nutmeg, baking soda, and baking powder into a medium bowl.
3. Beat the egg substitute in a large bowl until light and fluffy. Add the granulated and brown sugars and beat until well blended. Stir in the oil, applesauce, vanilla, zucchini, and chocolate morsels until well blended. Stir in the flour mixture until blended; avoid overmixing. Pour into the pan.
4. Bake for 60 minutes or until a knife inserted into the center comes out clean.

5. Cool in the pan on a wire rack for 5 minutes. Place the rack on top of the pan and carefully invert it so the cake is on the rack. Let cool to room temperature before cutting.

Nutritional Information per Serving
Calories 200 • CD 2.4 • Carbohydrate 30g • Fat 8g • Protein 4g • Fiber 2g

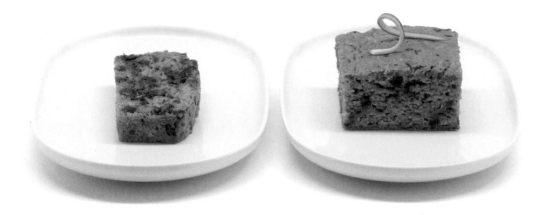

Traditional	How we lowered the CD	Volumetrics
Zucchini bread	• Used egg substitute instead of eggs • Substituted applesauce in place of some of the oil • Tripled the zucchini	Chocolate Chip–Zucchini Squares

Banana Cake

This moist cake is particularly flavorful when made with very ripe bananas. Dust with sifted powdered sugar and top with banana slices to make it a special party dessert. Any leftovers are delicious for breakfast the next day.

Makes 12 servings (120g each), one 3-inch square each

⌖ Vegetarian   ❄ Freezes well   🥘 Good for leftovers

2½ cups (300g) white whole-wheat flour

1 tablespoon (14g) baking soda

6 tablespoons (85g) salted butter, softened

½ cup (110g) packed light brown sugar

½ cup (100g) granulated sugar

1 teaspoon (4g) pure vanilla or almond extract

½ cup (122g) egg substitute

5 ripe small (590g) bananas, mashed (2½ cups)

⅔ cup (162g) low-fat buttermilk

1. Preheat the oven to 350°F. Spray a 9 by 13-inch glass baking pan with cooking spray.
2. Whisk together the flour and baking soda in a small bowl.
3. Beat the butter, brown and granulated sugars, and vanilla until light and fluffy. Add the egg substitute and continue to beat until well blended. Mix in the mashed bananas until well blended.
4. Add half of the flour mixture and beat on low until blended. Add ⅓ cup of buttermilk and beat on low until blended. Repeat with the remaining flour and the remaining buttermilk. Be careful not to overmix the ingredients. Pour into the prepared pan.
5. Bake for 35 minutes or until a knife inserted into the center comes out clean.
6. Allow the cake to cool in the pan for 15 minutes. Remove from the pan and cool on a rack until it is cool to the touch.

Nutritional Information per Serving
Calories 260 • CD 2.2 • Carbohydrate 46g • Fat 6g • Protein 5g • Fiber 4g

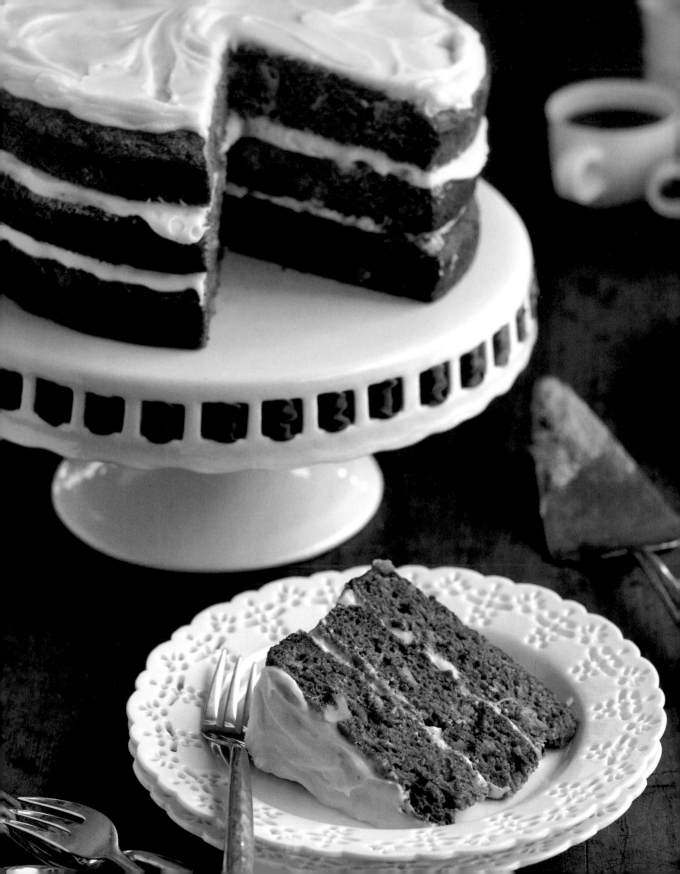

Alex's Three-Layer Carrot Cake

I love carrot cake and Alex, one of my graduate students, shows how delicious it can be when the CD is reduced by using plenty of carrots and applesauce in place of some of the oil or butter. This three-layer cake is a delicious treat for entertaining.

Makes 16 servings (140g each)

 Vegetarian

CAKE

1 cup (244g) egg substitute

¾ cup (165g) packed light brown sugar

¾ cup (150g) granulated sugar

1½ cups (366g) unsweetened applesauce

2 cups (240g) regular whole-wheat flour

2 teaspoons (9g) baking soda

2 teaspoons (5g) baking powder

2 teaspoons (5g) ground cinnamon

1½ teaspoons (3g) ground nutmeg

1 pound (454g) carrots, peeled or scrubbed and finely grated

One 8-ounce (227g) can crushed pineapple in juice, drained well

¾ cup (124g) golden raisins

½ cup (62g) walnuts, coarsely chopped

FROSTING

4 tablespoons (56g) butter, softened

4 ounces (113g) light cream cheese, softened

Half of a 1-pound package (227g) powdered sugar (about 2 cups)

1½ teaspoons (6g) pure vanilla extract

1. Preheat the oven to 325°F. Spray three 9-inch round cake pans with cooking spray.

2. Beat the egg substitute, brown and granulated sugars, and applesauce in a large bowl until well blended. Add the flour, baking soda, baking powder, cinnamon, and nutmeg and stir until smooth. Stir in the carrots, pineapple, raisins, and walnuts. Pour the batter into the prepared pans.

3. Bake for 40 minutes or until a toothpick comes out clean when inserted in the center of each cake.

4. Allow the layers to cool in the pans for 15 minutes. Remove from the pans and cool on a rack until they are cool to the touch.

5. When ready to frost the cake, mix the butter, cream cheese, powdered sugar, and vanilla extract in a medium bowl by hand until smooth.

6. Frost the top of each layer with a thin coat of frosting and assemble the layers.

NOTE: This cake has frosting between the layers and on top but not on the sides.

Nutritional Information per Serving
Calories 310 • CD 2.2 • Carbohydrate 59g • Fat 7g • Protein 6g • Fiber 4g

Fruit Desserts

Ginger Apple Crumble

I created this lower-CD gingersnap topping to take the place of traditional butter-flour-sugar crumbs. As the crumble bakes, some of the topping combines with the apples to thicken and flavor the cooking liquid.

Makes 6 servings (185g each), about 1 cup each

 Vegetarian

4 medium (587g) apples, cored and thinly sliced, skins on (see note)

½ cup (120g) water, apple juice, or cranberry juice

12 (85g) gingersnaps, broken into quarters

2 tablespoons (16g) all-purpose flour

2 tablespoons (32g) light brown sugar

1 tablespoon (14g) melted butter

1. Preheat the oven to 350°F. Spray an 8-inch square baking dish with cooking spray.
2. Place the apples and water or juice in the baking dish.
3. Blend or process the gingersnaps, flour, brown sugar, and butter to form coarse crumbs. Top the apples with the crumbs.
4. Bake for 45 minutes or until the apples are soft and the crumbs have darkened in color. Serve warm or at room temperature.

NOTE: Many apple varieties are suitable for cooking, including Granny Smith (tart), Golden Delicious (sweet-tart), and McIntosh (applesauce-like). Mix and match two or three varieties if you prefer a texture that is both smooth and chunky.

Nutritional Information per Serving

Calories 185 • CD 1.0 • Carbohydrate 39g • Fat 4g • Protein 4g • Fiber 4g

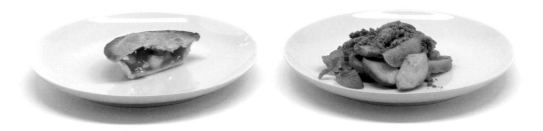

Traditional	How we lowered the CD	Volumetrics
Apple pie	• Increased the apples • Switched from pie crust to a crumb topping	Ginger Apple Crumble

Peach Bread Pudding

The recipe makes a delicious dessert or satisfying breakfast. I make it all year round by using frozen peaches when fresh are not available. It also is tasty with chopped apples or fresh or frozen berries. For an even moister pudding, bake it in a deep, round soufflé dish and increase the baking time to 60 minutes.

Makes 8 servings (160g each), 1½ cups each

 Vegetarian   Good for leftovers

2 cups (448g) fat-free milk

2 large (100g) eggs

2 large (66g) egg whites

⅓ cup (67g) sugar

2 teaspoons (18g) pure vanilla extract

1 teaspoon (2g) ground cinnamon

3 cups (462g) fresh or frozen peach slices

8 slices (192g) whole-grain or cinnamon raisin bread, toasted and cut into 1-inch cubes

1. Preheat the oven to 350°F. Spray a 9 by 13-inch baking pan with cooking spray.

2. Whisk together the milk, eggs, egg whites, sugar, vanilla, and cinnamon in a large bowl. Add the peaches and bread cubes and stir to combine. Pour into the prepared pan.

3. Bake for 30 to 45 minutes, until the custard is set. Serve warm or at room temperature.

Nutritional Information per Serving

Calories 170 • CD 1.1 • Carbohydrate 29g • Fat 3g • Protein 9g • Fiber 3g

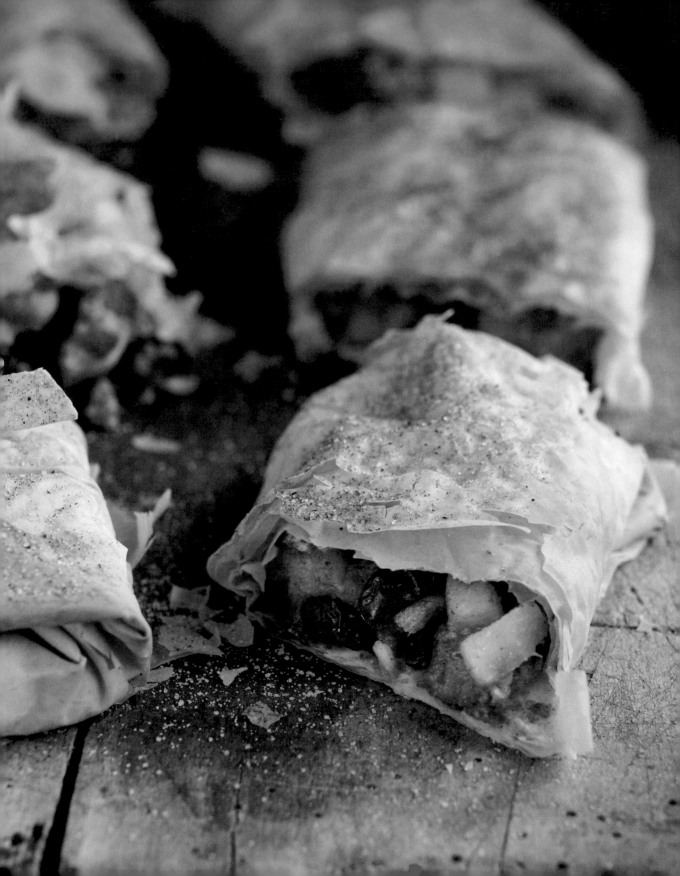

Pear Cranberry Strudel

This light and simple dessert works best with pears or apples—their relatively dry flesh allows the phyllo to get crisp. Look for the smaller size phyllo sheets as they are very easy to work with.

Makes 6 servings (100g each), 3-inch piece each

 Vegetarian

3 medium (444g) or 2 large pears (about 1 pound), peeled, cored, and chopped

2 (14g) graham cracker squares, crushed

¼ cup (15g) loosely packed dried cranberries

1 tablespoon (16g) light brown sugar

2 teaspoons (5g) ground cinnamon

1 teaspoon (3g) cornstarch

1 teaspoon (4g) granulated sugar

Eight 9 by 14-inch (90g) or four 14 by 18-inch sheets phyllo dough

1. Preheat the oven to 350°F. Spray a baking sheet with cooking spray.
2. Combine the pears, graham crackers, cranberries, brown sugar, 1 teaspoon of the cinnamon, and the cornstarch in a medium bowl.
3. If using the large size phyllo, cut in half to create eight 9 by 14-inch sheets. Working quickly to prevent the dough from drying out, stack 2 sheets on the baking sheet, spray lightly with cooking spray, and top with 2 more sheets. Place half of the pear mixture along the long edge of the phyllo stack about 2 inches from the edge and 2 inches from each side. Fold the edge over the filling, fold the side edges over the filling, then gently roll up. Position seam-side down, spray lightly with cooking spray, and sprinkle with ½ teaspoon each cinnamon and granulated sugar.
4. Repeat with the remaining phyllo dough and filling.
5. Bake for 40 minutes or until the phyllo is light brown and very crisp. Cut each strudel into 3 pieces and serve immediately.

Nutritional Information per Serving
Calories 120 • CD 1.2 • Carbohydrate 26g • Fat 1g • Protein 2g • Fiber 3g

Fruit Salads

Red, Black, and Blue Berry Medley

This salad is accented with the flavors of a Cosmo cocktail, cranberry and orange. I like the tart flavor of 100 percent cranberry juice as a perfect contrast to the sweet berries. Try other combinations of fresh berries, or use a frozen berry blend when fresh berries are not available.

Makes 4 servings (160g each), about 1 cup each

 Vegetarian

½ pint (123g) red raspberries

½ pint (144g) blackberries

1 pint (296g) blueberries

1 tablespoon (14g) sugar

2 tablespoons (32g) cranberry juice, preferably unsweetened

2 tablespoons (28g) orange liqueur or orange juice

1 tablespoon (6g) grated orange peel

Mint sprigs, for garnish

Gently combine the berries, sugar, and juices in a medium bowl. Garnish with the orange peel and mint sprigs.

Nutritional Information per Serving
Calories 115 • CD 0.72 • Carbohydrate 25g • Fat 1g • Protein 1g • Fiber 6g

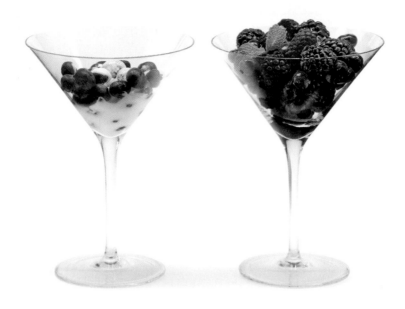

Traditional	How we lowered the CD	Volumetrics
Blueberries and cream	• Decreased the sugar • Increased the berries • Drizzled the berries with juice instead of serving in cream	Red, Black, and Blue Berry Medley

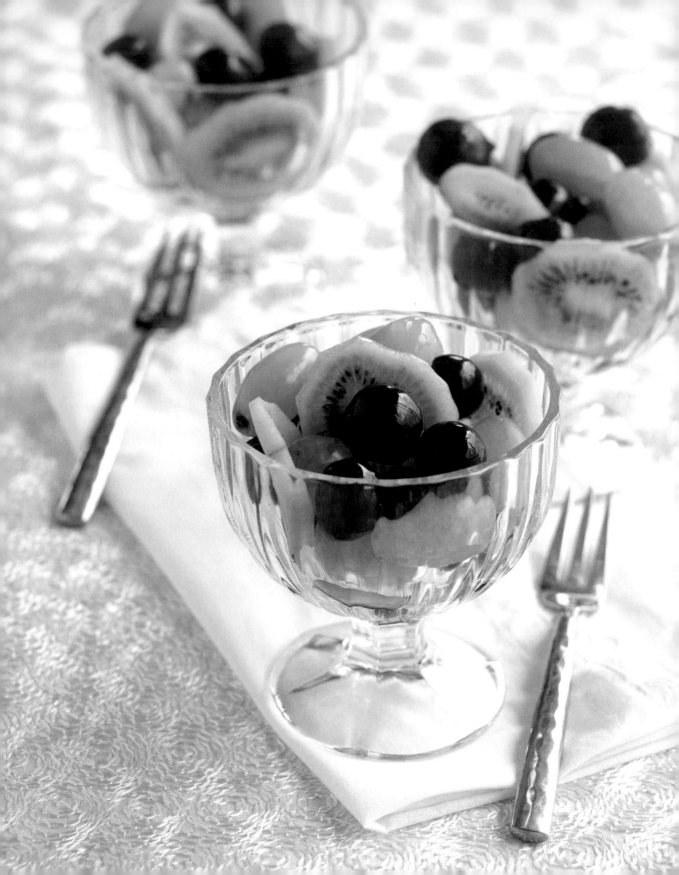

Holiday Balsamic Grape Salad

This red and green fruit salad looks beautiful on a winter holiday table. The balsamic vinegar is a surprising way to accent the flavor of fruit. In the summer, add strawberries or watermelon in addition to the grapes.

Makes 4 servings (205g each), about 1¼ cups each

 Vegetarian

2 cups (320g) red grapes

2 cups (320g) green grapes

2 medium (138g) kiwis, scooped into small balls or peeled and sliced

1 tablespoon (15g) white or regular balsamic vinegar

1 tablespoon (21g) honey

Combine the grapes, kiwis, vinegar, and honey in a medium bowl.

Nutritional Information per Serving

Calories 150 • CD 0.73 • Carbohydrate 39g • Fat 0g • Protein 2g • Fiber 2g

Retro Melon Ball Trio

To make this colorful combination of three different melons even more festive for guests, I serve it in scooped out cantaloupe halves or in a watermelon "basket."

Makes 4 servings (265g each), 1½ cups each

 Vegetarian

2 cups (354g) cantaloupe balls
(1 medium cantaloupe)

2 cups (354g) honeydew balls (½ small honeydew melon)

2 cups (308g) watermelon balls
(½ mini watermelon)

1 tablespoon (14g) sugar

Juice of ½ lime (22g)

2 tablespoons (10g) sweetened flaked coconut (optional)

Grated peel of 1 lime

Combine the melon balls, sugar, and lime juice in a medium bowl. Garnish with the coconut, if desired, and the lime peel.

Nutritional Information per Serving
Calories 100 • CD 0.38 • Carbohydrate 25g • Fat 0g • Protein 2g • Fiber 2g

Appendix

Modular Food Lists

You can use these lists to make substitutions for foods in the menu plan and when developing your personal diet plan. Within each modular list—breakfast foods, soups, side dishes, main dishes, snacks and desserts, and beverages—foods are grouped by category and listed by calorie level so you can easily determine which foods are interchangeable. The CD of each food is listed to help you make the most satiating choices. I've also included the weight of the foods in grams so you will see how the portion sizes compare when you are choosing foods. Weights of similar foods may very as a result of differences in databases.

Breakfast Food Modular List

Let's use the breakfast modular list to show you how to make the most satisfying choices. When choosing between foods with a similar calorie level, you will be able to have a larger portion if you choose the food with the lower CD. For example, two pancakes with butter and syrup (CD 2.8) contain about 320 calories. Light as a Feather Pancakes (CD 1.3) (page 179) have about the same calories as the traditional pancakes but weigh more than twice as much.

Cereal with fat-free milk is a good choice for breakfast. Pay attention to portion sizes. I list calories per cup of cereal, but that does not mean you should eat that amount. If you ate a cup of granola with fat-free milk, you would get 570 calories!

Breakfast Food Modular List

[Italicized items are Volumetrics recipes.]	CALORIES	WEIGHT (GRAMS)	CALORIE DENSITY
DAIRY			
Yogurt, light (nonfat, low-cal sweetener), 6 oz	80	170	0.44
Yogurt, Greek-style, nonfat, plain, 6 oz	90	170	0.53
Yogurt, nonfat, plain, 6 oz	95	170	0.56
Yogurt, low-fat, plain, 6 oz	115	170	0.68
Yogurt, low-fat, fruit, 6 oz	185	170	1.1
Greek Apple Parfait, page 190	260	300	0.87
Berry Parfait, page 186	265	370	0.72
Peach Melba Parfait, page 189	310	310	1.0
CEREALS AND GRAINS			
White bread, 1 slice	65	25	2.6
Whole-wheat bread, 1 slice	75	25	2.8
Pancake, buttermilk, 4-inch diameter, 1 each	85	40	2.1
Pancake, whole-wheat, 4-inch diameter, 1 each	90	45	2.0
Waffle, toasted from frozen, 4-inch square, 1 each	105	35	3.0
Bran muffin, toaster, 2½-inch diameter, 1 each	105	35	3.0
Apple Oatmeal Muffins, page 191	115	50	2.3
Hot wheat or farina cereal, 1 cup	125	250	0.5
1 biscuit, 2½-inch diameter, 1 each	130	35	3.7
English muffin, whole-wheat, toasted, 1 each	135	65	2.1
English muffin, plain, toasted, 1 each	135	55	2.5
Corn flakes cereal, 1 cup, with ½ cup fat-free milk	140	150	0.93
Crispy rice cereal, 1 cup, with ½ cup fat-free milk	140	145	0.97
Oat rings cereal, 1 cup, with ½ cup fat-free milk	145	150	0.97
Pumpkin Cranberry Bread, page 193	150	80	1.9
French toast, 1 slice made with 2% milk	150	65	2.3
High-fiber cereal, 1 cup, with ½ cup fat-free milk	160	180	0.89
Oatmeal, 1 cup	165	235	0.70
Wheat bran flakes cereal, 1 cup, with ½ cup fat-free milk	170	160	1.1
Blueberry Lemon Breakfast Loaf, page 195	170	90	1.9
Corn grits, 1 cup	180	255	0.70
All-bran cereal, 1 cup, with ½ cup fat-free milk	200	180	1.1
Shredded wheat cereal, spoon size, 1 cup, with ½ cup fat-free milk	210	170	1.2
Fruit pastry, toaster-type, 1 each	210	55	3.8
Cinnamon sweet roll with raisins, 2¾-inch, 1 each	225	60	3.8
Raisin bran cereal, 1 cup, with ½ cup fat-free milk	230	180	1.3
Croissant, 1 medium	230	55	4.2
Glazed donut, 1 medium	255	65	3.9
Cinnamon Danish pastry, 1 medium	260	65	4.0
Plain bagel, 3½-inch diameter, 1 each	290	105	2.8
Light as a Feather Pancakes with Berry Sauce, page 179	310	240	1.3
2 buttermilk pancakes with 2 pats butter, 1½ tbsp maple syrup	320	115	2.8
Cornmeal Pancakes with Cinnamon Apples, page 177	330	235	1.4
Cherry-Vanilla French Toast, page 175	385	320	1.2

[Italicized items are Volumetrics recipes.]	CALORIES	WEIGHT (GRAMS)	CALORIE DENSITY
Granola cereal, low-fat, 1 cup, with ½ cup fat-free milk	420	220	1.9
Granola cereal, 1 cup, with ½ cup fat-free milk	570	235	2.4
MEAT, POULTRY, FISH			
Veggie sausage links, 2 links	70	45	1.6
Canadian bacon, 2 slices	85	45	1.9
Pork bacon, 3 slices	130	25	5.2
Pork sausage, 4-inch patty, 1 each	215	55	3.9
EGGS			
Scrambled liquid egg substitute, ¼ cup	30	60	0.5
Boiled egg, 1 large egg	80	50	1.5
Fried egg, 1 large egg	90	45	2.0
Vegetable Denver Omelet, page 184	160	145	1.1
Greek Frittata, page 183	220	200	1.1
MIXED DISHES			
Fajita Breakfast Burrito, page 180	390	260	1.5
Butter croissant with bacon, eggs, and cheese	415	130	3.2
Biscuit with egg and sausage	505	160	3.2
Steak, egg, and cheese on a bagel	610	215	2.8

Soup Modular List

Keep appetizer soups to 150 calories or less. Soups that are higher in calories make a nutritious and filling main course at lunch or dinner. Soups also make good snacks. If you are buying prepared soup, check the label for calories since brands can differ considerably.

[Italicized items are Volumetrics recipes.]	CALORIES	WEIGHT (GRAMS)	CALORIE DENSITY
SOUPS			
Broth, 99% fat-free, 1 cup	10	225	0.04
Vegetable broth, 1 cup	15	235	0.06
Beef or chicken broth, 1 cup	40	240	0.17
Gazpacho, canned, ready-to-serve, 1 cup	45	245	0.18
Onion, prepared with water, 1 cup	55	245	0.22
Chicken noodle, 1 cup	60	250	0.31
Chicken, rice and vegetable, canned, ready-to-serve, 1 cup	60	245	0.24
Vegetarian vegetable, prepared with water, 1 cup	70	245	0.29
Tomato, prepared with water, 1 cup	75	250	0.30
Cream of potato, prepared with water, 1 cup	75	245	0.31
Minestrone, prepared with water, 1 cup	80	240	0.33
New England clam chowder, prepared with water, 1 cup	85	250	0.34

[Italicized items are Volumetrics recipes.]	CALORIES	WEIGHT (GRAMS)	CALORIE DENSITY
Butternut squash, ready-to-serve, 1 cup	90	245	0.37
Chunky chicken noodle, canned, ready-to-serve, 1 cup	90	245	0.37
Cream of mushroom, prepared with water, 1 cup	105	250	0.42
Black bean, prepared with water, 1 cup	115	245	0.47
Vegetable beef, canned, ready-to-serve, 1 cup	120	245	0.49
The Volumetrics Soup, page 196	130	390	0.33
Chilled Cucumber and Summer Vegetable Soup, page 198	135	305	0.44
Lentil and ham, canned, ready-to-serve, 1 cup	140	250	0.56
Tomato, prepared with milk, 1 cup	140	250	0.56
Red Lentil Soup, page 200	150	250	0.60
Chunky beef, canned, ready-to-serve, 1 cup	160	245	0.65
Chunky vegetable, canned, ready-to-serve, 1 cup	165	240	0.69
Bean with bacon, prepared with water, 1 cup	170	265	0.64
Split pea, prepared with water, 1 cup	180	255	0.71
Chicken corn chowder, canned, ready-to-serve, 1 cup	200	245	0.82
Vegetable Barley Soup, page 203	225	400	0.56
Chunky bean with ham, canned, ready-to-serve, 1 cup	230	245	0.94
Chicken Tortilla Soup, page 205	320	550	0.58
Caribbean Bean and Squash Soup, page 201	340	505	0.67

Side Dish Modular List

This list contains an assortment of side dishes such as vegetables, grains, salads, and legumes. You will find many dishes with less than 100 calories as well as many in the 100- to 200-calorie range.

[Italicized items are Volumetrics recipes.]	CALORIES	WEIGHT (GRAMS)	CALORIE DENSITY
VEGETABLES			
Spinach, raw, 1 cup	5	30	0.17
Arugula, raw, 1 cup	5	20	0.25
Mixed salad greens, 1 cup	10	55	0.18
Mushrooms, raw, ½ cup	10	35	0.29
Zucchini, cooked, ½ cup	15	90	0.17
Swiss chard, cooked, ½ cup	15	85	0.18
Green cabbage, cooked, ½ cup	15	75	0.20
Roasted red peppers, jarred, ½ cup	15	70	0.21
Cauliflower, cooked, ½ cup	15	60	0.25
Bean sprouts, raw, ½ cup	15	50	0.30
Summer squash, cooked, ½ cup	20	90	0.22
Spinach, cooked, ½ cup	20	90	0.22

[Italicized items are Volumetrics recipes.]	CALORIES	WEIGHT (GRAMS)	CALORIE DENSITY
Asparagus, cooked, ½ cup	20	90	0.22
Okra, cooked, ½ cup	20	80	0.25
Broccoli florets, raw, 1 cup	20	70	0.29
Fennel, raw, 1 cup	25	85	0.29
Beets, cooked, ½ cup	25	80	0.31
Green beans, cooked, ½ cup	25	65	0.38
Broccoli, cooked, ½ cup	30	80	0.38
Brussels sprouts, cooked, ½ cup	30	80	0.38
Carrots, cooked, ½ cup	30	80	0.38
Snow peas, cooked, ½ cup	35	80	0.44
Winter squash, baked, ½ cup	40	105	0.38
Artichoke hearts, canned, drained, ½ cup	45	85	0.53
Asparagus with Tarragon-Mustard Vinaigrette, page 215	55	105	0.52
Parsnips, cooked, ½ cup	55	80	0.69
Asian Sesame Slaw, page 211	60	130	0.46
Asian Green Beans, page 294	65	130	0.50
Green peas, cooked, ½ cup	65	80	0.81
Grilled Portobello Mushroom Caps, page 298	75	85	0.86
Corn, frozen, cooked, ½ cup	80	85	0.94
Classic Spinach Salad, page 206	85	150	0.57
Balsamic-Glazed Carrots, page 301	85	130	0.65
Baby Arugula Salad, page 210	90	155	0.58
Creamed corn, canned, ½ cup	90	130	0.69
Ear of corn, cooked, 1 medium	90	100	0.90
Mixed Greens with Strawberries, Pears, and Walnuts, page 209	105	200	0.53
South-of-France Ratatouille, page 297	110	225	0.49
Persian-Style Grilled Vegetables, page 283	110	175	0.63
Mashed potatoes with milk and butter, ½ cup	120	105	1.1
Sweet potato, cooked, mashed, ½ cup	125	165	0.76
Creamy Broccoli-Feta Salad, page 307	125	160	0.78
Lemony New Potato Salad, page 304	125	135	0.93
Succotash Salad, page 308	125	105	1.2
Sweet Potato Casserole, page 299	140	100	1.4
Coleslaw, ½ cup	145	95	1.5
Baked potato with skin, 1 medium	160	175	0.91
Potato salad, ½ cup	165	145	1.1
Onion rings, batter-dipped, fried, 7 rings	170	40	4.2
Roasted Diced Fall Vegetables, page 303	180	180	1.0
Volumetrics Vegetable Fried Rice, page 313	210	230	0.91
Hash browns, ½ cup	235	70	3.4
French fries, 4 oz	330	115	2.9
GRAINS			
Bulgur, cooked, ½ cup	75	90	0.83
Buckwheat groats (kasha), cooked, ½ cup	75	85	0.88
Wild rice, cooked, ½ cup	85	80	1.1
Spaghetti, whole-wheat, cooked, ½ cup	85	70	1.2

[Italicized items are Volumetrics recipes.]	CALORIES	WEIGHT (GRAMS)	CALORIE DENSITY
Pearled barley, cooked, ½ cup	95	80	1.2
Millet, cooked, ½ cup	105	90	1.2
White rice, cooked, ½ cup	105	80	1.3
Quinoa, cooked, ½ cup	110	95	1.2
Brown rice, cooked, ½ cup	110	95	1.2
Spaghetti, regular, cooked, ½ cup	110	70	1.6
Quinoa Tabbouleh Salad, page 289	125	210	0.6
Cauliflower Rice, page 311	135	165	0.82
Wheatberry Salad, page 293	155	160	0.97
Squash Risotto, page 309	160	190	0.84
LEGUMES			
Tofu, firm, ½ cup	90	125	0.72
Black-eyed peas, canned, drained, ½ cup	90	120	0.75
Refried beans, canned, fat-free, ½ cup	90	115	0.78
Pinto beans, canned, ½ cup	105	120	0.88
Lima beans, cooked, ½ cup	105	85	1.2
Kidney beans, canned, ½ cup	110	130	0.85
Black beans, canned, ½ cup	110	120	0.92
Refried beans, canned, ½ cup	110	120	0.92
Lentils, cooked, ½ cup	115	100	1.2
Split peas, cooked, ½ cup	115	100	1.2
Vegetarian baked beans, canned, ½ cup	120	125	0.96
Chickpeas (garbanzo beans), canned, ½ cup	145	120	1.2
Navy or white beans, canned, ½ cup	150	130	1.2
Spicy Lentil Salad, page 213	235	285	0.82
Kim's Black Bean and Barley Salad, page 291	280	255	1.1
BREADS			
Corn tortilla, 1 each	55	25	2.2
White bread, 1 slice	65	25	2.6
Whole-grain bread, 1 slice	70	25	2.8
Whole-wheat pita, 4-inch	75	30	2.5
Flatbread, 1.9 oz	90	55	1.6
Whole-grain roll, medium	95	35	2.7
Whole-wheat tortilla, 2 oz	120	55	2.2
Hamburger bun, 1 each	120	45	2.7
Flour tortilla, 7-inch	145	45	3.2
Cornbread, 2½-inch square	150	65	2.3
Croissant, medium	230	55	4.2

Main Dish Modular List

In this list you will find a variety of dishes that serve as the main course. They include meat, poultry, and fish, as well as pizza, sandwiches, large salads, and Volumetrics entrées. Add side dishes and starters that fit your calorie level and balance your meal nutritionally.

[Italicized items are Volumetrics recipes.]	CALORIES	WEIGHT (GRAMS)	CALORIE DENSITY
MEAT, POULTRY, FISH			
Lobster, steamed, 3oz	75	85	0.88
Alaskan king crab, steamed, 3oz	80	85	0.94
Cod, baked, 3oz	90	85	1.1
Halibut, baked, 3oz	95	85	1.1
Scallops, steamed, 3oz	95	85	1.1
Tuna, yellowfin, raw (sashimi), 3oz	95	85	1.1
Perch, baked, 3oz	100	85	1.2
Tuna, light, canned in water, drained, 3oz	100	85	1.2
Shrimp, steamed, 3oz	100	85	1.2
Snapper, baked, 3oz	110	85	1.3
Tilapia, baked, 3oz	110	85	1.3
Chicken Breast Strips with Smoky Orange Dipping Sauce, page 318	110	75	1.5
Turkey breast, skinless, roasted, 3oz	115	85	1.4
Turkey, ground, 99% fat-free, 4oz before cooking	120	115	1.0
Salmon, wild, baked, 3oz	120	85	1.4
Ham, extra lean (5% fat), roasted, 3oz	125	85	1.5
Chicken breast, skinless, roasted, 3oz	140	85	1.6
Ground beef, extra lean (5% fat), broiled, 3oz	145	85	1.7
Turkey, ground, 7% fat, 4oz before cooking	150	115	1.3
Ham, 11% fat, roasted, 3oz	150	85	1.8
Buffalo chicken wings, 3 each, without sauce	150	50	3.0
Top sirloin steak, lean, broiled, 3oz	155	85	1.8
Turkey breast, skin-on, roasted, 3oz	160	85	1.9
Turkey, dark, skinless, roasted, 3oz	160	85	1.9
Greek Tilapia Fillets with Olives and Oregano, page 278	165	150	1.1
Chicken breast, skin-on, roasted, 3oz	170	85	2.0
Clams, breaded and fried, 3oz	170	85	2.0
Duck, skinless, roasted, 3oz	170	85	2.0
Oysters, breaded and fried, 3oz	170	85	2.0
Tuna, light, canned in oil, drained, 3oz	170	85	2.0
Roast beef, lean, braised, 3oz	175	85	2.1
Salmon, farmed, baked, 3oz	175	85	2.1
Turkey, ground, cooked, 3oz	175	85	2.1
Anne's Sautéed Sea Scallops with Radishes and Spring Onions, page 277	180	265	0.68
Chicken and Seasonal Tomatoes in a Packet, page 271	185	295	0.63
Ground beef, lean (10% fat), broiled, 3oz	185	85	2.2
Pork rib chop, lean, broiled, 3oz	185	85	2.2

[Italicized items are Volumetrics recipes.]	CALORIES	WEIGHT (GRAMS)	CALORIE DENSITY
Turkey, dark, skin-on, roasted, 3 oz	190	85	2.2
Catfish, breaded and fried, 3 oz	195	85	2.3
Korean-Style Steak Fajitas, page 279	205	275	0.75
Chicken breast, skin-on, batter-fried, 3 oz	220	85	2.6
Crab-Asparagus Quiche, page 274	225	190	1.2
Turkey Piccata with Broccoli, page 267	230	210	1.1
Steak and Onions in a Packet, page 269	230	210	1.1
Ground beef, 20% fat, broiled, 3 oz	230	85	2.7
Chicken and Zucchini Skewers with Peanut Dipping Sauce, page 281	245	175	1.4
Chicken nuggets, boneless, breaded and fried, 3 oz	255	85	3.0
Rib-eye steak, broiled, 3 oz	265	85	3.1
Beef bologna, 3 oz	270	85	3.2
Irish Lamb Stew, page 258	280	320	0.88
Jennifer's Orange Chicken, page 268	290	170	1.7
Italian sausage, cooked, 3 oz	295	85	3.5
French Beef Stew, page 254	300	410	0.73
Cheeseburger, fast-food	305	100	3.0
Asian Salmon in a Packet, page 273	315	255	1.2
Volumetrics Gumbo, page 259	320	450	0.71
Chicken-Broccoli Stir-Fry with Water Chestnuts and Carrots, page 248	330	390	0.85
Pork Stir-Fry with Asian Cabbage and Red Pepper page 251	345	385	0.90
Volumetrics Chicken Cacciatore, page 264	360	395	0.91
Creamy Pork Tenderloin with Mushrooms over Egg Noodles, page 241	450	345	1.3
MIXED DISHES (INCLUDING PASTAS AND SALADS)			
Rainbow Chef's Salad, page 216	230	385	0.60
Fettuccine Alfredo reduced-calorie frozen entrée	240	260	0.92
Melissa's Peanut-Udon Salad, page 319	260	190	1.4
Enchilada Casserole, page 261	265	365	0.73
Salade Niçoise, page 220	270	290	0.93
Chili-Rubbed Steak on a Deconstructed Guacamole Salad, page 219	270	210	1.3
Beef ravioli in tomato sauce, 6 oz	270	170	1.6
Spicy Tofu with Peppers and Snow Peas, page 253	275	285	0.96
Pasta with Exploding Tomatoes and Arugula, page 245	275	280	0.98
Asian Chicken Salad, page 323	275	165	1.7
Ziti marinara reduced-calorie frozen entrée	290	255	1.1
Lasagna with meat, frozen entrée, 8 oz	290	225	1.3
Lasagna with meat sauce, reduced-calorie frozen entrée	300	295	1.0
Pasta Tricolore, page 242	310	255	1.2
Volumetrics Macaroni and Cheese, page 321	315	240	1.3
Vegetarian lasagna, 1 cup	315	225	1.4
Baked Potato with Black Bean and Pepper Salsa, page 263	325	360	0.90

[Italicized items are Volumetrics recipes.]	CALORIES	WEIGHT (GRAMS)	CALORIE DENSITY
Volumetrics Spaghetti Bolognese, page 236	335	340	0.98
Couscous with Middle Eastern Vegetable Stew, page 257	355	600	0.59
Juliet's Vegetarian Chili, page 287	375	465	0.81
Macaroni and cheese, prepared with 2% milk and margarine, 1 cup	395	225	1.8
Volumetrics Chili con Carne, page 284	425	445	0.96
Melissa's Leek Lasagna, page 246	425	425	1.0
White Turkey Chili, page 288	440	520	0.85
Diane's Basil Shrimp and Pasta, page 239	440	500	0.88
SANDWICHES AND PIZZAS			
Hawaiian Pizza, page 233	165	120	1.4
Cheese pizza, thin crust, 1/8 of 14-inch pie	240	80	3.0
Chicken Caesar Panini, page 226	290	250	1.2
Hummus and Veggies Sandwich, page 229	290	225	1.3
Zesty Roast Beef and Veggie Pocket, page 230	290	205	1.4
Pesto Pizza with Chicken and Vegetables, page 235	300	160	1.9
Egg and Veggie Salad Sandwich, page 223	305	205	1.5
Cheese pizza, thick crust, 1/8 of 14-inch pie	330	120	2.8
Pepperoni pizza, 1/8 of 14-inch pie	330	120	2.8
Tuna-Apple Salad Sandwich, page 221	350	235	1.5
Meat and vegetable pizza, 1/8 of 14-inch pie	355	145	2.4
Very Veggie Pizza, page 231	360	275	1.3
Chicken Salad Sandwich, page 225	400	235	1.7

Snacks and Desserts Modular List

This list contains a wide variety of foods that can be eaten between meals or for dessert. You can also snack on foods from other lists, such as soup or cereal. Choose your snacks wisely! Although I have included foods with a high CD, they are not your best choices. They are too easy to overeat and are less filling than foods with a low CD.

[Italicized items are Volumetrics recipes.]	CALORIES	WEIGHT (GRAMS)	CALORIE DENSITY
VEGETABLES			
Celery, 1 stalk	5	40	0.12
Cucumber slices, 1 cup	15	120	0.12
Tomato, 1 medium	20	125	0.16
Broccoli florets, 1 cup	20	70	0.28
Marinated Mushrooms, page 338	25	75	0.33
Tomato, cherry, 10 each	30	170	0.18
Red bell pepper slices, 1 cup	30	90	0.33
Jicama slices, 1 cup	45	120	0.38

[Italicized items are Volumetrics recipes.]	CALORIES	WEIGHT (GRAMS)	CALORIE DENSITY
Baby carrots, 15	50	150	0.33
Crudités with Cilantro-Lime Ranch Dip, page 317	75	155	0.48
FRUITS			
Plum, 1 medium	30	65	0.46
Mandarin oranges, canned, drained, ½ cup	35	95	0.37
Clementine, 1 medium	35	75	0.47
Kiwi, 1 medium	40	70	0.57
Watermelon balls, 1 cup	45	155	0.29
Tangerine, 1 medium	45	90	0.50
Grapefruit, ½ medium	50	125	0.40
Applesauce, unsweetened, ½ cup	50	120	0.42
Strawberries, 1 cup	55	165	0.33
Canned fruit cocktail, in juice, drained, ½ cup	55	120	0.46
Cantaloupe balls, 1 cup	60	175	0.34
Peach, 1 medium	60	150	0.40
Blackberries, 1 cup	60	145	0.41
Orange, 1 medium	60	130	0.46
Honeydew balls, 1 cup	65	175	0.37
Raspberries, 1 cup	65	125	0.52
Pineapple chunks, 1 cup	80	165	0.48
Dried apricots, ¼ cup	80	30	2.7
Blueberries, 1 cup	85	150	0.57
Apple, 1 medium	95	180	0.53
Retro Melon Ball Trio, page 354	100	265	0.38
Baked apple, unsweetened, 1 medium	100	160	0.62
Pear, 1 medium	105	180	0.58
Banana, 1 medium	105	120	0.88
Grapes, seedless, 1 cup	110	160	0.69
Raisins, ¼ cup	110	35	3.1
Red, Black, and Blue Berry Medley, page 350	115	160	0.72
Avocado, California (Hass), ½ each	115	70	1.6
Banana, 1 medium	120	105	1.1
Figs, dried, ¼ cup	125	50	2.5
Holiday Balsamic Grape Salad, page 353	150	205	0.73
Avocado, Florida, ½ each	180	150	1.2
DAIRY			
Cheese, spread, light, wedge	35	20	1.8
Pudding, sugar-free, snack cup	60	105	0.57
Vanilla pudding, sugar-free, prepared with fat-free milk, ½ cup	65	130	0.50
Cheese, American, ⅔ oz slice	70	20	3.5
Chocolate pudding, sugar-free, prepared with fat-free milk, ½ cup	75	130	0.58
Cheese, feta, 1 oz	75	30	2.5
Yogurt, flavored, nonfat, low-cal sweetener, 6 oz	80	170	0.44
Cottage cheese, 1% fat, ½ cup	80	115	0.70
Cheese, string, 1 oz	80	30	2.7
Cheese, cheddar, reduced-fat, 1 oz	80	30	2.7

[Italicized items are Volumetrics recipes.]	CALORIES	WEIGHT (GRAMS)	CALORIE DENSITY
Yogurt, Greek-style, nonfat, plain, 6 oz	90	170	0.53
Cheese, swiss, reduced-fat, 1 oz	90	30	3.0
Yogurt, nonfat, plain, 6 oz	95	170	0.56
Vanilla ice cream, fat-free, ½ cup	95	70	1.4
Cheese, Jack, 1 oz	105	30	3.5
Frozen yogurt, ½ cup	110	85	1.3
Yogurt, low-fat, plain, 6 oz	115	170	0.68
Frozen yogurt, soft-serve, ½ cup	115	70	1.6
Cheese, cheddar, 1 oz	115	30	3.8
Vanilla ice cream, ½ cup	135	65	2.1
Vanilla pudding, prepared with 2% milk, ½ cup	140	140	1.0
Chocolate pudding, prepared with 2% milk, ½ cup	145	140	1.0
Yogurt, low-fat, fruit, 6 oz	185	170	1.1
Rice pudding, ½ cup	185	125	1.5
Vanilla ice cream, premium, ½ cup	290	105	2.8
DESSERTS, PASTRIES, CANDY			
Gelatin snack cup, sugar-free	10	90	0.11
Hard candy, 1 piece	25	5	0.5
Popsicle, 1.75 oz	40	50	0.80
Fudgsicle, no-sugar-added, 1.5 oz	45	40	1.1
Fudgsicle, low-fat, 1.75 oz	60	45	1.3
Gelatin snack cup	70	100	0.70
Angel food cake, 1 oz slice, approximately 1/12 cake	70	30	2.3
Fruit sorbet, ½ cup	80	100	0.80
Frozen fruit and juice bar, 3 oz	80	90	0.89
Vanilla wafers, 5 each	80	20	4.0
Marshmallows, 4 each	90	30	3.0
Graham cracker crisps, 100-calorie pack	100	25	4.0
Orange sherbet, ½ cup	105	75	1.4
Fig bar cookies, Newton type, 2 each	110	30	3.7
Animal crackers, 10 each	110	25	4.4
Cookies, creme-filled chocolate sandwich, 2	110	25	4.4
Pound cake, 1 oz slice	115	30	3.8
Pear Cranberry Strudel, page 349	120	100	1.2
Caramel corn, 1 oz	120	30	4.0
Graham cracker squares, 4 each	120	30	4.0
Granola bar, hard, 7/8 oz	120	25	4.8
Italian ice, 1 cup	125	230	0.54
Chocolate, milk, 1 oz	150	30	5.0
Cookies, chocolate chip, 2-inch, homemade, 2	155	30	5.2
Jelly beans, 15 large	160	40	4.0
Granola bar, chocolate chip, chocolate-covered, 1.25 oz	165	35	4.7
Peach Bread Pudding, page 347	170	160	1.1
Chocolate, dark, 1 oz	170	30	5.7
Coffee cake with crumb topping, 1/8 of 8-inch cake	180	55	3.3
Ginger Apple Crumble, page 345	185	185	1.0
Chocolate Chip–Zucchini Squares, page 339	200	85	2.4
Chocolate cupcake, cream-filled, frosted	200	50	4.0

[Italicized items are Volumetrics recipes.]	CALORIES	WEIGHT (GRAMS)	CALORIE DENSITY
Doughnut, cake, medium	225	55	4.1
Brownie, 2-inch square	245	60	4.1
German chocolate cake with frosting, ⅛ of 8-inch cake	250	70	3.6
Cheesecake, ⅙ of 6-inch cake	255	80	3.2
Banana Cake, page 341	260	120	2.2
Pie, apple, ⅛ of 9-inch pie	295	125	2.4
Alex's Three-Layer Carrot Cake, page 343	310	140	2.2
Pie, pumpkin, ⅛ of 9-inch pie	315	155	2.0
Pie, cherry, ⅛ of 9-inch pie	325	125	2.6
Pie, banana cream, ⅛ of 9-inch pie	385	145	2.7
Pie, apple, ⅛ of 9-inch pie	410	155	2.6
Carrot cake with cream cheese frosting, 1/12 of a 9-inch cake	435	110	4.0
SNACK FOODS			
Rice cake, plain	35	10	3.5
Olives, green, 10	40	30	1.3
Olives, black, 10	50	45	1.1
Hard-cooked egg	80	50	1.6
Apple–Goat Cheese Dip with Endive Leaves, page 327	85	165	0.51
Mozzarella cheese, part-skim, 1 oz	85	30	2.8
Tomato and Mozzarella Mini Sticks , page 333	95	75	1.3
Popcorn, air-popped, 3 cups	95	25	3.8
Potato chips, baked, 100-calorie pack	100	25	4.0
Cheese puffs, baked, crunchy, 100-calorie pack	100	20	5.0
Potato crisps, 100-calorie pack	100	18	5.6
Curried Chicken Lettuce Cups, page 337	105	75	1.4
Hummus, ¼ cup	105	60	1.8
Pretzels, 1 oz	105	30	3.5
Soy chips, 1 oz	110	30	3.7
Soy nuts, 1 oz	130	30	4.3
Tortilla chips, baked, 1 oz	130	30	4.3
Trail mix, 1 oz	130	30	4.3
Wheat crackers, thin, 1 oz	130	30	4.3
Potato chips, baked, 1 oz	135	30	4.5
Spinach-Cheese Balls, page 334	140	115	1.2
Tortilla chips, 1 oz	140	30	4.7
Potato chips, 1 oz	155	30	5.2
Cheese puffs, 1 oz	160	30	5.3
Corn chips, 1 oz	160	30	5.3
Jennifer's Buffalo Party Dip, page 314	165	185	0.89
Zesty Vegetable Pinwheels, page 331	165	125	1.3
Popcorn, oil-popped, 3 cups	165	35	4.7
Roasted Eggplant and Fennel Caponata, page 329	195	280	0.70
Volumetrics Spinach-Artichoke Dip, page 324	215	240	0.9
Kim's Cantina Night Bean Dip, page 328	225	205	1.1
Soft pretzel, medium 4 oz	390	115	3.4

[Italicized items are Volumetrics recipes.]	CALORIES	WEIGHT (GRAMS)	CALORIE DENSITY
NUTS (SHELLED)			
Walnuts, ¼ cup	165	25	6.6
Pecans, ¼ cup	170	25	6.8
Sunflower seed kernels, ¼ cup	185	30	6.2
Almonds, ¼ cup	205	35	5.9
Peanuts, ¼ cup	215	35	6.1

Condiments and Spreads Modular List

Remember to add the calories from toppings, spreads, and condiments when budgeting your calories. Notice how many calories the high-fat, high-CD condiments such as regular mayonnaise can add to a dish.

	CALORIES	WEIGHT (GRAMS)	CALORIE DENSITY
CONDIMENTS			
Vinegar, 1 tbsp	5	15	0.33
Salsa, 1 tbsp	5	15	0.33
Mustard, 1 tsp	5	5	1.0
Fat-free milk, 2 tbsp	10	30	0.33
Sour cream, fat-free, 1 tbsp	10	15	0.67
Soy sauce, 1 tbsp	10	15	0.67
Italian dressing, fat-free, 2 tbsp	15	30	0.5
Cream cheese, fat-free, 1 tbsp	15	15	1.0
Ketchup, 1 tbsp	15	15	1.0
Sugar, 1 tsp	15	5	3.0
Whole milk, 2 tbsp	20	30	0.61
Half-and-half, fat-free, 2 tbsp	20	30	0.67
Olives, green, 5 each	20	15	1.3
Sour cream, light, 1 tbsp	20	15	1.3
Honey, 1 tsp	20	5	4.0
Jam, 1 tsp	20	5	4.0
Marshmallow topping, 1 tbsp	20	5	4.0
Barbeque sauce, 1 tbsp	25	15	1.7
Pancake syrup, light, 1 tbsp	25	15	1.7
Margarine spread, reduced-fat, 1 tsp	25	5	5.0
Cream cheese, light, 1 tbsp	30	15	2.0
Sour cream, regular, 1 tbsp	30	15	1.0
Guacamole, 2 tbsp	35	30	1.2
Ranch dressing, fat-free, 2 tbsp	35	30	1.2
Butter, 1 tsp	35	5	7.0

	CALORIES	WEIGHT (GRAMS)	CALORIE DENSITY
Margarine, 1 tsp	35	5	7.0
Blue cheese dressing, fat-free, 2 tbsp	40	35	1.1
Half-and-half, 2 tbsp	40	30	1.3
Canola oil, 1 tsp	40	5	9.0
Olive oil, 1 tsp	40	5	9.0
Pancake syrup, regular, 1 tbsp	45	20	2.2
Parmesan cheese, grated, 2 tbsp	45	10	4.5
Nondairy creamer, fat-free, hazelnut, 2 tbsp	50	35	1.4
Maple syrup, 1 tbsp	50	20	2.5
Mayonnaise, light, 1 tbsp	50	15	3.3
Cream cheese, regular, 1 tbsp	50	15	3.3
Italian dressing, light, 2 tbsp	55	30	1.8
Olives, Kalamata, 5 each	55	20	2.8
Ranch dressing, reduced-fat, 2 tbsp	60	30	2.0
Chocolate topping, 1 tbsp	65	20	3.2
Nondairy creamer, hazelnut, 2 tbsp	70	35	2.0
Peanut butter, reduced-fat, 1 tbsp	75	15	5.0
Italian dressing, 2 tbsp	85	30	2.8
Pasta sauce, tomato and basil, ½ cup	90	125	0.72
Almond butter, 1 tbsp	95	15	6.3
Peanut butter, regular, 1 tbsp	95	15	6.3
Mayonnaise, regular, 1 tbsp	100	15	6.7
Frosting, vanilla, 2 tbsp	120	30	4.0
Blue cheese dressing, regular, 2 tbsp	145	30	4.8
Ranch dressing, regular, 2 tbsp	145	30	4.8

Beverages Modular List

You will notice that, with the exception of milk, beverages were not included in the menu plan. This does not mean that you are not "allowed" to have beverages. Just make sure that you budget in the calories. So if you want a glass of wine with dinner, skip dessert or save some calories from snack time. Remember that beverage calories add on to food calories, so substitute low-calorie or zero-calorie beverages whenever you can.

	CALORIES	WEIGHT (GRAMS)	CALORIE DENSITY
WATER			
Tap water, unflavored sparkling water, seltzer, 8 fl oz	0	235	0
Sweetened flavored water, 12 fl oz	80	355	0.22
TEA			
Tea, brewed, without sugar, 8 fl oz	0	235	0
Tea, bottled, sweetened, 12 fl oz	120	370	0.32

	CALORIES	WEIGHT (GRAMS)	CALORIE DENSITY
COFFEE AND COFFEE DRINKS			
Coffee, black, unsweetened, 8 fl oz	5	235	0.02
Coffee, with fat-free milk, 8 fl oz	10	240	0.04
Coffee, with whole milk, 8 fl oz	20	240	0.08
Coffee, with half-and-half, 8 fl oz	40	240	0.17
Cappuccino, with fat-free milk, 8 fl oz	40	115	0.35
Cappuccino, with 2% milk, 8 fl oz	60	115	0.52
Latte or café au lait, with fat-free milk, 8 fl oz	65	240	0.27
Cappuccino, with whole milk, 8 fl oz	75	115	0.65
Latte or café au lait, with 2% milk, 8 fl oz	100	240	0.42
Latte or café au lait, with whole milk, 8 fl oz	115	240	0.48
SODA			
Diet soda, 12 fl oz	0	360	0
Ginger ale, 12 fl oz	125	365	0.34
Regular cola, lemon-lime soda, 12 fl oz	155	370	0.42
MILK, MILK DRINKS, AND NONDAIRY MILK ALTERNATIVES			
Soy milk, 8 fl oz	80	245	0.33
Fat-free milk, 8 fl oz	80	245	0.33
1% milk, 8 fl oz	100	245	0.41
2% milk, 8 fl oz	120	245	0.49
Rice milk, 8 fl oz	145	245	0.59
Whole milk, 8 fl oz	150	245	0.61
Fast-food vanilla milkshake, 12 fl oz	505	340	1.49
VEGETABLE AND FRUIT JUICES			
Tomato juice, 6 fl oz	30	180	0.17
Light cranberry juice, 6 fl oz	35	180	0.19
Vegetable juice, 6 fl oz	40	180	0.22
Grapefruit juice, 6 fl oz	70	185	0.38
Orange juice, 6 fl oz	90	185	0.49
Cranberry juice cocktail, 6 fl oz	105	190	0.55
Lemonade, sugar-sweetened, 12 fl oz	160	370	0.43
SPORTS AND ENERGY DRINKS			
Sports drink, sugar-sweetened, 12 fl oz	95	365	0.26
Energy drink, sugar-sweetened, 12 fl oz	145–210	360	0.40–0.58
ALCOHOLIC BEVERAGES			
Sangria, 4 fl oz	80	120	0.67
Sherry, dry, 4 fl oz	80	120	0.67
Champagne, 4 fl oz	85	120	0.71
Whiskey, rum, vodka, gin, 1.5 fl oz	95	40	2.4
Wine, 4 fl oz	100	120	0.83
Light beer, 12 fl oz	105	355	0.30
Gin and tonic, 6 fl oz (1 oz gin, 5 oz tonic)	115	170	0.68
Beer, 12 fl oz	155	355	0.44
Eggnog, 4 fl oz	200	130	1.5
Piña colada, 6 fl oz	330	190	1.7
Daiquiri, 6 fl oz	335	180	1.9
Margarita, 6 fl oz	375	170	2.2

Suggested Food Group Servings

The Dietary Guidelines recommend a number of servings per day from each food group for different daily calorie levels. Find the calorie level that is closest to your daily goal and use this chart to make sure that you're choosing the right balance of foods.

FOOD GROUP	DAILY CALORIES				SERVING SIZE
	1,400	1,600	1,800	2,000	
Grains	5–6	6	6	6–8	• 1 slice bread • 1 oz dry cereal • ½ cup cooked rice, pasta, or cereal
Vegetables	3–4	3–4	4–5	4–5	• 1 cup raw leafy vegetable • ½ cup cut-up raw or cooked vegetable • ½ cup vegetable juice
Fruits	4	4	4–5	4–5	• 1 medium fruit • ¼ cup dried fruit • ½ cup fresh, frozen, or canned fruit • ½ cup fruit juice

FOOD GROUP	DAILY CALORIES				SERVING SIZE
	1,400	**1,600**	**1,800**	**2,000**	
Fat-free or low-fat milk and milk products	2–3	2–3	2–3	2–3	• 1 cup milk or yogurt • 1 ½ oz cheese
Lean meats, poultry, and fish	3–4 or less	3–4 or less	6 or less	6 or less	• 1 oz cooked meats, poultry, or fish • 1 egg
Nuts, seeds, and legumes	3 per week	3–4 per week	4 per week	4–5 per week	• ⅓ cup or 1½ oz nuts • 2 tbsp peanut butter • 2 tbsp or ½ oz seeds • ½ cup cooked legumes (beans, peas)
Fats and oils	1	2	2–3	2–3	• 1 tsp soft margarine • 1 tsp vegetable oil • 1 tbsp mayonnaise • 1 tbsp salad dressing
Sweets and added sugars	3 or less per week	3 or less per week	5 or less per week	5 or less per week	• 1 tbsp sugar • 1 tbsp jelly or jam • 1 cup lemonade

Adapted from the Dietary Guidelines for Americans 2010, *Appendix 10. The* DASH Diet Eating Plan at Various Calorie Levels, *www.dietaryguidelines.gov*

Kitchen Conversion Charts

WEIGHT MEASURES OF COMMON DRY INGREDIENTS

Ingredient	Grams per cup
Flour, white	125
Flour, whole-wheat	120
Macaroni, whole-wheat	105
Oats, rolled	80
Rice, brown	185
Sugar, granulated	200

WEIGHT MEASURES

Ounces	Pounds	Grams
1	1/16	28
4	1/4	112
8	1/2	224
12	3/4	336
16	1	448

VOLUME MEASURES (LIQUID)

MEASURE	EQUIVALENT	GRAMS
1 teaspoon	1/3 tablespoon	5
1 tablespoon	1/2 fluid ounce	15
1/8 cup	1 fluid ounce	30
1/4 cup	2 fluid ounces	60
1/2 cup	4 fluid ounces	120
3/4 cup	6 fluid ounces	180
1 cup	8 fluid ounces	240
2 cups or 1 pint	16 fluid ounces	480
4 cups or 2 pints or 1 quart	32 fluid ounces	960

Selected References

Week 0

Butryn, M.L., Phelan, S., Hill, J.O., and Wing, R.R. 2007. "Consistent self-monitoring of weight: a key component of successful weight loss maintenance." *Obesity*, 15: 3091–3096.

Drapeau,V., King, N., Hetherington, M., Doucet, E., Blundell, J., and Tremblay, A. 2007. "Appetite sensations and satiety quotient: predictors of energy intake and weight loss." *Appetite*, 48: 159–166.

Nonas, C.A., and Foster, G.D. 2005. "Setting achievable goals for weight loss." *Journal of the American Dietetic Association*, 105: S118–123.

"Position of the American Dietetic Association: Weight Management." 2009. *Journal of the American Dietetic Association*, 109: 330–346.

U.S. Department of Agriculture and U.S. Department of Health and Human Services. *Dietary Guidelines for Americans, 2010.* 7th Edition. Washington, D.C.: U.S. Government Printing Office, December 2010.

U.S. Department of Health and Human Services. *2008 Physical Activity Guidelines for Americans.* www.health.gov/paguidelines

VanWormer, J.J., Martinez, A.M., Martinson, B.C., Crain, A.L., Benson, G.A., Cosentino, D.L., and Pronk, N.P. 2009. "Self-weighing promotes weight loss for obese adults." *American Journal of Preventive Medicine*, 36: 70–73.

Week 1

Bell, E.A., Castellanos, V.H., Pelkman, C.L., Thorwart, M.L., and Rolls, B.J. 1998. "Energy density of foods affects energy intake in normal-weight women." *American Journal of Clinical Nutrition*, 67: 412–420.

Bell, E.A., and Rolls, B.J. 2001. "Energy density of foods affects energy intake across multiple levels of fat content in lean and obese women." *American Journal of Clinical Nutrition*, 73: 1010–1018.

Bes-Rastrollo, M., van Dam, R.M., Martinez-Gonzalez, M.A., Li, T.Y., Sampson, L.L., and Hu, F.B. 2008. "Prospective study of dietary energy density and weight gain in women." *American Journal of Clinical Nutrition*, 88: 769–777.

Ello-Martin, J.A., Roe, L.S., Ledikwe, J.H., Beach, A.M., and Rolls, B.J. 2007. "Dietary energy density in the treatment of obesity: A year-long trial comparing two weight-loss diets." *American Journal of Clinical Nutrition*, 85: 1465–1477.

Garber, C.E., Blissmer, B., Deschenes, M.R., Franklin, B.A., Lamonte, M.J., Lee, I.M., Nieman, D.C., and Swain, D.P. 2011. "Quantity and quality of exercise for developing and maintaining cardiorespiratory, musculoskeletal, and neuromotor fitness in apparently healthy adults: guidance for prescribing exercise." *Medicine & Science in Sports & Exercise*, 43: 1334–1359.

Kant, A.K., and Graubard, B.I. 2005. "Energy density of diets reported by American adults: association with food group intake, nutrient intake, and body weight." *International Journal of Obesity*, 29: 950–956.

Ledikwe, J.H., Blanck, H.M., Kettel Khan, L., Serdula, M.K., Seymour, J.D., Tohill, B.C., and Rolls, B.J. "Reductions in dietary energy density as a weight management strategy." In *Contemporary Endocrinology: Treatment of the Obese Patient*. Edited by R.F. Kushner and D.H. Bessesen. Totowa, New Jersey: Humana Press Inc., 2007.

Rolls, B.J. 2009. "The relationship between dietary energy density and energy intake." *Physiology & Behavior*, 97: 609–615.

Rolls, B.J. 2010. Plenary Lecture 1: Dietary strategies for the prevention and treatment of obesity. *Proceedings of the Nutrition Society*, 69: 70–79.

Savage. J.S., Marini, M., and Birch, L.L. 2008. "Dietary energy density predicts women's weight change over 6 y." *American Journal of Clinical Nutrition*, 88: 677–684.

Week 2

DellaValle, D.M., Roe, L.S., and Rolls, B.J. 2005. "Does the consumption of caloric and non-caloric beverages with a meal affect energy intake?" *Appetite*, 44: 187–193.

Epstein, L.H., Paluch, R.A., Beecher, M.D., and Roemmich, J.N. 2008. "Increasing healthy eating vs. reducing high energy-dense foods to treat pediatric obesity." *Obesity*, 16: 318–326.

Ledikwe, J.H., Rolls, B.J., Smiciklas-Wright, H., Mitchell, D.C., Ard, J.D., Champagne, C., Karanja, N., Lin, P., Stevens, V.J., and Appel, L.J. 2007. "Reductions in dietary energy density are associated with weight loss in overweight and obese participants in the PREMIER trial." *American Journal of Clinical Nutrition*, 85: 1212–1221.

McCaffrey, T.A., Rennie, K.L., Kerr, M.A., Wallace, J.M., Hannon-Fletcher, M.P., Coward, W.A., Jebb, S.A., and Livingstone, M.B. 2008. "Energy density of the diet and change in body fatness from childhood to adolescence; is there a relation?" *American Journal of Clinical Nutrition*, 87: 1230–1237.

Rolls, B.J., Roe, L.S., Beach, A.M., and Kris-Etherton, P.M. 2005. "Provision of foods differing in energy density affects long-term weight loss." *Obesity Research*, 13: 1052–1060.

The Food Processor® Nutrition and Fitness Software (version 10.8), ESHA Research, Inc., 2011.

Week 3

Kral, T.V.E., and Rolls, B.J. 2011. "Portion size and the obesity epidemic." In *Handbook of Social Science of Obesity—The Causes and Correlates of Diet, Physical Activity, and Obesity*. Edited by John Cawley. Oxford: Oxford University Press, pp. 367–384.

McGaffey, A., Hughes, K., Fidler, S.K., D'Amico, F.J., and Stalter, M.N. 2010. "Can Elvis Pretzley and the Fitwits improve knowledge of obesity, nutrition, exercise, and portions in fifth graders?" *International Journal of Obesity*, 34: 1134–1142.

Osterholt, K.M., Roe, L.S., and Rolls, B.J. 2007. "Incorporation of air into a snack food reduces energy intake." *Appetite*, 48: 351–358.

Rolls, B.J., Castellanos, V.H., Halford, J.C., Kilara, A., Panyam, D., Pelkman, C.L., Smith, G.P., and Thorwart, M.L. 1998. "Volume of food consumed affects satiety in men." *American Journal of Clinical Nutrition*, 67: 1170–1177.

Rolls, B.J., Morris, E.L., and Roe, L.S. 2002. "Portion size of food affects energy intake in normal-weight and overweight men and women." *American Journal of Clinical Nutrition*, 76: 1207–1213.

Rolls, B.J., Roe, L.S., and Meengs, J.S. 2007. "The effect of large portion sizes on energy intake is sustained for 11 days." *Obesity*, 15: 1535–1543.

Rolls, B.J., Roe, L.S., and Meengs, J.S. 2010. "Portion size can be used strategically to increase vegetable consumption in adults." *American Journal of Clinical Nutrition*, 91: 913–922.

Rolls, B.J., Roe, L.S., Meengs, J.S., and Wall, D.E. 2004. "Increasing the portion size of a sandwich increases energy intake." *Journal of the American Dietetic Association*, 104: 367–372.

Rolls, B.J., Roe, L.S., and Meengs, J.S. 2006. "Reductions in portion size and energy density of foods are additive and lead to sustained decreases in energy intake." *American Journal of Clinical Nutrition*, 83: 11–17

Steenhuis, I.H., and Vermeer, W.M. 2009. "Portion size: review and framework for interventions." *International Journal of Behavioral Nutrition and Physical Activity*, 6: 58.

Young, L.R., and Nestle, M. 2007. "Portion sizes and obesity: responses of fast-food companies." *Journal of Public Health Policy*, 28: 238–248.

Week 4

Flood, J.E., and Rolls, B.J. 2007. "Soup preloads in a variety of forms reduce meal energy intake." *Appetite*, 49: 626–634.

Flood-Obbagy, J.E., and Rolls, B.J. 2009. "The effect of fruit in different forms on energy intake and satiety at a meal." *Appetite*, 52: 416–422.

Hill, J.O. 2009. "Can a small-changes approach help address the obesity epidemic? A report of the Joint Task Force of the American Society for Nutrition, Institute of Food Technologists, and International Food Information Council." *American Journal of Clinical Nutrition*, 89: 477–484.

O'Neil, C.E., Zanovec, M., Cho, S.S., and Nicklas, T.A. 2010. "Whole grain and fiber consumption are associated with lower body weight measures in US adults: National Health and Nutrition Examination Survey 1999–2004." *Nutrition Research*, 30: 815–822.

Ratliff, J., Leite, J.O., de Ogburn, R., Puglisi, M.J., VanHeest, J., and Fernandez, M.L. 2010. "Consuming eggs for breakfast influences plasma glucose and ghrelin, while reducing energy intake during the next 24 hours in adult men." *Nutrition Research*, 30: 96–103.

Rolls, B.J., Bell, E.A., and Thorwart, M.L. 1999. "Water incorporated into a food but not served with a food decreases energy intake in lean women." *American Journal of Clinical Nutrition*, 70: 448–455.

Song, W.O., Chun, O.K., Obayashi, S., Cho, S., and Chung, C.E. 2005. "Is consumption of breakfast associated with body mass index in U.S. adults?" *Journal of the American Dietetic Association*, 105: 1373–1382.

Wyatt, H.R., Grunwald, G.K., Mosca, C.L., Klem, M.L., Wing, R.R., and Hill, J.O. 2002. "Long-term weight loss and breakfast in subjects in the National Weight Control Registry." *Obesity Research*, 10: 78–82.

Week 5

Blatt, A.D., Roe, L.S., and Rolls, B.J. 2011. "Hidden vegetables: an effective strategy to reduce energy intake and increase vegetable intake in adults." *American Journal of Clinical Nutrition*, 93: 756–763.

Kral, T.V.E., Kabay, A.C., Roe, L.S., and Rolls, B.J. 2010. "Effects of doubling the portion size of fruit and vegetable side dishes on children's intake at a meal." *Obesity*, 18: 521–527.

Leahy, K.E., Birch, L.L., Fisher, J.O., and Rolls, B.J. 2008. "Reductions in entrée energy density increase children's vegetable intake and reduce energy intake." *Obesity*, 16: 1559–1565.

Rolls, B.J., Roe, L.S., and Meengs, J.S. 2004. "Salad and satiety: energy density and portion size of a first course salad affect energy intake at lunch." *Journal of the American Dietetic Association*, 104: 1570–1576.

Rolls, B.J., Ello Martin, J.A., and Tohill, B.C. 2004. "What can intervention studies tell us about the relationship between fruit and vegetable consumption and weight management?" *Nutrition Reviews*, 62: 1–17.

Spill, M.K., Birch, L.L., Roe, L.S., and Rolls, B.J. 2010. "Eating vegetables first: the use of portion size to increase vegetable intake in preschool children." *American Journal of Clinical Nutrition*, 91: 1237–1243.

Spill, M.K., Birch, L.L., Roe, L.S., and Rolls, B.J. 2011. "Hiding vegetables to reduce energy density: an effective strategy to increase children's vegetable intake and reduce energy intake." *American Journal of Clinical Nutrition*, 94: 735–741.

Week 6

Blatt, A.D., Roe, L.S., and Rolls, B.J. 2011. "Increasing the protein content of meals and its effect on daily intake." *Journal of the American Dietetic Association*, 111: 290–294.

Gilbert, J.A., Bendsen, N.T., Tremblay, A., Astrup, A. 2011. "Effect of proteins from different sources on boby composition." *Nutrition, Metabolism & Cardiovascular Diseases*, 21 (suppl 2): B16–B31.

Harland, J.I., and Garton, L.E. 2008. "Whole-grain intake as a marker of healthy body weight and adiposity." *Public Health Nutrition*, 11: 554–563.

Hartman, T.J., Zhang, Z., Albert, P.S., Bagshaw, D., Mentor-Marcel, R., Mitchell, D.C., Colburn, N.H., Kris-Etherton, P.M., and Lanza, E. 2011. "Reduced energy intake and weight loss on a legume-enriched diet lead to improvements in biomarkers related to chronic disease." *Topics in Clinical Nutrition*, 26: 208–215.

Jonnalagadda, S.S., Harnack, L., Liu, R.H., McKeown, N., Seal, C., Liu, S., and Fahey, G.C. 2011. "Putting the whole grain puzzle together: health benefits associated with whole grains—summary of American Society for Nutrition 2010 satellite symposium." *The Journal of Nutrition*, 141: 1011S–1022S.

McCrory, M.A., Hamaker, B.R., Lovejoy, J.C., and Eichelsdoerfer, P.E. 2010. "Pulse consumption, satiety, and weight management." *Advances in Nutrition*, 1: 17–30.

"Position of the American Dietetic Association: Health Implications of Dietary Fiber." 2008. *Journal of the American Dietetic Association*, 108: 1716–1731.

Wanders, A.J., van den Borne, J.J., de Graaf, C., Hulshof, T., Jonathan, M.C., Kristensen, M., Mars, M., Schols, H.A., and Feskens, E.J. 2011. "Effects of dietary fibre on subjective appetite, energy intake and body weight: a systematic review of randomized controlled trials." *Obesity Reviews,* 12: 724–739.

Williams, P.G., Grafenauer, S.J., and O'Shea, J.E. 2008. "Cereal grains, legumes, and weight management: a comprehensive review of the scientific evidence." *Nutrition Reviews*, 66: 171–182.

Week 7

Aston, L.M., Stokes, C.S., and Jebb, S.A. 2008. "No effect of a diet with a reduced glycaemic index on satiety, energy intake and body weight in overweight and obese women." *International Journal of Obesity*, 32: 160–165.

Bellisle, F., and Drewnowski, A. 2007. "Intense sweeteners, energy intake and the control of body weight." *European Journal of Clinical Nutrition*, 61: 691–700.

Drewnowski, A., and Almiron-Roig, E. "Human perceptions and preferences for fat-rich foods." In *Fat Detection: Taste, Texture, and Post Ingestive Effects*. Edited by J.P. Montmayeur and J. le Coutre. Boca Raton: CRC Press, 2010.

Foster, G.D., Wyatt, H.R., Hill, J.O., Makris, A.P., Rosenbaum, D.L., Brill, C., Stein, R.I., Mohammed, B.S., Miller, B., Rader, D.J., Zemel, B., Wadden, T.A., Tenhave, T., Newcomb, C.W., and Klein, S. 2010. "Weight and metabolic outcomes after 2 years on a low-carbohydrate versus low-fat diet: a randomized trial." *Annals of Internal Medicine*, 153: 147–157.

Howard, B.V., Manson, J.E., Stefanick, M.L., Beresford, S.A., Frank, G., Jones, B., Rodabough, R.J., Snetselaar, L., Thomson, C., Tinker, L., Vitolins, M., and Prentice, R. 2006. "Low-fat dietary pattern and weight change over 7 years: the Women's Health Initiative Dietary Modification Trial." *Journal of the American Medical Association*, 295: 39–49.

Sacks, F.M., Bray, G.A., Carey, V.J., Smith, S.R., Ryan, D.H., Anton, S.D., McManus, K., Champagne, C.M., Bishop, L.M., Laranjo, N., Leboff, M.S., Rood, J.C., de Jonge, L., Greenway, F.L., Loria, C.M., Obarzanek, E., and Williamson, D.A. 2009. "Comparison of weight-loss diets with different compositions of fat, protein, and carbohydrates." *New England Journal of Medicine*, 360: 859–873.

Shikany, J.M., Vaughan, L.K., Baskin, M.L., Cope, M.B., Hill, J.O., and Allison, D.B. 2010. "Is dietary fat 'fattening'? A comprehensive research synthesis." *Critical Reviews in Food Science and Nutrition*, 50: 699–715.

van Baak, M.A., and Astrup, A. 2009. "Consumption of sugars and body weight." *Obesity Reviews*, 10 Suppl 1: 9–23.

Week 8

Chapelot, D. 2011. "The role of snacking in energy balance: a biobehavioral approach." *The Journal of Nutrition*, 141: 158S–162S.

Leidy, H.J., and Campbell, W.W. 2011. "The effect of eating frequency on appetite control and food intake: brief synopsis of controlled feeding studies." *The Journal of Nutrition*, 141: 154S–157S.

McCrory, M.A., Howarth, N.C., Roberts, S.B., and Huang, T.T.-K. 2011. "Eating frequency and energy regulation in free-living adults consuming self-selected diets." *The Journal of Nutrition*, 141: 148S–153S.

Ovaskainen, M.-L., Reinivuo, H., Tapanainen, H., Hannila, M.-L., Korhonen, T., and

Pakkala, H. 2006. "Snacks as an element of energy intake and food consumption." *European Journal of Clinical Nutrition,* 60: 494–501.

Palmer, M.A., Capra, S., and Baines, S.K. 2009. "Association between eating frequency, weight, and health." *Nutrition Reviews*, 67: 379–390.

Rolls, B.J., Roe, L.S., Kral, T.V., Meengs, J.S., and Wall, D.E. 2004. "Increasing the portion size of a packaged snack increases energy intake in men and women." *Appetite*, 42: 63–69.

Scott, M.L., Nowlis, S.M., Mandel, N., and Morales, A.C. 2008. "The effects of reduced food size and package size on the consumption behavior of restrained and unrestrained eaters." *Journal of Consumer Research*, 35: 391–405.

Stroebele, N., Ogden, L.G., and Hill, J.O. 2009. "Do calorie-controlled portion sizes of snacks reduce energy intake?" *Appetite*, 52: 793–796.

Week 9

Caton, S.J., Bate, L., and Hetherington, M.M. 2007. "Acute effects of an alcoholic drink on food intake: aperitif versus co-ingestion." *Physiology & Behavior*, 90: 368–375.

Chen, L., Appel, L.J., Loria, C., Lin, P.H., Champagne, C.M., Elmer, P.J., Ard, J.D., Mitchell, D., Batch, B.C., Svetkey, L.P., and Caballero, B. 2009. "Reduction in consumption of sugar-sweetened beverages is associated with weight loss: the PREMIER trial." *American Journal of Clinical Nutrition*, 89: 1299–1306.

de Graaf, C. 2011. "Why liquid energy results in overconsumption." *Proceedings of the Nutrition Society*, 70: 162–170.

Dennis, E.A., Dengo, A.L., Comber, D.L., Flack, K.D., Savla, J., Davy, K.P., and Davy, B.M. 2009. "Water consumption increases weight loss during a hypocaloric diet intervention in middle-aged and older adults." *Obesity*, 18: 300–307.

Flood, J.E., Roe, L.S., and Rolls, B.J. 2006. "The effect of increased beverage portion size on energy intake at a meal." *Journal of the American Dietetic Association*, 106: 1984–1990.

Kant, A.K., Graubard, B.I., and Atchison, E.A. 2009. "Intakes of plain water, moisture in foods and beverages, and total water in the adult US population—nutritional, meal pattern, and body weight correlates: National Health and Nutrition Examination Surveys 1999–2006." *American Journal of Clinical Nutrition*, 90: 655–663.

Mattes, R.D., Shikany, J.M., Kaiser, K.A., and Allison, D.B. 2011. "Nutritively sweetened beverage consumption and body weight: a systematic review and meta-analysis of randomized experiments." *Obesity Reviews*, 12: 346–365.

Yeomans, M.R. 2010. "Alcohol, appetite and energy balance: is alcohol a risk factor for obesity?" *Physiology & Behavior*, 100: 82–89.

Week 10

Chandon, P., and Wansink B. 2007. "The biasing health halos of fast food restaurant health claims: Lower calorie estimates and higher side-dish consumption intentions." *Journal of Consumer Research*, 34: 301–314.

Condrasky, M., Ledikwe, J.H., Flood, J.E., and Rolls, B.J. 2007. "Chefs' opinions of restaurant portion sizes." *Obesity*, 15: 2086–2094.

Diliberti, N., Bordi, P., Conklin, M.T., Roe, L.S., and Rolls, B.J. 2004. "Increased portion size leads to increased energy intake in a restaurant meal." *Obesity Research*, 12: 562–568.

Keystone Center. *The Keystone Forum on away-from-home foods: opportunities for preventing weight gain and obesity*. Washington, D.C.: The Keystone Center, 2006. keystone.org/files/file/about/publications/Forum_Report_FINAL_5–30–06.pdf.

Obbagy, J.E., Condrasky, M., Roe, L.S., Sharp, J.L., and Rolls, B.J. 2011. "Chefs' opinions about reducing the calorie content of menu items in restaurants." *Obesity*, 19: 332–337.

Robert Wood Johnson Foundation. *Menu Labeling: Does Providing Nutrition Information at the Point of Purchase Affect Consumer Behavior?* June 2009. rwjf.org/files/research/20090630her menulabeling.pdf.

Week 11

Cappelleri, J.C., Bushmakin, A.G., Gerber, R.A., Leidy, N.K., Sexton, C.C., Karlsson, J., and Lowe, M.R. 2009. "Evaluating the Power of Food Scale in obese subjects and a general sample of individuals: development and measurement properties." *International Journal of Obesity*, 33: 913–922.

Christakis, N.A., and Fowler, J.H. 2007. "The spread of obesity in a large social network over 32 years." *New England Journal of Medicine*, 357: 370–379.

Fay, S.H., Ferriday, D., Hinton, E.C., Shakeshaft, N.G., Rogers, P.J., and Brunstrom, J.M. 2011. "What determines real-world meal size? Evidence for pre-meal planning." *Appetite*, 56: 284–289.

Hetherington, M.M. 2007. "Cues to overeat: psychological factors influencing overconsumption." *Proceedings of the Nutrition Society*, 66: 113–123.

Higgs, S., and Woodward, M. 2009. "Television watching during lunch increases afternoon snack intake of young women." *Appetite*, 52: 39–43.

Jones, K.E., Otten, J.J., Johnson, R.K., and Harvey-Berino, J.R. 2010. "Removing the bedroom television set: a possible method for decreasing television viewing time in overweight and obese adults." *Behavior Modification*, 34: 290–298.

Koh, J., and Pliner, P. 2009. "The effects of degree of acquaintance, plate size, and sharing on food intake." *Appetite*, 52: 595–602.

Pedersen, S.D., Kang, J., and Kline, G.A. 2007. "Portion control plate for weight loss in obese patients with type 2 diabetes mellitus: a controlled clinical trial." *Archives of Internal Medicine*, 167: 1277–1283.

Rolls, B.J. "Sensory-specific satiety and variety in the meal." In *Dimensions of the Meal: The Science, Culture, Business and Art of Eating*. Edited by H.L. Meiselman. Gaithersburg, Md.: Aspen Publishers, Inc., 2000.

Rolls, B.J., Roe, L.S., Halverson, K.H., and Meengs, J.S. 2007. "Using a smaller plate did not reduce energy intake at meals." *Appetite*, 49: 652–660.

Wansink, B. 2010. "From mindless eating to mindlessly eating better." *Physiology & Behavior*, 100: 454–463.

Week 12

Bartfield, J.K., Stevens, V.J., Jerome, G.J., Batch, B.C., Kennedy, B.M., Vollmer, W.M., Harsha, D., Appel, L.J., Desmond, R., and Ard, J.D. 2011. "Behavioral transitions and weight change patterns within the PREMIER Trial." *Obesity*, 19: 1609–1615.

Catenacci, V.A., Ogden, L.G., Stuht, J., Phelan, S., Wing, R.R., Hill, J.O., and Wyatt, H.R. 2008. "Physical activity patterns in the National Weight Control Registry." *Obesity*, 16: 153–161.

Cox, T.L., Malpede, C.Z., Desmond, R.A., Faulk, L.E., Myer, R.A., Henson, C.S., Heimburger, D.C., and Ard, J.D. 2007. "Physical activity patterns during weight maintenance following a low-energy density dietary intervention." *Obesity*, 15: 1226–1232.

Greene, L.F., Malpede, C.Z., Henson, C.S., Hubbert, K.A., Heimburger, D.C., and Ard, J.D. 2006. "Weight maintenance 2 years after participation in a weight loss program promoting low-energy density foods." *Obesity*, 14: 1795–1801.

Phelan, S., Lang, W., Jordan, D., and Wing, R.R. 2009. "Use of artificial sweeteners and fat-modified foods in weight loss maintainers and always-normal weight individuals." *International Journal of Obesity*, 33: 1183–1190.

Raynor, H.A., Van Walleghen, E.L., Bachman, J.L., Looney, S.M., Phelan, S., and Wing, R.R. 2011. "Dietary energy density and successful weight loss maintenance." *Eating Behavior*, 12: 119–125.

Sciamanna, C.N., Kiernan, M., Boan, J., Miller, C.K., Rolls, B.J., Jensen, G., and Hartman, T.J. 2011. "Are the practices associated with weight loss different from those associated with weight loss maintenance? Results of a national survey." *American Journal of Preventive Medicine*, 41: 159–166.

Wing, R.R., and Phelan, S. 2005. "Long-term weight loss maintenance." *American Journal of Clinical Nutrition*, 82: 222S–225S.

Wing, R.R., Papandonatos, G., Fava, J.L., Gorin, A.A., Phelan, S., McCaffery, J., and Tate, D.F. 2008. "Maintaining large weight losses: the role of behavioral and psychological factors." *Journal of Consulting and Clinical Psychology*, 76: 1015–1021.

Index

Note: Page references in *italics* indicate recipe photographs.